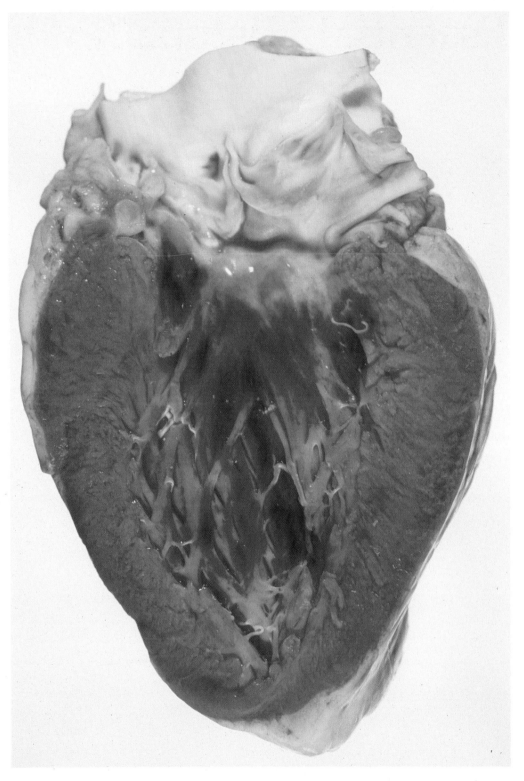

Frontispiece. Endocardial surface of the left ventricle with widespread subendocardial haemorrhage, a complication of severe head injuries. The patient had died following a road traffic accident.

Essential Histopathology

Peter R. Millard
MD, FRCPath
Consultant Histopathologist
The John Radcliffe Hospital
Oxford

BLACKWELL SCIENTIFIC PUBLICATIONS

OXFORD LONDON

EDINBURGH BOSTON MELBOURNE

© 1990 by
Blackwell Scientific Publications
Editorial offices:
Osney Mead, Oxford OX2 oEL
8 John Street, London WC1N 2ES
23 Ainslie Place, Edinburgh EH3 6AJ
3 Cambridge Center, Suite 208
   Cambridge, Massachusetts 02142, USA
107 Barry Street, Carlton
   Victoria 3053, Australia

First published 1990

Set by Setrite Typesetters, Hong Kong;
Printed and bound in Hong Kong
by Dah Hua Printing Co. Ltd

DISTRIBUTORS

Marston Book Services Ltd
PO Box 87
Oxford OX2 oDT
(*Orders*: Tel: 0865 791155
       Fax: 0865 791927
       Telex: 837515)
USA
   Year Book Medical Publishers
   200 North LaSalle Street
   Chicago, Illinois 60601
   (*Orders*: Tel: (312) 726−9733)

Canada
   The C.V. Mosby Company
   5240 Finch Avenue East
   Scarborough, Ontario
   (*Orders*: Tel: 416 298−1588)

Australia
   Blackwell Scientific Publications
   (Australia) Pty Ltd
   107 Barry Street
   Carlton, Victoria 3053
   (*Orders*: Tel: (03) 347−0300)

British Library
Cataloguing in Publication Data

Millard, P.R.
   Essential histopathology
   1. Medicine, histopathology
   I. Title
   611′.018

ISBN 0−632−02238−8

Contents

Preface

The majority of medical students will not become histopathologists, a specialty confined to about 1% of medical practitioners, but all medical students have to know some histopathology. This is because the subject is fundamental to an understanding of many branches of medicine and consequently holds an integral place in pre- and postgraduate medical courses. The discipline provides knowledge of the basic processes involved in disorders and aids in appreciating their evolution. The hope behind this text is that by concentrating mainly on common disorders, essentials of the discipline are covered and that by applying pre-clinical knowledge some clinical observations become comprehensible. The possibilities and factors producing the tissue changes of these disorders are outlined, including admissions of ignorance and opposing and alternative views — too many medical students assume uncritically that all is black and white. In the first two chapters there is a brief reiteration of the more important tissue reactions and only here are histological details given; subsequent chapters assume that these reactions in specific organs can then be worked out. Later chapters hence rely almost entirely on gross descriptions of disorders but do refer to jargon histopathology phrases and to important diagnostic techniques used. Some knowledge of all of these is important if clinicians are to interpret clinical appearances and to assess and understand histopathologists' reports. The finer points of histopathological events are the essence of histopathology practice and can be found in appropriate texts given at the end of each chapter, but are not required from medical students. Consequently, detailed subclassifications of tumours and some other diseases, the fascination of many histopathologists, are not presented and nor are all disorders of any one organ exhaustively discussed or even mentioned. If these reservations are understood, this text should provide the histopathology essential for the medical student and may even help postgraduate students in a range of major medical and surgical subspecialties.

Acknowledgements

Without the very considerable secretarial skills of Mrs Rachel Hunt, and also her seemingly endless patience, this text would never have developed. Morticians, MLSOs and photographers have all given substantial help over the years in the collection and preparation of many of the specimens illustrated while others have been generously provided by a variety of colleagues. The penultimate draft was read by Dr J.F.R. Flint, in part while coping with his final examinations. Dr Flint provided many constructive criticisms and sound comments. Early drafts of individual chapters were kindly read by Professor S.M. Cobbe and Drs J. Arno, N.J. Barnard, M.K. Bennett, D.R. Davies, M.M. Esiri, P.F. Jenkins, R.R. Millis, G.H. Millward-Sadler, J. Piris and R.C. Turner and numerous others provided individual comments and help. Dr Victoria Reeders skilfully guided the early developmental stages for Blackwell Scientific Publications Ltd., while Peter Saugman was a source of enthusiastic support and Karen Anthony bore the burden of subediting.

1 Tissue responses and skin disorders

Table 1.1 Sources for histopathological diagnoses

Tissues	Cell preparations
Biopsies	Fluid aspirates
Shave	Smears
Punch	Brushings
Needle	Fine needle
Excision	aspirates
Resected organs	
Partial	
Complete	
Autopsy	

Histopathology is the part of pathology concerned with the structural effects of disease and how these come about. The subject cannot, however, be divorced from other facets of pathology or medicine since most diseases involve or are affected by other processes. Malignant tumours, as an example, can be recognized from their structural appearances but the factors influencing their development and their impact on the body can include genetic, immune, haematological and biochemical changes as well as microbial infection, each forming a subspeciality of pathology.

Histopathology makes two important contributions to clinical medicine. First, it corroborates or provides a diagnosis, and secondly it gives insight into how a disease originates, progresses and is affected by therapy. This second aspect may in turn help in the prevention of some disease states.

Histopathology diagnosis involves the examination of tissues and cells and the recognition of alterations from the normal. Abnormalities may either be evident to the naked eye (*macroscopic* or *gross appearances*) or only appreciated from light microscopy (*microscopic appearance*). The microscopic features may be supplemented by special staining procedures, immunohistology and electron microscopy. In whole tissues, diagnosis is reached predominantly from recognition of changes in pattern or architecture, whereas in cell preparations (Table 1.1), with no intact tissue, diagnosis rests upon cytological changes. Ideally for diagnosis a combination of macroscopic and microscopic appearances should be available together with clinical details (Fig. 1.1), but often the histopathologist sees only microscopic features. Macroscopic abnormalities may be unavailable because the specimen is obtained as a closed biopsy, or they may only reach the histopathologist at second-hand from the clinician, illustrating the importance of some knowledge of macroscopic appearances.

Tissue reactions

Abnormal appearances are recognized from a knowledge of the normal and their interpretation from an appreciation of the potential reactions of tissues to a wide variety of stimuli (Table 1.2). Normal appearances are maintained in the absence of non-physiological or extraneous stimuli but should these occur diseases may develop

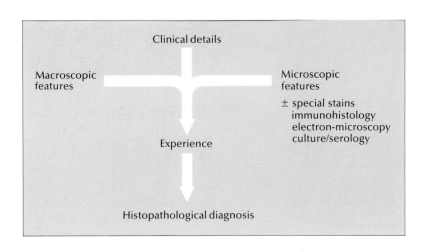

Fig. 1.1 Elements of diagnosis.

Table 1.2 Causes of tissue responses

Micro-organisms	Bacteria
	Viruses
	Fungi
	Protozoa
Physical	Trauma
	Heat and cold
	Ultraviolet light
	X-irradiation
Chemical	Drugs
	Microbial toxins
	Poisons
	Food elements
	including
	deficiencies
Genetic	Predisposition
	Inherited defect
	Acquired defect
Immune	Hypersensitivity
	reactions
	Deficiencies
Tissue damage	

and, in an attempt to restore normality, reactions aimed at protecting the body as well as destroying the stimulus. As a part of these, body tissues may also be destroyed and will need replacing. Microbial infection is the most important stimulus to disease although there are many diseases for which no clear cause emerges. Inflammation and repair are the main protective responses and death of tissues and growth disorders, including tumour formation, the principal destructive results. These responses are modified in individual tissues by the different cellular constituents and also by the defence mechanisms of each tissue. The natural defence mechanisms depend upon an underlying normal physiology and anatomy, which apart from specific disease can be adversely influenced by impaired oxygen and nutrition, age, an abnormal immune system and the genetic make-up of the individual.

The normal skin

The skin, with its two main divisions, epidermis and dermis, envelops the body and helps to provide individual identity by maintaining shape and appearance. It is also important in controlling body temperature and fluid content and in warding off physical trauma, as well as attracting sexual partners. Modifications from the basic structure in different areas are adaptations assisting these functions which also influence the distribution of some skin diseases. The concentration of the apocrine sweat glands in the axilla, genital and breast regions governs the site of sweat gland tumours, as does the hair distribution that of many forms of hair loss, *alopecia*. Direct exposure to the environment, sexual differences, ageing and the impact of impaired venous and lymphatic drainage also affect the pattern of skin disorders. Common skin cancers related to sun exposure all predominate on the face and exposed areas; baldness is mainly a male phenomenon, acne is a disorder of puberty and stasis or varicose ulcers are found around the ankles. The immediate contact of the skin with the environment also provides easy access for noxious stimuli as well as a way in which the skin's anatomy and physiology is altered. Sun tanning illustrates both of these phenomena; tanning involves the redistribution of melanin and increased melanocytic activity but, done to excess, burns the skin and may provoke formation of the tumour, melanoma.

Natural defence mechanisms

These include:

1 Epidermal stratification, keratinization and hairs, all providing waterproofing and protection from physical injury and micro-organisms. Wounds, dirt, retained moisture and vitamin A and C deficiency will all impair these functions.

2 Bacterial commensals that compete for nutrients with pathogenic organisms and release toxic metabolites against infecting organisms.

3 Glandular secretions which inhibit bacterial colonization by acidifying sweat secretions and destroying bacteria via lysosomal digestion.

4 Phagocytic cells (*Langerhan's cells*) in the epidermis and dermis that process antigen and affect immune responses.

5 A well-developed vascular and lymphatic system.

Inflammation

Inflammation is the most common tissue response and is usually indicated by the suffix *itis*. Although many of the underlying factors are understood, there are many which remain unclear. The end point is the protection of the body, but sometimes the reaction ensures the preservation of the stimulus and so continuing harm. Inflammation separates into acute and chronic stages depending on its duration as well as the type of stimulus and the tissue involved. It is important to realize that chronic inflammation is not an invariable sequel to acute inflammation and that much acute inflammation is short-lived.

Acute inflammation

This was recognized by Celsus over 2000 years ago from four basic signs: calor (heat), rubor (redness), dolor (pain) and tumor (swelling) to which has been added loss or impairment of function. The presentation of each sign reflects the interaction of the stimulus, the response and the affected tissue. The main phenomena underlying acute inflammation are a vascular response, interstitial fluid changes and a cellular infiltrate (Fig. 1.2).

Vascular response

The vascular component contributes to increase in temperature and redness and, to a lesser degree, swelling. An initial reaction in the skin is blanching, which is a transitory change and seen after firm stroking, but one that may occur with other stimuli and in other organs. This momentary vasoconstriction is rapidly succeeded by a

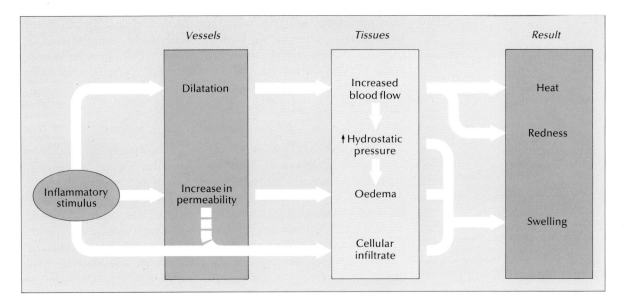

Fig. 1.2 Acute inflammation.

more prolonged interval of vasodilatation producing redness (Fig. 2.1). For minor degrees of injury, vasodilatation persists for 10−15 min but with more severe injury it may extend over several hours. Dilatation affects the small arterioles and fills a greater proportion of the capillary bed than normal, thus creating the false impression of an increase in vasculature. The reaction is partly due to a local axon response and histamine release but is independent of the central nervous system, since it persists following denervation. A marked increase in blood flow results, which may be ten times that of normal. This in turn alters the normal pattern of the blood constituents from that of peripheral plasma and a central core of white cells to one with cells at the perimeter, a phenomenon referred to as *pavementation* or *margination* of white cells. As part of this the red cells clump together (*rouleaux formation*) and the rate of blood flow diminishes and may even cease. The endothelial cells contribute to sludging of the blood by swelling and obstructing the lumen of the vessel and becoming sticky.

Interstitial fluid changes

Swelling, or inflammation, is often the most conspicuous feature and one that is largely a reflection of fluid changes. These involve the increase in the local volume of blood and that in the interstitial tissue fluid from disruption of the normal balance in the blood of osmotic and hydrostatic pressures. Osmotic pressure relates to the protein concentration of the plasma and is normally higher in the blood than the interstitial tissues; fluid therefore flows from the interstitium into the blood. Hydrostatic pressure, in part reflecting systemic blood pressure, has the reverse effect. Inflammation increases the permeability of the endothelial cells, mainly those in the capillaries, and thereby gives fluid and protein easier access to the

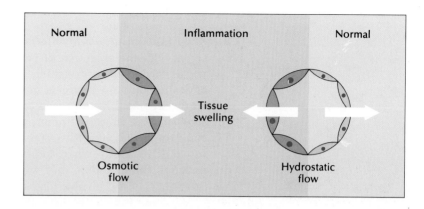

Fig. 1.3 Interstitial fluid changes.

interstitium (Fig. 1.3). This reverses the osmotic pressure gradient which then, like the hydrostatic pressure, forces fluid from the vessels. Proteins that escape into the interstitium include fibrinogen and immunoglobulins and are accompanied by red and white blood cells. Red blood cells are carried passively into the interstitium but white cells actively migrate via the spaces separating the endothelial cells. Fluid exudate may also include antibacterial substances, drugs and antibiotics, complement components and any circulating irritants stimulating the inflammatory response. Increase in interstitial fluid is actively maintained since there is a concomitant increase in lymph flow.

The effects of the fluid exudate are to:

1 Alter the texture of the tissues and make them stiffer if dense and more fluid if loose.

2 Dilute toxins and harmful substances.

3 Confine toxins and harmful substances to the area via fibrin clot formation.

4 Assist phagocytosis by providing a medium for cells to reach micro-organisms and other particles.

5 Bring immunoglobulins and complement to the area.

6 Provide nutrients to the affected tissues.

7 Encourage immune responses following lymphatic transport of antigens to the local lymph nodes.

Cellular infiltrate

This is formed predominantly from *polymorphoneutrophil leucocytes* or *neutrophil polymorphs*. These cells in tissue sections have lobed and irregular nuclei with indistinct and poorly defined cytoplasm and inconspicuous granules (Fig. 1.4). Influx of these cells adds to the swelling of inflammation and is almost exclusively an active process, independent of the fluid exudate. Active attraction occurs within minutes and probably involves mediators arising from the plasma and released by cells in the inflamed area. The neutrophil polymorphs phagocytose foreign particles, digest cellular debris by releasing lysosomes from their granules and contribute to pus formation.

Tissue responses and skin disorders/**5**

Acute inflammation is manifest macroscopically by the basic cardinal signs, with the exception of pain. (Pain remains poorly explained and is attributed to stretching of nerve endings and accumulation of toxins and end products of the increased metabolism.) Microscopically (Fig. 1.5) capillaries are dilated and their endothelial cells swollen and, in some, neutrophil polymorphs line their lumen. Neutrophil polymorphs are also evident within the surrounding tissue. This tissue when loose includes amorphous eosinophilic material, fluid exudate, but when compact is swollen with slight separation of the involved components.

All these features occur with most acute inflammatory skin disorders including the common viral infections such as measles, some

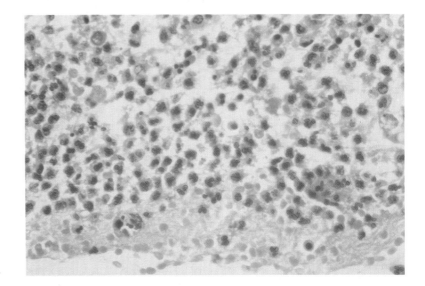

Fig. 1.4 Neutrophil polymorphs in the subserosal tissue of an acutely inflamed appendix. The irregular nuclei are surrounded by indistinct cytoplasm which is enclosed by a poorly defined cell membrane.

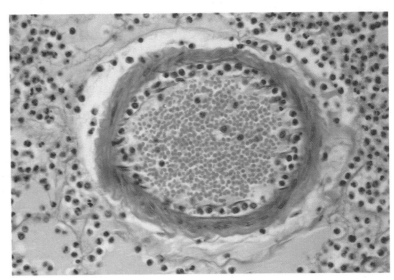

Fig. 1.5 Acute inflammation. The vessel is dilated with swelling of the endothelial cells and some white cells adherent to the endothelium. The surrounding tissue is oedematous with an infiltrate of neutrophil polymorphs present.

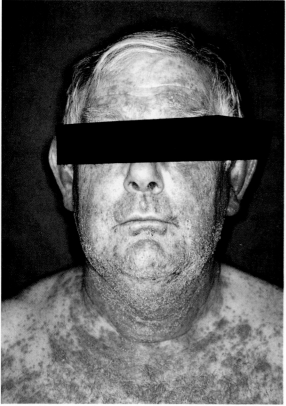

Fig. 1.6 Acute eczematous response due to drugs. There is redness and swelling to the skin.

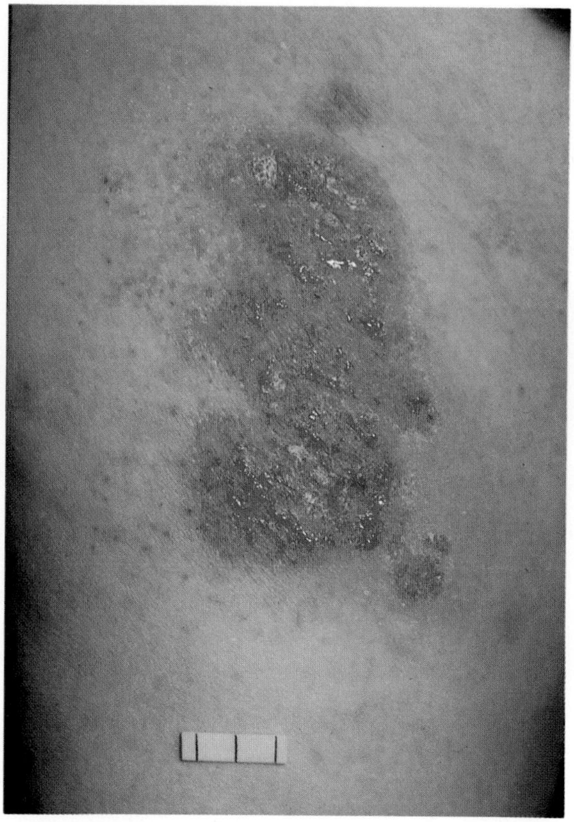

Fig. 1.7 Vesicles: acute eczema following nickel sensitivity. The acute inflammatory reaction includes vesicle formation in the epidermis.

Table 1.3 Examples of bullous disorders with the site of the bullae

Bullous pemphigoid	Subepidermal
Pemphigus	Intra-epithelial
Dermatitis herpetiformis	Subepidermal
Bullous disorders of pregnancy	Subepidermal
Epidermolysis bullosa	Subepidermal

drug eruptions (Fig. 1.6) and mild sunburn as well as around cuts and abrasions. With other inflammatory disorders fluid exudate is more conspicuous and focal small blisters (*vesicles*) and large blisters (*bullae*) form in the epidermis (Fig. 1.7). This reaction may accompany some forms of eczema but is also characteristic of the bullous group of skin disorders which are thought to depend upon immune reactions (Table 1.3).

Course of acute inflammation

Acute inflammation can follow a number of courses:

1 The process can counter the stimulus, resolve and the tissue assume its normal appearance (*resolution*).

2 Healing with fibrosis and scarring of the tissue develops. This may involve regeneration of some cellular components.

3 Death of the tissues follows, complicated by microbial infection and pus formation (*suppuration*).

4 The acute inflammatory response, either because of the tissue involved or from persistence of the cause, progresses to a chronic reaction (chronic inflammation).

Resolution

This reaction restores the tissue from one of acute inflammation to normal with no loss of tissue or residual tissue injury. The neutrophil polymorphs and macrophages are the cells responsible but fibrinolysins and the lymphatics also contribute. Cellular infiltration and activation of macrophages involves a range of products from host tissues and micro-organisms closely linked, via lymphokines, with immune responses which release products aiding resolution. Fibrinolysins originate from the inflammatory exudate and the tissues and their release and inactivation contribute to the removal of the fluid exudate. The lymphatics have a supporting role and remove the exudate and transport antigens to the local lymph nodes where an immune response is initiated.

Macrophages are larger than neutrophil polymorphs with a single nucleus, which in tissue sections can be bean-shaped and vacuolated. Their cytoplasm is pale, sometimes eosinophilic and usually with an irregular outline and a poorly defined cell membrane. Because of these variable appearances recognition may depend upon engulfed or phagocytosed material within the cell or the use of labelled antibodies (Fig. 1.8). Macrophages are derived from the blood monocytes as well as from phagocytic cells dormant in the tissue (*histiocytes*) and are attracted to areas of inflammation by chemotatic forces similar to those attracting neutrophil polymorphs. They appear at the end of an acute inflammatory reaction and herald the potential onset of resolution. For phagocytosis to occur the cells must be activated either by complement, antigen or products of infection. Their membrane receptors bind to the noxious material which is then engulfed and destroyed by lysosomal enzymes. Smaller and soluble particles enter the cell by *pinocytosis*, a process enclosing the particle within a part of the cell membrane which then herniates into the cytoplasm and becomes detached. Macrophages are more effective at phagocytosis than neutrophil polymorphs because they ingest large particles and have a longer life span. They also divide and replace their intracellular enzymes and organelles.

APPEARANCES

Distinguishing between acute inflammation and resolution hinges upon identifying a substantial infiltrate of macrophages. The two processes overlap and in early phases of resolution, features of acute inflammation persist. Towards the end of resolution there are only macrophages within otherwise normal tissue. Once resolution is complete the tissue is structurally and functionally entirely normal.

Fibrosis and scarring

These reactions are a much more common sequel of acute inflammation than resolution. They are not, however, always apparent macroscopically and the functional deficit may also be minimal.

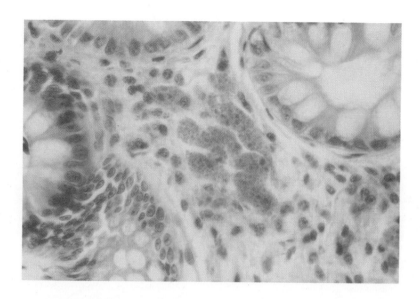

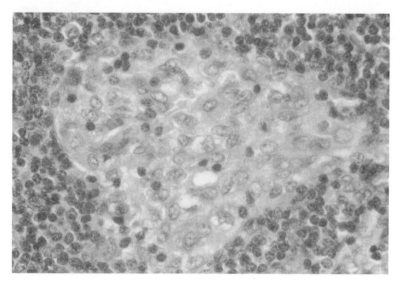

Fig. 1.8 Macrophages (top) in the colon filled with brown pigment, a condition known as melanosis coli. The engulfed material identifies the macrophage. Macrophages (bottom) in the medullary sinus of a lymph node. Antibody markers provide the only proof in tissue sections of the identity of these cells.

Acute inflammation proceeds to granulation tissue which in turn culminates in fibrosis. The persistence of the fibrous tissue and contraction of the tissue together produce a scar.

Granulation tissue is the combination of proliferating endothelial cells and fibroblasts with infiltrates of plasma cells (Fig. 1.9).

Endothelial cells and *fibroblasts* may derive from a common primitive mesenchymal cell, the *myofibroblast* (Fig. 1.10) which, ultrastructurally, combines the features of both. Endothelial cells appear initially as single cells and lie in small tight clusters. After a few days capillary loops form and then venules and arterioles, some joined by arteriovenous shunts, and later lymphatics. Fibroblasts are plump and fusiform and produce *collagen* which provides the scaffolding for tissues, although varying biochemically in different sites. The important property of collagen is its tensile strength. Accumulated collagen, the result of granulation tissue, is *fibrosis*

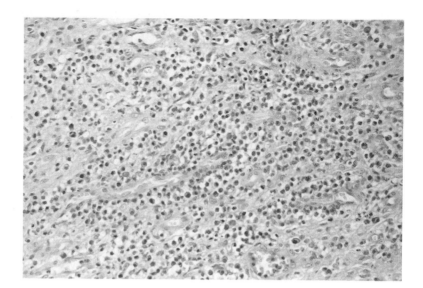

Fig. 1.9 Granulation tissue. The proliferating endothelial cells have formed many vascular channels. The cellular infiltrate includes lymphocytes and plasma cells.

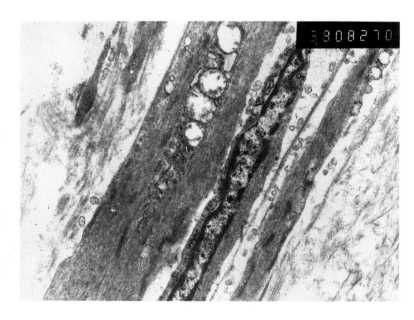

Fig. 1.10 Parts of three myofibroblasts, electron microscopy features. There are filaments with focal densities and similar densities along parts of the cell membrane, features seen in smooth muscle cells. The vesicles and plentiful rough endoplasmic reticulum present in the cell on the left are features characteristic of fibroblasts.

and *fibrous tissue*, which has the structural appearance of collagen but not its functional properties. As fibrous tissue accumulates the newly formed vessels disappear and the region becomes relatively avascular.

Plasma cells are attracted by lymphokines and provide antibody. They are characterized by a prominent nucleus with irregular chromatin aggregates around the circumference simulating a clock-face or hot cross bun (Fig. 1.11). The nucleus lies towards one pole of the cells which are ovoid and include a moderate amount of strikingly eosinophilic cytoplasm. They appear in variable numbers for short periods, reappearing if the reaction proceeds to chronic inflammation.

Contraction is integral to the development of granulation tissue

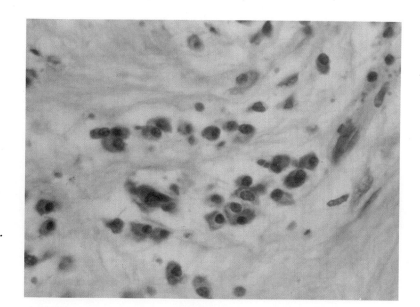

Fig. 1.11 Plasma cells. The cytoplasm is eosinophilic and the nucleus displaced to one pole. The irregular dispersal of the nuclear chromatin is apparent in some cells.

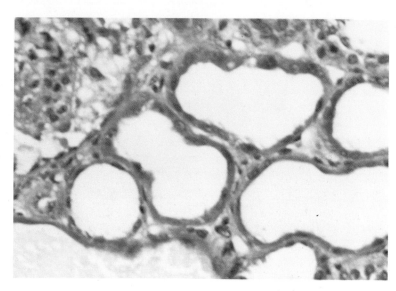

Fig. 1.12 Regeneration of the epithelium of the proximal convoluted tubules following acute tubular necrosis. The normal epithelium is more columnar and all the cells share the same appearances. In these tubules there is variation in the size and shape of the cells and most are markedly flattened.

and fibrosis. This occurs independently of scar formation and may be initiated by the myofibroblasts.

Regeneration can accompany scar formation and is the replacement of lost epithelial cells or specialized cells by similar cells (Fig. 1.12). This only occurs if the cells are able to divide and is in response to growth factors from macrophages and fibroblasts. Regeneration may also be influenced by the loss of contact inhibition that follows tissue injury. *Contact inhibition* is seen in cell cultures where migration occurs until cells come into contact with one another.

Delayed healing results from inadequate oxygen and nutrition. Protein and vitamin C deficiency both impair collagen formation and increasing age, infection, foreign material, excessive movement and malignant tumours all disrupt healing, as do systemic steroids and ultraviolet light.

When a scar is present the area is puckered and denser and tougher than the surrounding tissues. Depending upon the interval after formation it may include obvious vessels or be avascular. Microscopic examination in the early stages reveals capillaries and a few formed venules and arterioles with cells and fibroblasts amongst the stromal tissues (Fig. 1.13). Many of the cells and vessels may be aligned in one direction, particularly if there are stresses applied in these directions. At later stages the tissues include few vessels and collagen is predominant with only occasional fibroblasts.

In the skin when a sterile surgical incision is sutured a minimal scar results and the fibrous tissue is distributed uniformly along the depth of the incision (Fig. 1.14). Re-epithelialization at the

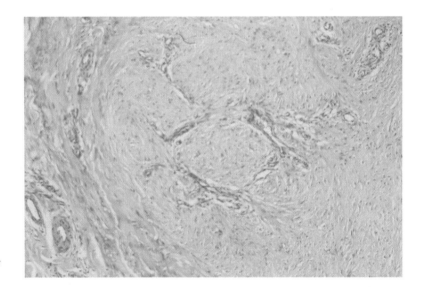

Fig. 1.13 Scar tissue within the abdominal wall. Normal tissue is seen on the left. The fibrous tissue is arranged haphazardly and vessels are prominent within this tissue.

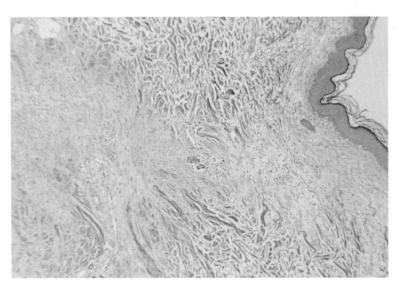

Fig. 1.14 Healed surgical incision. The scar is linear in contrast to the pattern in Fig. 1.13.

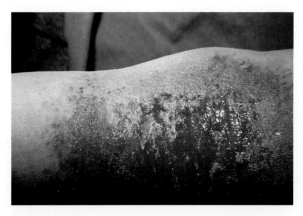

Fig. 1.15 Granulation tissue with small islands of re-epithelialization lying within the area.

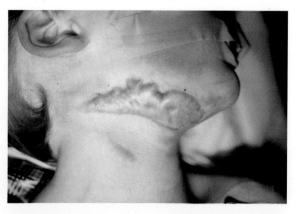

Fig. 1.16 Keloid following a burn on a young boy's neck.

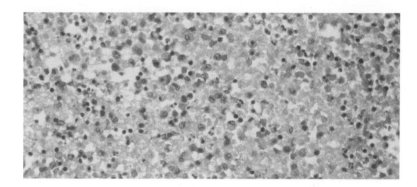

Fig. 1.17 Pus. The amorphous eosinophilic material is the dead cells. The infiltrating cells are principally neutrophil polymorphs.

surface is an early event. If the edges of a wound are not closely apposed or if infection supervenes, fibrosis is initiated at the base of the wound and slowly extends to the surface. Granulation tissue at the base is easily seen if the serum and coagulated blood that form the scab are removed (Fig. 1.15). The eventual scar is prominent with a greater amount of fibrous tissue at the surface than at the base and re-epithelialization is the final event. This type of wound healing is often referred to as *healing by second intention* and that following a surgical incision as *healing by first intention*. But despite this division there are patients, particularly black, who respond to all wounds with florid scar formation (*keloids*) (Fig. 1.16). Scar formation in the skin is also seen as part of the connective tissue disorder, progressive systemic sclerosis or scleroderma, where the stimulus might be immune.

Suppuration

Formation of pus within an area of acute inflammation is known as suppuration. *Pus* is formed from dead and dying cells associated with micro-organisms and supported by inflammatory exudate (Fig. 1.17). The predominant cells are neutrophil polymorphs but cells of the inflamed tissue as well as lymphocytes and macrophages occur.

Tissue responses and skin disorders/**13**

Bacteria are the most common micro-organisms but fungus and even protozoa are found, which may be viable or dead. Pus spreads through pathways of least resistance which within tissues is along tissue planes or towards a free surface. Pus within a confined area produces an abscess and, if an epithelial surface is involved, ulceration.

The essential factor for suppuration is microbial destruction of tissue. Some bacteria also release enzymes which promote tissue digestion. These in turn free lysosomal enzymes, encouraging further destruction. If microbial inflammation is confined by dense tissues and there is no easy drainage route suppuration is almost inevitable. Poor lymphatic drainage can play an important role by aiding stagnation of the inflammatory exudate and other factors, including the virulence, dose and type of the organism, the resistance of the host, and, in particular, the effectiveness of the inflammatory and immune responses, all affect suppuration.

APPEARANCES

Pus varies in consistency from fluid to thick, almost solid material and also has a range of colours (Fig. 1.18). These properties reflect the micro-organisms involved and will further vary if there is more than one organism. When *Staphylococcus aureus* is present the pus is yellowish, while pus associated with *Pseudomonas* species is green. *Candida* infections produce a creamy white pus and *Amoebae* brown. None of these appearances are absolute and culture and microscopy are essential to identify the causative organism.

Chronic inflammation

With this form of inflammation, healing and inflammation coexist (Fig. 1.19). Healing includes granulation tissue and fibrosis, the balance between the two varying with the cause, the host response

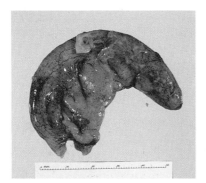

Fig. 1.18 Acute appendicitis with yellowish pus covering parts of the tip. The organ is enlarged and reddened.

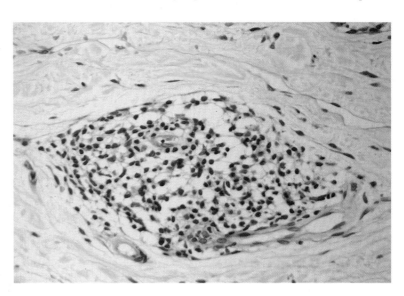

Fig. 1.19 Focal infiltrate of lymphocytes. The conspicuous features are the round deeply basophil nuclei.

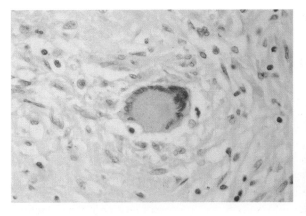

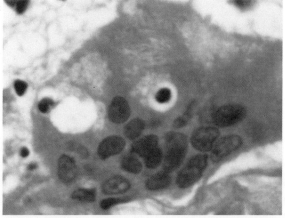

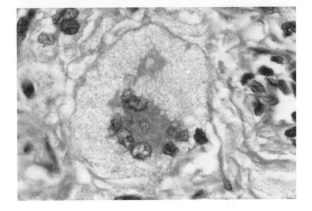

Fig. 1.20 Giant cells. (*Above left*) Langerhan, typical of Mycobacteria tuberculosis infection; (*above right*) foreign body giant cell; (*right*) Touton, a feature of some benign dermal tumours (dermatofibromas).

and the presence or absence of infection. Inflammatory features differ from those found in acute inflammation in that:

1 Vascular response is less evident and consists of formed vessels rather than developing capillaries.

2 Fluid exudate is not so apparent and may be replaced by pus.

3 Cellular response changes from one of phagocytic cells to one in which there are lymphocytes, plasma cells and macrophages reflecting a greater role for the immune system and antigenic sensitization. *Lymphocytes* are identified by their round uniformly basophilic nuclei. Their cytoplasm is not readily apparent (Fig. 1.19). Antibodies can be used to distinguish the T- and B-cell types.

Granuloma formation is a variant of the chronic inflammation response. Granulomas are aggregates of macrophages, either mildly infiltrated or surrounded by lymphocytes. Additionally there may be small numbers of *giant cells* which may arise from the fusion of macrophages and include several different types, mostly multinucleate (Fig. 1.20). A granulomatous response occurs in a large number of chronic inflammatory reactions of which the best known is that following infection by *Mycobacteria* including tuberculosis and leprae (Fig. 1.21). Other examples are to foreign bodies, sarcoidosis (Fig. 1.22) and a range of infections, but few of these include unique or diagnostic appearances. The lack of specificity makes it essential that every ancillary means is used to identify the

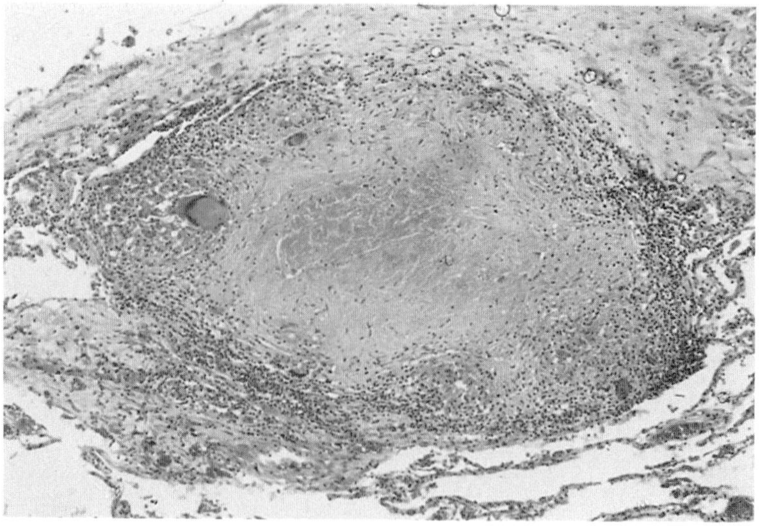

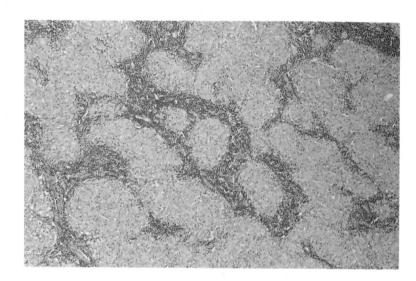

Fig. 1.21 Typical tuberculous granuloma. The centre is necrotic material and around this are macrophages, a Langerhan's giant cell and some lymphocytes.

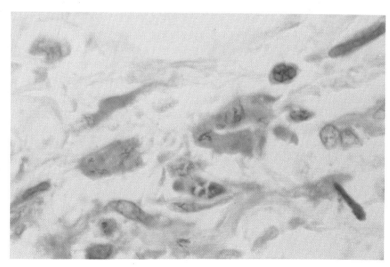

Fig. 1.22 Granulomas associated with sarcoidosis in a lymph node. Each granuloma is an aggregate of macrophages. Sarcoidosis is a disorder characterized by these appearances in any of the tissues involved and with no recognized cause.

Fig. 1.23 Mycobacteria within a granuloma stained by the Ziehl–Nielsen technique. Recognition of these organisms identifies the cause of the granuloma.

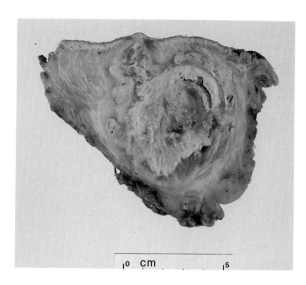

Fig. 1.25 Abscess. The centre is filled with pus and this is encased by thick grey-white fibrous tissue. There is a tract forming towards the skin surface.

cause including a careful clinical history, microbial cultures, serology and special staining procedures (Fig. 1.23).

Chronic inflammation follows acute inflammation usually because the stimulus persists. Impaired body responses and delayed healing are other causes. Inflammation can, however, develop without any preceding acute phase and in these circumstances aberrant immune responses, hypersensitivity reactions, are possibly responsible. These reactions are suggested particularly when the cause is unclear and when there is substantial fibrosis. Fibrosis of this type is found as a part of some connective tissue disorders and in some forms of tuberculosis and syphilis.

APPEARANCES

These mirror those of fibrosis and scarring and may include suppuration. When extensive there is widespread destruction of tissues and consequent functional impairment (Fig. 1.24).

In the skin chronic inflammation is typified by a *chronic abscess* or *boil* (Fig. 1.25). The centre is filled with pus and within the immediately adjacent tissue there is a layer of granulation tissue supported by a fibrous capsule of variable thickness. The capsule may, in long-standing examples, include only small numbers of lymphocytes but in the earlier stages these cells are more numerous.

Granulomas occur in the skin in a wide variety of circumstances, including local disorders and systemic diseases. They are seen as part of acne and in response to insect bites and foreign bodies (Fig. 1.26). Granulomas also form part of the cutaneous manifestations of rheumatoid arthritis (*rheumatoid nodules*), diabetes mellitus (*necrobiosis lipoidica*) and sarcoidosis (Fig. 1.27).

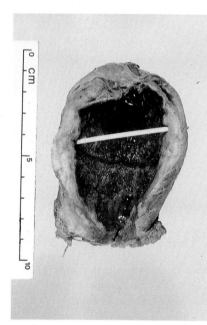

Fig. 1.24 Gall bladder with chronic cholecystitis. There were gall-stones present that resulted in obstruction. The wall of the gall bladder is markedly thickened and replaced by white fibrous tissue. The lining is reddened and oedematous.

Tissue responses and skin disorders/**17**

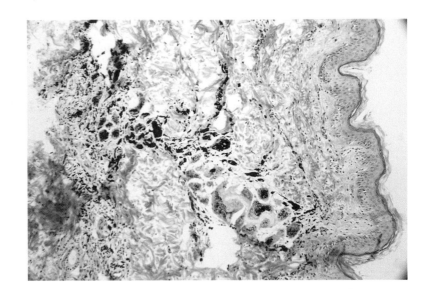

Fig. 1.26 Granuloma following tattooing.

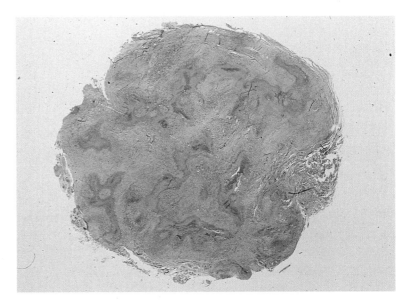

Fig. 1.27 Rheumatoid nodule. The striate brightly eosinophilic areas are necrotic tissue and the blue halo around these is formed by macrophages and some lymphocytes. This type of nodule is found subcutaneously in patients with the joint disease rheumatoid arthritis.

Death of tissues

Necrosis or cell death is the inevitable end point of many disorders. The initial injury is biochemical following anoxia, direct poisoning, complement digestion or mechanical rupture of the cell. This is followed by irreversible changes affecting the cell membrane, cytoplasm, micro-organelles and nucleus which may excite an inflammatory response. The features are rarely confined to single cells but affect all or part of an organ (Fig. 1.28). A similar spectrum of changes, *autolysis*, involves the entire body after death but without any inflammatory response, an important contrast from necrosis and one which may help the forensic pathologist to distinguish between injury caused before and after death.

Degeneration is injury to cells that is insufficient to cause necrosis.

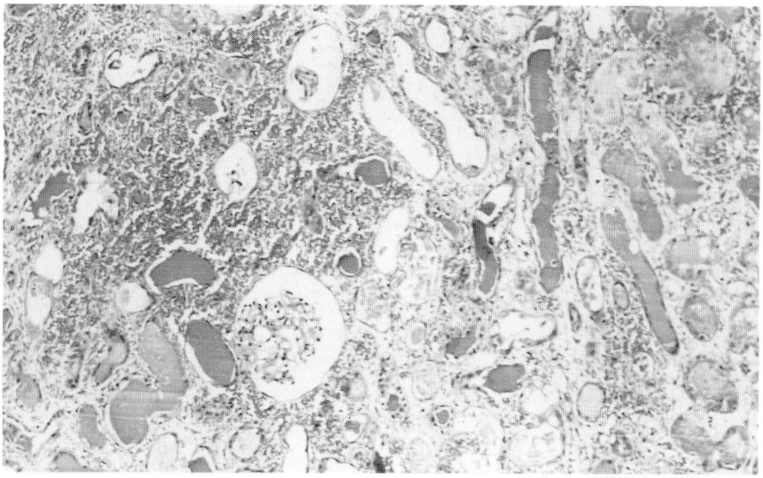

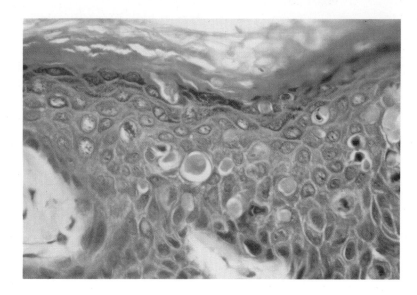

Fig. 1.28 Area of necrosis within a rejected renal transplant. The tubular and glomerular structure is still identifiable but these no longer include a full complement of cells. The interstitial tissue is oedematous and includes haemorrhage, evidence of involvement of the vessels.

Fig. 1.29 Apoptosis within skin involved by in situ carcinoma. The round pink foci are the apoptotic cells.

A sequence of intracytoplasmic events is initiated but the nucleus is not affected. As with necrosis an inflammatory response can occur.

Apoptosis is the third process involved in cell death. This can follow injury but is also physiological and not associated with an inflammatory reaction. Physiologically, there is active cell deletion which models the embryo during development and counters the continuous replacement of adult tissues such as the skin (Fig. 1.29), liver and intestinal mucosa. Apoptosis also plays a part in atrophy and the involution of tissues, control of tumour growth and in cell mediated immune responses.

APPEARANCES

Degenerative and apoptotic changes have no macroscopic counterparts. Necrotic tissue is soft, even to the point of forming fluid, and

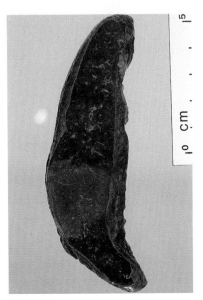

Fig. 1.30 Infarct in the spleen. This is red and the tissues are necrotic.

swollen in contrast to its surroundings. The tissue may be paler or darker than normal depending mainly upon the blood supply (Fig. 1.30). In organs with a plentiful blood supply the affected areas are dark red, even black, while in poorly vascularized regions the tissue is pale. Haemolysis is an important part of these colour differences. Infection and pus formation may supervene in any necrotic tissue.

Necrosis involves a series of changes culminating in cell rupture. These reflect an alteration in the permeability of the cell membrane and also that of the micro-organelles, most importantly the mito-chondria and lysosymes. The cell's cytoplasm may undergo

• either *cloudy swelling* which is a finely vacuolar change from an influx of fluid;

• or *fatty change*, seen as intracytoplasmic vacuoles of fat, due to the unmasking of the fat that provides the energy source for the cell;

• or *hyaline degeneration* in which the cytoplasm becomes finely granular and eosinophilic with an increase in micro-organelles.

The nucleus at first contracts and becomes more deeply stain-ing (*pyknosis*) and then breaks up into chromatin fragments (*karyorrhexis*). The final event in the nucleus is that it disappears (*karyolysis*). If the general architecture of the tissue remains the necrosis is referred to as *coagulative* but when the basic tissue pattern is lost, the necrosis is *liquefactive* or *colliquative*. Liquefactive necrosis is seen in the brain which naturally has a high water content and is also associated with pus but is otherwise uncommon. Coagulative necrosis is best seen after ischaemia but even in these circumstances it may not be as distinctive as is implied (Fig. 1.31).

Degeneration is recognized by the same cytoplasmic changes as necrosis. With degeneration, however, these do not progress to cell rupture and none of the nuclear changes appear.

Apoptosis is completed within hours via a series of stages but,

Fig. 1.31 Necrosis within the mesentery. In the lower part the fat cells are swollen and the cytoplasm is basophilic. Above this many of the cells are entirely necrotic with rupture of the cell membranes and release of the basophilic chromatin and cell constituents.

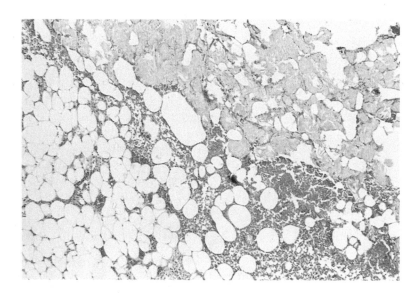

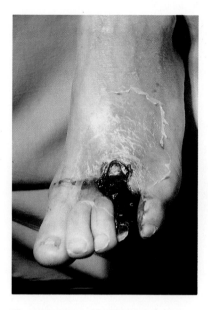

Fig. 1.32 Gangrene. This developed in a diabetic with peripheral vascular disease.

because of the speed of the process, affected cells are rarely seen in normal tissues although in disease they are more readily identified. First, the cell loses contact with its neighbours and any intercellular junctions are broken. The cell then shrinks irregularly so that parts protrude from the main mass and concurrently the nucleus shrinks and breaks up. The micro-organelles and cell membrane remain intact although some of the protruding parts break off. The fragments are finally ingested and degraded by neighbouring cells, which in some tissues will involve macrophages.

In the skin, necrosis is sometimes referred to as *gangrene* (Fig. 1.32). The area is black and, if infected, offensive. The organisms involved are anaerobic, particularly Clostridia species but also Streptococci and Bacteroidaceae. Without infection there is an underlying peripheral vascular disease with obliteration of the blood supply. Gangrene is a gross example of necrosis in the skin and less conspicuous examples accompany a wide range of other skin diseases, some preceded by degeneration. The development of the vesicles in eczema and the lesions of chickenpox (Fig. 1.33) and smallpox are changes of this type. Apoptosis is seen in skin exposed to ultraviolet light and skin in diseases such as lichen planus when injury is allied with altered cellular immunity (Fig. 1.34).

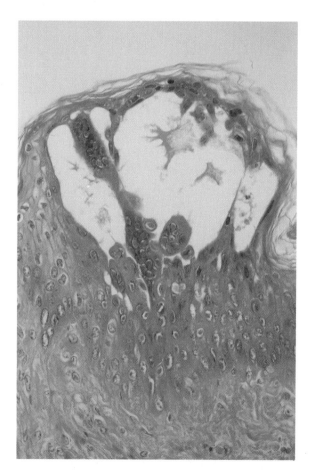

Fig. 1.33 Chickenpox in the late eruptive stage with vesicles coalescing, multinucleate giant cells and inclusions within some cells.

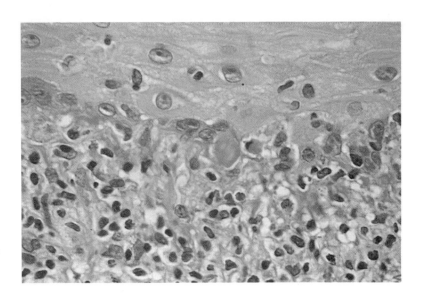

Fig. 1.34 Apoptotic cell at the base of the epidermis in lichen planus, an irritant, often diffuse disorder.

Further reading

Chapel, H. and Haeney, M. (1988). *Essentials of Clinical Immunology* (2nd Edition). Blackwell Scientific Publications: Oxford and London.

Johnston, R.B. (1988). Monocytes and macrophages. *New Eng. J. Med.* **318**, 747–52.

Kerr, J.F.R., Bishop, C.J. and Searle, J. (1984). Apoptosis. In: *Recent Advances in Histopathology*. 12. Ed. by P.P. Anthony and R.N.M. MacSween, pp 1–15. Churchill Livingstone: Edinburgh, London.

Mackie, R.M. (1984). *Milne's Dermatopathology*. Edward Arnold: London.

Anderson, J.R. *Muir's Textbook of Pathology* (12 Edition). Edward Arnold: London.

Rook, A., Wilkinson, D.S., Ebling, F.J.G., Champion, R.H. and Burton, J.L. (1986). *Textbook of Dermatology* (4th Edition). Volumes 1–4. Blackwell Scientific Publications: Oxford.

Walter, J.B. and Israel, M.S. (1987). *General Pathology* (6th Edition). Churchill Livingstone: Edinburgh, London and New York.

Weatherall, D.J. (1985). *The New Genetics and Clinical Practice* (2nd Edition). Oxford University Press: Oxford and New York.

Williams, G.T. and Williams, W.J. (1983). Granulomatous inflammation — a review. *J. Clin. Path.* **36**, 723–33.

Woolf, N. (1986). *Cell, Tissue and Disease: the Basis of Pathology* (2nd Edition). Bailliere Tindall: London, Philadelphia and Toronto.

2 Tumour diagnosis

A *tumour* is a swelling. The term incorporates a range of lesions including abscesses, areas of bruising or inflammation and also cancers. *Cancer* is a widely used term for a harmful or malignant tumour of any type and any cancer is a *neoplasm* or new growth. Neoplasms grow independently of their parent tissues but are not necessarily malignant. Neoplasms, growths or tumours should therefore be prefixed with 'benign' or 'malignant'. Attempts at defining benign and malignant neoplasms have never met with universal agreement because there are neoplasms which are neither clearly benign nor malignant and others that alter their behaviour or do not have their predicted effects. Therapy for example can completely cure some highly malignant tumours of the testes and lymph nodes while any neoplasm within the skull and compressing the brain is potentially lethal. There are also no absolute histopathological appearances peculiar to either type of tumour although their behavioural pattern is suggestive. A tumour that spreads is unequivocally malignant, but if spread is absent the possibility of a malignant tumour still exists since the diagnosis may have preceded recognizable dissemination.

Causes of neoplasia

No single cause for all neoplasms is known although for individual tumours there are some distinct risk factors, such as cigarettes for lung cancer. All agents producing inflammatory and destructive tissue changes have been implicated as carcinogenic and present knowledge suggests that for any neoplasm there are multiple causative factors, specific and shared. Examples of these and their role for individual tumours are presented in subsequent chapters. Viruses and particular genes (*oncogenes*) are currently under intense investigation. All cells include genes affecting growth and differentiation (*proto-oncogenes*) and if these are modified to oncogenes neoplasia can follow. Such somatic mutations may appear spontaneously or be induced by external agents including radiation, chemical carcinogens and viruses. Other oncogenes arise from the incorporation of viral oncogenes into cells which then persist in the altered and malignant progeny. A balance may exist between these oncogenes and other tumour suppressing genes, or *anti-oncogenes*, which if upset results in cancer. A further postulate is that there are cancer predisposing genes which determine the direction of this balance.

Most tumour research involves malignant neoplasms, mainly because these rapidly growing tumours yield quick results, but whether these observations are applicable to benign tumours is not clear. The end result is that a large number of potential avenues have been studied as causes of many malignant tumours, but for the majority of benign tumours virtually nothing is known. Studies are often restricted to laboratory animals and the observations then directly substituted to man, a jump that may be inappropriate. The experimental rat has a known and mapped pedigree, it can be restrained in a controlled environment and submitted to potential carcinogenic stimuli of known doses for definite periods. The short life span, in contrast to that of man, makes it possible for any latent period between tumour induction and development to be bridged and for the type of tumour produced to be defined. Man, in contrast, with an impure and often imprecise genetic background, a long life span, free in his environment and exposed continuously to multiple carcinogens of unknown strength, as well as to non-carcinogenic stimuli with potential additive effects, is less easily studied.

Tumour diagnosis

This involves the histopathologist in recognizing premalignant states, classifying, staging and grading tumours and knowing how neoplasms spread and behave as well as being aware of their appearances.

Premalignant states

The histopathologist recognizes conditions which may proceed to malignancy including cellular changes and disease states.

1   The cellular changes preceding epithelial tumours are referred to as *intraepithelial neoplasia* or *carcinoma in situ*. The epithelium is replaced by malignant cells and any semblance of normal maturation and the presence of specialized cells is lost. The changes are limited to the epithelium and there is no invasion into the underlying tissue (Fig. 2.1). This state may be maintained for short periods or for years but eventually an invasive carcinoma will appear. Carcinoma-in-situ can develop within any epithelium and its natural history can be monitored by biopsies or cytology, as is done in the cervix.

2   Disease states that may progress to malignancy include some benign tumours (large intestinal adenomas (Fig. 2.2) and skin naevi), chronic inflammatory conditions (chronic skin ulcers and inflammatory bowel disease (ulcerative colitis)) and rare genetic disorders (xeroderma pigmentosa associated with all common skin malignancies and the genetic defects underlying the ´childhood renal malignancy, Wilm's tumour and immunodeficiency syndromes that progress to lymphomas).

Most premalignant states involve epithelial malignancies and with this knowledge and their accessibility, effective monitoring and potential preventative measures are possible.

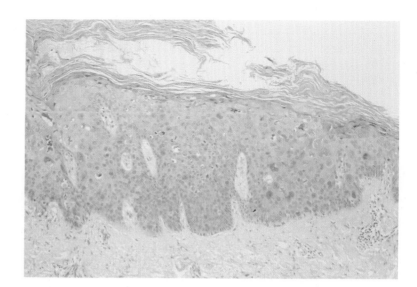

Fig. 2.1 Intra-epithelial neoplasia. A biopsy from the vulva in which the normal maturation pattern of the epithelium is lost. Large basophilic cells and pleomorphic cells are lying both near the surface and at the base of the epithelium.

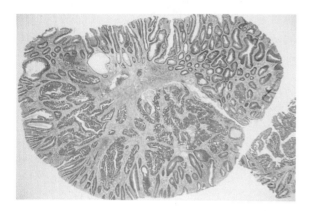

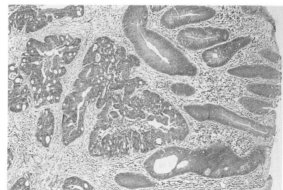

Fig. 2.2 Tubulovillous adenoma from the colon; (*above left*) a tumour that while usually benign, can be a precursor to an adenocarcinoma. In this example malignant change has developed on the left side with (*above right*) a change in the appearance of the epithelium immediately below the surface.

Tumour classifications

1 Benign and malignant is a useful prognostic division. This ultimately depends upon differences in behaviour, i.e., the potential to spread, but can be inferred from a number of appearances (Table 2.1). These, however, are generalizations and for each statement there are always exceptions. Mitotic rate provides an illustration in that in malignant tumours this is usually high and greater than that of benign tumours. There are nonetheless malignant tumours such as some skin tumours arising from melanocytes (melanomas) where mitoses are not widespread, and occasional benign tumours with many mitoses. The more useful observation is that aberrant mitoses (Fig. 2.3) characterize malignant tumours but these may be few or totally absent because of the speed of the cell cycle.

2 *Primary* is used to refer to the site of origin of any malignant tumour and *secondary* or *metastasis* to tumour that has spread from this site to other tissues. An adenocarcinoma of the stomach is a primary tumour and tumour from this in lymph nodes or liver is

Table 2.1 Comparisons between benign and malignant tumours

	Neoplasms	
	Benign	Malignant
Site	Localized growth	Spread locally and systemically
Growth	Slow	Rapid
Size	Small	Large
Metastatic potential	None	Inherent
Tumour edge	Abrupt and encapsulated	Infiltrating
Cell differentiation	Good	Poor
Mitoses	Few and normal	Many and aberrant
Intratumour complications	None	Haemorrhage and necrosis
Systemic effects	Local compression	Destruction locally and systemically
Mortality	None	Inevitable

secondary or metastatic tumour. Identical microscopic features are shared by both tumours (Fig. 2.4). Primary growths are often amenable to therapy, particularly surgery, but metastatic disease requires chemotherapy or irradiation which is often only palliative. Recognizing the origin of a metastasis without knowledge of the primary site is often impossible because many tumours share similar appearances.

3   According to the cell of origin:
(a) epithelium — *carcinomas* (malignant); *adenomas* (benign);
(b) connective tissues — *sarcomas* (malignant); *lipomas, fibromas,* etc. (benign);
(c) totipotential tissues — *teratomas* (malignant and benign);
(d) mononuclear cells — *lymphomas* and *leukaemias* (malignant).

Malignant epithelial tumours subdivide into those originating from squamous, mucous and transitional cells, respectively known as *squamous carcinomas, adenocarcinoma* and *transitional cell carcinomas.* Connective tissue tumours embrace every facet of connective tissue including fat, fibrous tissue, nerves and vessels. These all share a common mesenchymal origin and an individual tumour may include more than one component. Thus, fat and vessels can be the principal constituents producing *angiolipomas* or *angiolipo-sarcomas.* The testicular and ovarian epithelial cells are prime sources of teratomas and T- and B-lymphocytes, and macrophages the cells forming mononuclear cell tumours.

Carcinomas are more amenable to surgery than lymphomas but are less affected by chemotherapy and many sarcomas carry a worse outlook than either carcinomas or lymphomas.

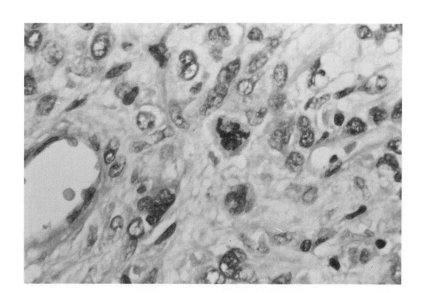

Fig. 2.3 Bizarre mitosis within a tumour. This observation is more suggestive that the tumour is malignant than the presence of numerous normal mitoses.

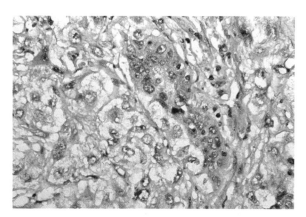 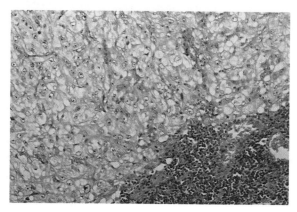

Fig. 2.4 Clear cell carcinoma of the kidney; (*above left*) in the kidney and (*above right*) in a lymph node in the same patient. There is striking similarity in the appearances of the tumour cells in both sites.

Divisions are made from knowledge of the site of the tumour and of its gross and microscopic appearances. Ancillary investigations using special staining techniques for mucus, melanin and other cell products, also electron microscopy to define ultrastructure and labelled antibodies to cell components, can confirm and, in some examples, indicate the cell of origin. Nevertheless, there are sporadic tumours which after light microscopy complemented by these special techniques defy categorization. Characteristically such tumours are malignant and are described as *anaplastic* (Fig. 2.5). If it is probable that these lesions are carcinomas rather than sarcomas or vice versa they can then be referred to as anaplastic carcinomas or sarcomas, respectively.

4 Further subclassifications used by histopathologists arise from those of the WHO and Armed Forces Institute of Pathology. These split tumours extensively according to their cellular appearances, again with an aim of reflecting prognosis and therapy, but are often self-defeating because of their complexity and ultimate dependence upon personal interpretation and experience. A more recent approach, successful with a tumour of infancy, the neuroblastoma, is

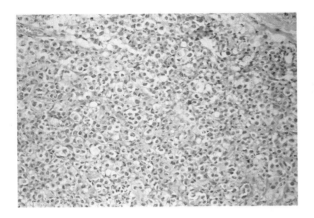 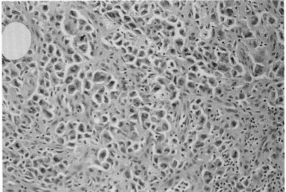

Fig. 2.5 Undifferentiated tumour; (*above left*) involving skeletal muscle and (*above right*) in a different patient, in the retroperitoneal tissues.

to grade tumours according to their oncogene content but whether this will be widely applicable is as yet uncertain.

Tumour staging

The mass of the primary malignant tumour and the extent and localization of metastatic spread, particularly the number of lymph nodes involved, all indicate the total tumour load and can be used to assess prognosis and therapy. The approach is the basis of the Tumour, Nodes, Metastases (TNM) staging of tumours (Table 2.2) which is extensively used in the USA but has not been so widely adopted in the UK. The final TNM category combines histopathological, clinical and investigative findings and varies between centres depending on the different investigative tools used and the thoroughness with which clinical and histopathological investigation is performed.

Tumour grading

Grading malignant tumours is highly subjective and open to error. Grading systems depend upon choosing microscopic criteria such as keratin formation and separating the tumours according to how well these are represented (Fig. 2.6). The main shortcomings are that the greater the amount of tumour examined the wider the variation in appearances found and that, in practice, it is not feasible to cut serial sections of entire tumours, the only absolute method of examining all parts of any tumour. Nevertheless, histo-

Table 2.2 TNM classification

	Grades
T: size and extent of tumour locally	1–4
N: number of involved regional lymph nodes	0–3
M: presence of distant metastases	0–1

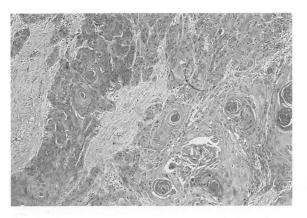

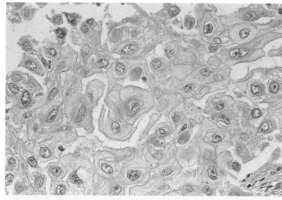

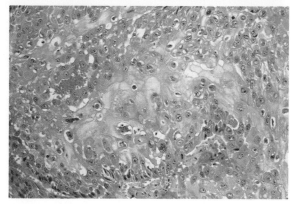

Fig. 2.6 Examples of squamous carcinomas; (*above left*) includes easily recognized and numerous round red masses of keratin (keratin pearls) lying amongst the tumour islands; (*above right*) with keratin restricted to within the tumour cells, the darker red material; (*right*) with no keratin.

pathologists commonly describe tumours as *well differentiated*, *moderately well differentiated* and *poorly differentiated*, so making a subjective judgement from the overall appearances of the parts they have selected. Implicit in these decisions is that well differentiated tumours will behave less aggressively than poorly differentiated ones, and so carry a better prognosis, conclusions that in practice are not always true. The poorly differentiated tumours may be more amenable to therapy than their well differentiated counterparts and so have a good prognosis.

Spread of malignant tumours

A tumour is indisputably malignant once it has spread from its site of origin to distant tissues. Metastases develop either by direct invasion into surrounding tissue or by embolization via blood vessels or lymphatic vessels or by spread across cavities (transcoelomic).

Invasion in surrounding tissues usually involves following a path of least resistance, including natural tissue planes, such as between muscle bundles or around nerves and vessels (Fig. 2.7). Within vessels the tumour may either grow along the lumen to other sites or parts may break off forming emboli, which are then carried to distant organs (Fig. 2.8). The tumour enters the vessels by invading newly formed vessels within and around the tumour and in lymphatics this may be facilitated by their incomplete basement

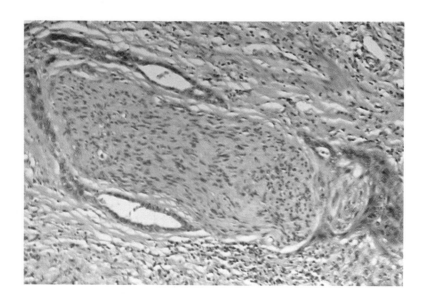

Fig. 2.7 Adenocarcinoma spreading through tissues with a nerve acting as the pathway.

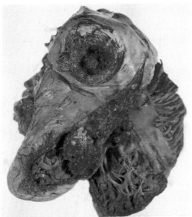

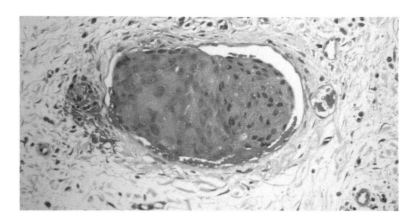

Fig. 2.8 Tumour spreading within vessels; (*above right*) a breast carcinoma with tumour within a lymphatic and (*above left*) an adenocarcinoma from the colon entering the right atrium and right ventricle of the heart. The vena cava was filled with tumour and this had spread via the liver.

membrane. Only lymphatics and veins are involved. Arterioles and larger arteries are only very rarely infiltrated, although why this is so is unresolved. Once within lymphatics tumour cells are carried to the nearest lymph node and once in venules to the most immediate organ but at these new sites the tumour cells will not always immediately proliferate and establish a metastasis. The lymph node or organ may be skipped and the next tissue in line provide the seat for a metastasis. Alternatively no immediate metastasis may develop at any site, the secondary tumour appearing months or years after the primary is recognized and even after this has been removed.

The stimulus for a tumour to spread is unclear. Loss of adhesion between tumour cells, active motility of tumour cells, secretion of substances promoting spread and the handling of tumours have all been suggested and the last certainly proved. Equally unclear is how the dispersed tumour cells establish metastasis and why some produce secondary growth in some sites in preference to others. Differences in venous and lymphatic drainage are not sufficient

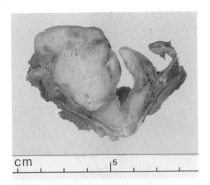

Fig. 2.9 Carcinoma of the larynx which by extending into the lumen of the larynx obstructs this and embarrasses breathing.

explanations and undoubtedly only a very small proportion of disseminated cells successfully produce a metastatic lesion.

Effects of tumours

Benign and malignant tumours both exert functional changes but these are generally more dramatic and serious with the malignant growths.

1 All tumours have the facility to destroy tissues. Some benign tumours do this because space for growth is restricted, as within the skull, but with malignant tumours there is active replacement of tissues.

2 Any tumour can mechanically obstruct drainage pathways, for example benign and malignant tumours in the bronchus, ureter or gastrointestinal tract (Fig. 2.9).

3 Pain, haemorrhage and infection locally can each be associated with tumours but more especially with malignant neoplasms.

4 Nutritional effects including disproportionate wasting equivalent to starvation (*cachexia*) are almost entirely confined to malignancy.

5 Persistent and intermittent fever, independent of infection, is characteristic of many malignant tumours.

6 Secondary immunosuppression is a phenomenon of malignant growths but it is also contributed to by antitumour therapy.

7 Secretion of hormones, enzymes and proteins is seen, most notably with malignant tumours. This may be appropriate to the tissue, as ACTH from a pituitary tumour, or inappropriate, ACTH from a lung tumour, and may occur in amounts sufficient to produce effects or remain clinically silent. The formation of foetal antigens (*oncofoetal proteins*) and hormones assists in the diagnosis clinically and histopathologically since antibodies can be prepared to these antigens.

8 Haemolytic anaemia, polycythaemia, thrombocytopenia, increased clotting and migratory thrombophlebitis are some of the haematological manifestations characterizing certain malignant tumours.

9 Other malignant tumours result in amyloid deposition and renal, neurological and skin disorders.

The mechanisms producing most of these effects are largely unknown. Some are the direct result of the release of substances by the tumour, others arise from changes in the body's physiology and others from the anti-tumour therapy received. Autoimmune responses may be the underlying cause in a few patients.

APPEARANCES

Benign tumours

These are usually well localized, slowly growing masses, often knowingly tolerated by the patient. They gradually achieve a maximum size and then maintain this. The ultimate size is generally

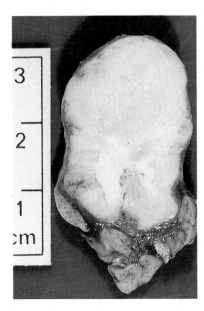

Fig. 2.10 Benign tumour in the parotid salivary gland, a pleomorphic adenoma. The uninvolved salivary gland is compressed and embraces the tumour but is clearly separate from this.

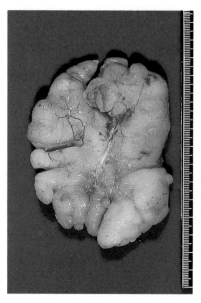

Fig. 2.11 Typical lipoma, presenting as a soft-to-firm subcutaneous swelling.

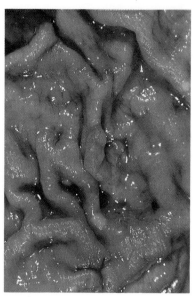

Fig. 2.12 Tubular villous adenoma in the colon. The difference in colour from the surrounding mucosa reflects the cellularity and vascularity of the tumour. Tumour is projecting into the lumen of the bowel.

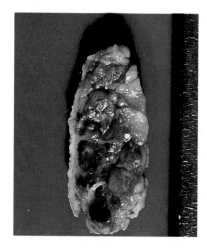

Fig. 2.13 Haemangioma. This benign tumour is not encapsulated and not well circumscribed.

less than that of their malignant counterpart although very large benign tumours are found. The tumour may be surrounded by a capsule or by compressed tissue forming a pseudocapsule (Fig. 2.10). Necrosis, ulceration and haemorrhage are not commonly seen. The colour and consistency reflect the cell of origin although epithelial tumours are softer than most benign connective tissue tumours with tumours of fat (lipomas) (Fig. 2.11) providing an obvious exception. Epithelial tumours project from the surface with or without a stalk forming *adenomas* and *papillomas* (Fig. 2.12), respectively, while benign connective tissue tumours tend to lie within the involved organ and are often poorly circumscribed (Fig. 2.13).

Microscopic features. These mimic those of the parent tissue. For example, benign adenomas of the large intestine have very similar appearances to the normal large bowel epithelium but differ in that there is a greater concentration of epithelial cells at one site. The benign tumour may also mimic the normal function of the parent tissue by producing mucus, hormones or other substances.

Malignant tumours

These are often rapidly growing with focal haemorrhage and necrosis as common complications. Symptoms alter with the site and size of the tumour and also the tolerance of the patient. Occasional patients

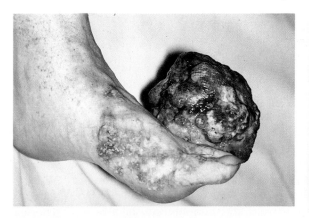

Fig. 2.14 (*Above left*) Melanoma that has reached an enormous size and must have caused inconvenience. The patient presented only because of repeated bleeding from

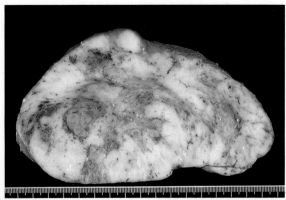

the tumour that was difficult to stem; (*above right*) a huge fibromyosarcoma from the peritoneal cavity. The increase in girth was misinterpreted as an increase in weight.

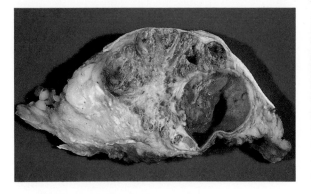

Fig. 2.15 (*Above left*) Carcinoma of the breast. The breast tissue has been destroyed and it is difficult to be sure where the tumour ends and normal breast tissue survives.

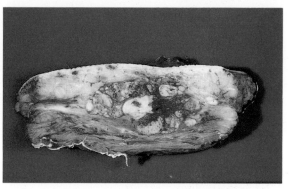

Much of the tumour is necrotic and haemorrhage has occurred; (*above right*) a leiomyosarcoma in the subcutaneous tissues with similar features to the breast carcinoma.

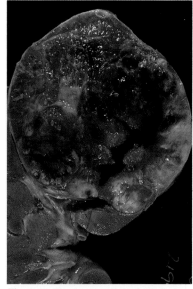

Fig. 2.16 Carcinoma of the kidney with haemorrhage and necrosis.

will be seen with gross tumours, some accepted for months despite their physical inconvenience and disfiguring effects (Fig. 2.14). The size of the tumour reflects the rate of growth rather than its duration but may be contributed to by haemorrhage, necrosis and inflammation. A rapid growth rate is also inferred from the lack of a true or pseudocapsule. No clear-cut separation exists between the tumour and the parent tissue and the periphery of the tumour is irregular and infiltrative (Fig. 2.15). If a free surface is involved the tumour will ulcerate and fungate from this. The consistency is softer than that of the surrounding tissues and the tumour is often paler. Haemorrhage and necrosis both result in further softening and produce discoloration (Fig. 2.16). Old haemorrhage and necrosis cause grey/black areas and recent haemorrhage dark red regions; vascular sarcomas (*angiosarcomas*) share many of these features.

A distinction between primary and secondary growths can be made if both are present in the same tissue. The primary is often larger and the secondary growths lie as satellites around this. Distinguishing individual primary and secondary tumour

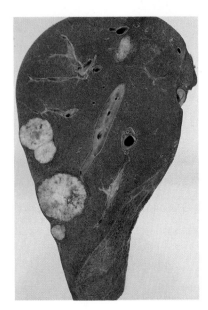

Fig. 2.17 Secondary tumour in the liver. All the deposits are of comparable size and there is no one deposit around which the others are clustered to suggest a primary liver cell carcinoma. The primary growth was in the colon.

macroscopically is otherwise difficult but any organ including many similar sized tumours is almost certainly involved by metastatic tumour (Fig. 2.17).

Microscopic features. The features that are useful for the microscopic diagnosis of malignancy are:

1 Invasion into any surrounding tissues, including vessels.

2 Architectural changes. These amongst carcinomas include an epithelium proliferating into and over the underlying tissue instead of simply lining it; glands that no longer retain a clear pattern between their acini and ducts; and islands and strands of epithelial cells lying in tissues where none are normally found (Fig. 2.18). With other malignancies the tumour cells take over the normal tissue, destroying and replacing it, and, in all examples, there is no uniform or regular pattern to these cells.

3 Cellular features. These include differences in the size and shape of cells and their nuclei (*pleomorphism*) (Fig. 2.19). A further character is *dysplasia* which is a subjective observation involving the recognition of differences in the cytoplasm and nucleus from those of normal cells (Fig. 2.20). The cell is also enlarged and the cytoplasm basophilic and any specialized function such as mucus production lost. The nucleus, too, is basophilic and may be dividing. The proportion of dividing cells, the *mitotic index*, is high and mitoses include normal patterns and, more significantly, bizarre forms. These cytological features are often the only ones that the cytologist has on which to form a diagnosis.

4 Stroma enveloping the tumour. This is more apparent in carcinomas than other malignancies and includes vessels and fibrous tissue which if abundant may, at low power microscopy, mask the tumour cells (Fig. 2.21). Infiltrating the stroma and malignant cells are variable numbers of mononuclear cells indicating both an inflammatory and an immune response. Attempts to quantify the

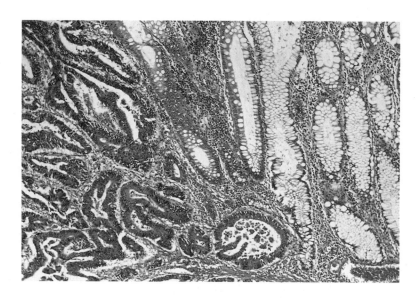

Fig. 2.18 Colonic carcinoma. The change from the normal architecture and histology on the right side contrasts with the loss of these in the tumour on the left side.

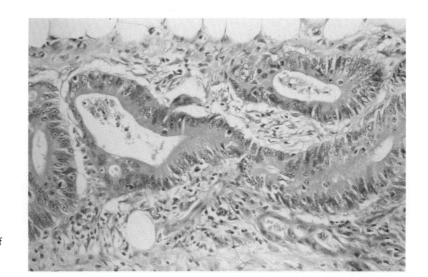

Fig. 2.19 Colonic carcinoma with variation amongst the appearances of the cells including their size and the size of their nuclei.

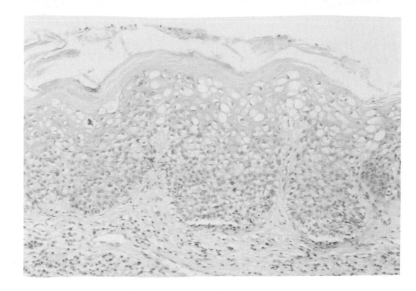

Fig. 2.20 Dysplasia within the vocal cord epithelium. The dysplastic cells fill the lower part of the epithelium and have different staining properties and appearances from the mature surface cells. This change occurs in smokers and heavy drinkers.

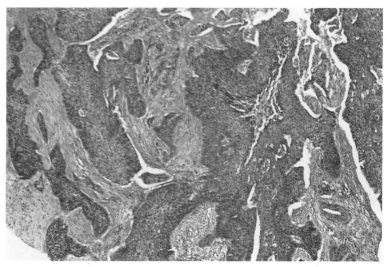

Fig. 2.21 Squamous cell carcinoma with bands of fibrous tissue around the islands of tumour cells.

number of these cells with prognosis have not fulfilled the initial claims that substantial mononuclear cell infiltrates correlated with a good prognosis and small numbers a bad prognosis. Necrosis is another feature especially in rapidly growing and larger tumours, including sarcomas, and haemorrhage may develop in the same regions.

Naming the tumour

This rests upon the histopathologist recognizing the origin of the tumour cells, which is rarely difficult with benign tumours. Well differentiated malignancies may also be so like their parent tissue that no difficulty arises, but with other tumours this may not be the case.

A *carcinoma* may be suspected if the malignant cells are cuboidal or columnar and have a moderate amount of cytoplasm. These cells are usually closely packed but, more helpfully, lines of closely apposed cells may also be present. Strands, the desmosomes and tonofibrils, extend between the cells in many squamous carcinomas but in other carcinomas the cell junctions can only be appreciated by electron microscopy. Adenocarcinomas produce mucin which can be stained (Fig. 2.22) and some melanomas and liver cell carcinomas, melanin and bile, respectively (Fig. 2.23). Labelled antibodies to cytokeratins provide a further means for identifying some carcinomas.

Sarcomas are more difficult to characterize and, in many, the tissue origin may never be found. Well differentiated sarcomas include some of the features of their cell of origin (Fig. 2.24) recognized by light or electron microscopy or displayed by labelled antibodies to intermediate filaments and basement membrane components. Such ancillary studies are essential if poorly differentiated sarcomas are to be categorized. The light microscopy diagnosis in such examples depends on the recognition of malignant cells

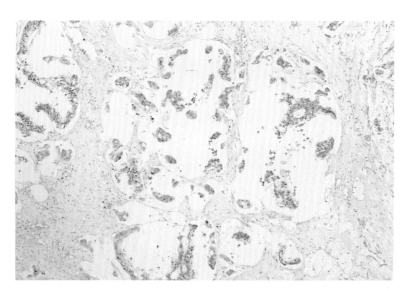

Fig. 2.22 Adenocarcinoma of the maxillary sinus with substantial mucus production.

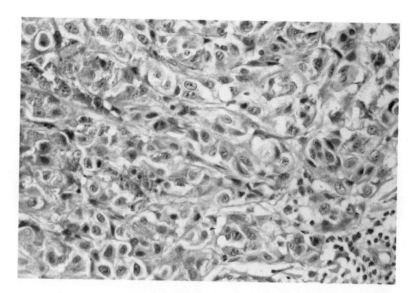

Fig. 2.23 Melanoma with melanin (brown pigment) within some of the tumour cells.

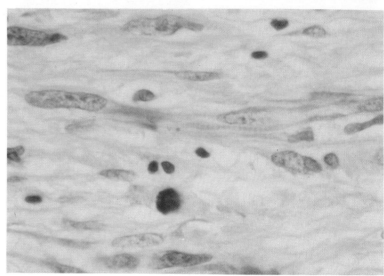

Fig. 2.24 Rhabdomyosarcoma. This skeletal muscle tumour is recognized by the striations (centre) within some tumour cells. These can also be seen at electron microscopy but in their absence the sarcoma may well be classified simply as a spindle cell sarcoma.

which are often haphazardly arranged and include none of the features suggestive of a carcinoma. Distinguishing between undifferentiated sarcomas and some lymphomas by light microscopy alone may also be impossible.

A *lymphoma* can often only be confidently diagnosed with the support of labelled antibodies to T-cells, B-cells and macrophages. The lymphoma cells can vary from almost normal to strikingly malignant and in all these tumours there is often no pattern and very little stroma (Fig. 2.25).

Further reading

Anderson, J.R. (Editor) (1985). *Muir's Textbook of Pathology* (12th Edition). Edward Arnold: London.

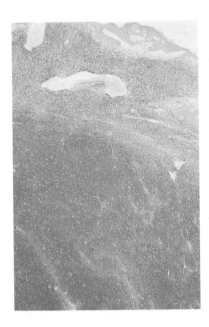

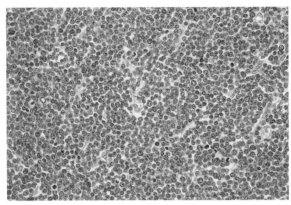

Fig. 2.25 Lymphoma of the tonsil; (*above left*) the contrast between the tumour and the normal tissue (top) is evident at low power; (*above right*) high power reveals a diffuse cellularity with little stroma.

Armed Forces Institute of Pathology: Washington DC. *Atlas of Tumour Pathology*

Friend, S.H., Dryja, T.P. and Weinberg, R.A. (1988). Oncogenes and tumour-suppressing genes. *New Eng. J. Med.* **318**, 618–22.

Ghadially, F.N. (1985). *Diagnostic Electron Microscopy of Tumours* (2nd Edition). Butterworths: London and Boston.

Slamon, D.J. (1987). Proto-oncogenes and human cancers. *New Eng. J. Med.* **317**, 955–7.

Walter, J.B. and Israel, M.S. (1987). *General Pathology* (6th Edition). Churchill Livingstone: Edinburgh and London.

World Health Organisation: Geneva. *International Histological Classification of Tumours.*

3 Heart and vessels

Heart disease is the major cause of death in the Western world accounting for over 160 000 deaths per annum in the UK. The main cause is coronary artery atherosclerosis with or without ischaemic heart disease. Other important causes of mortality and morbidity are endocarditis and, especially in developing countries, rheumatic heart disease and its sequelae, mitral and aortic valve disease. Cardiac disorders can also arise from diseases primarily affecting other organs such as the lung, producing cor pulmonale, and also as part of systemic diseases; for example, systemic lupus erythematosus (Table 3.1). These disorders as well as primary heart diseases can produce acute or chronic cardiac failure with changes including oedema and infarction in other organs.

Cardiac failure, whatever the cause (Table 3.2), is characterized by organ changes which reflect stasis of blood and decreased tissue perfusion associated with fluid accumulation. The heart itself may undergo dilatation with or without hypertrophy which will be most evident in the chambers mainly at fault. The affected fibres are elongated and compressed which may mask any coincident hypertrophy but if the process has been gradual and a raised systolic pressure has been maintained, cardiac hypertrophy develops.

Cardiac hypertrophy

This is seen as an increase in size of the muscle fibres and their organelles. In the adult, there is no hyperplasia since adult myocardial cells do not divide. Muscle hypertrophy is accompanied by an equal increase in capillary size and number and so does not result in ischaemia. Oedema and an increase in connective tissue also contribute to increased heart weight.

Hypertrophy may be uniform, as in response to hypertension or aortic valve disease, or focal, as is seen after myocardial infarction. It can also be induced by heavy manual labour or rigorous athletic training as well as by hypoxia associated with high altitudes. Virtually all congenital and acquired heart disease can evoke the response and common causes are included in Table 3.2. Clinically these separate into those due to pressure overload and those due to volume overload. Hypertrophy in the former is concentric and reduces the lumen of the ventricular chambers, while in volume

Table 3.1 Systemic disorders with specific cardiac features

Amyloid	(a) Old patients — confined to the heart; normal sized heart
	(b) As part of systemic deposition; enlarged heart
Rheumatoid arthritis	Only worst affected patients
	Pancarditis including granulomas and fibrosis
Ankylosing spondylitis	Late complication (>15 years)
	Aortic valve and ascending aorta dilate; fibrosis replaces the elastic tissue
Systemic lupus erythematosus	Pancarditis with non-bacterial endocarditis (Libman–Sacks)
Carcinoid syndrome	Endocardial fibrosis of right-sided chambers and valves
Sarcoidosis	Myocardial granulomas affecting the conduction tissue

Table 3.2 Causes of heart failure and myocardial hypertrophy

Common	Myocardial infarction
	Valvular defects (mitral and aortic)
	Systemic hypertension
	Congestive cardiomyopathy
Less common	Chronic diffuse lung disease
	Prolonged arrhythmias
	Anaemia
	Congenital heart defects
	Thyrotoxicosis
	Rheumatic carditis
Unusual	Arterio-venous aneurysms
	Cardiac trauma
	Chest deformities
	Cardiac tumours

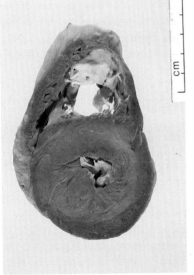

Fig. 3.1 Cardiac hypertrophy associated with hypertension. The left ventricle was 222 g and the right 52 g with a total heart weight of 405 g. The patient was an elderly female of below average weight and height.

overload the hypertrophy is marked by dilatation. Hypertrophy is potentially reversible but it can take months or even years before normality is restored.

APPEARANCES

Macroscopically, hypertrophy is often suspected but it can only be confidently quantitated if the individual chambers are weighed separately. The normal weight of the left ventricle (defined as the left ventricular free wall, freed of epicardial fat, and entire interventricular septum) is below 225 g, and of the right ventricle (defined as the right ventricular free wall devoid of epicardial fat) is below 80 g; the normal ratio is between 2:1 and 3:1, varying, as do the ventricular weights, in proportion to the body weight. Alterations in this ratio will indicate hypertrophy of a particular chamber and provide a more useful implication of pathology than an increase in total heart weight, particularly if there is only slight hypertrophy of one or other chamber (Fig. 3.1).

Cardiac atrophy

Atrophy is a condition theoretically incompatible with normal cardiac function; old people often have very small hearts, although in proportion to their short and reduced stature. Reduction in heart size does not have any functional significance and arises from a combination of age and degeneration.

APPEARANCES

The heart is uniformly small. The myocardium is brown and includes deposits of lipofuscin within the myocardial fibres. These reflect the age of the patient and associated chronic disorders including malignancy.

Coronary artery atherosclerosis and ischaemic heart disease

These two disorders are the principal causes of death from heart disease in the affluent societies of the Western hemisphere. They are also a major cause of morbidity. The arterial disorder and its complications result in ischaemic injury to the myocardium and so embarrass its function. Their effects in males are manifest at times of maximum proficiency and productivity and result in significant economic hardship to the individual, his family and the community. For these reasons immense efforts have been made to unveil the cause of these disorders as well as to find ways of preventing them. Unfortunately, much of this research is questionable since it pivots on feeding animals abnormal diets and extrapolating the results to man. Direct studies on humans, relating a specific factor with the development of these disorders, are fraught because it is difficult to isolate the important variables and to establish methods to measure their unmodified and modified effects. The student is consequently faced with a mass of literature, often dogmatically expressed and based upon conflicting data, and including all too often unjustified and later disproven claims. Nevertheless, it has become apparent that a small number of factors are unquestionably associated with the development of atherosclerosis and ischaemic heart disease.

1 Age and sex: an increasing incidence occurs with age and this is most marked in the male. After the menopause the differences between the sexes are less apparent.

2 Cigarette smoking: smoking, especially if over 20 cigarettes per day, and in young persons, is contributory.

3 High plasma lipoprotein levels: elevated lipoprotein, particularly high density types and cholesterol are involved. The high density lipoproteins in contrast to cholesterol and low density lipoproteins exert a protective effect.

4 Family history of these conditions.

5 Diabetes mellitus.

More contentious is the role of hypertension, chronic renal failure, obesity, shortness of stature, physical inactivity, oral contraceptives, a competitive personality and living in areas with soft water.

The diseases are, therefore, multifactorial but there are many elderly patients in whom none of these features can be identified. How each factor exerts its influence is conjectural but effects on blood clotting, blood flow and pressure and alterations in the cells and constituents of the vessel wall are all implicated. The mechanism triggering atherosclerosis, however, is not necessarily the same as that precipitating ischaemic heart disease and either disorder may appear without the other. However, both disorders have the same end result, namely the disruption of the normal myocardial blood supply.

Normal myocardial blood supply

Adequate blood, and thereby oxygen and nutritional supply is essential for normal cardiac function. The blood supply arises from two main coronary arteries and their three principal branches. Although these supply broadly constant regions of the myocardium (Table 3.3), they overlap in different subjects. Disease affecting one branch may be accompanied by compensatory changes in the others and by the appearance of collateral branches. The main coronary arteries provide blood for most of the myocardium and communicate directly with the cavities of the heart by endothelial lined sinuses. Nutrients and oxygen reach the endocardial regions through these sinuses as well as by perfusion from the blood within the ventricular chambers but the principal blood supply to all parts depends on adequate blood flow in the coronary arteries. This occurs during diastole and is in turn influenced by the systemic blood pressure and peripheral resistance of the myocardial vasculature. Filling is impeded by profound hypotension, aortic valve incompetence and obstructive lesions within the lumen of the coronary vessels as well as by changes in their contractility or, less commonly, that of the coronary ostia. Any impairment in systole adversely affects the emptying of the coronary arteries and promotes stasis.

Oxygenation directly from the blood within the cavities of the heart is probably slight. Although substances can diffuse directly and enter via the endothelial sinuses, constant contraction and accompanying changes in endothelial surface area restrict these

Table 3.3 Main coronary artery distribution regions

Main coronary artery	Main branches	Area of left ventricle supplied
Left	Anterior descending	Anterior wall Anterior of septum Bundle of His; right bundle branch
	Left circumflex	Posterior wall AV node
Right		Posterior wall SA, AV node, bundle of His

processes, as will any local disorder. Oedema and tissue deposits, principally fibrosis, will impede local diffusion as will many disorders of the blood. The subendocardial myocardium is therefore surprisingly exposed to ischaemic damage. This vulnerability is worsened by a redistribution of blood from the subendocardium to the main mass of the myocardium in conditions such as profound hypotension.

Coronary artery atherosclerosis

Definition

Atherosclerosis embraces atheroma and arteriosclerosis and like these terms does not have an agreed definition. It has been defined as 'The widely prevalent arterial lesion characterised by patchy thickening of the intima, the thickening comprising accumulations of fat and layers of collagen-like fibres, both being present in widely varying proportions' (Crawford). This definition makes the point that the disorder is not confined to the coronary arteries and that it embraces the simultaneous occurrence of proliferative and degenerative changes. It also implies that the lesions are seen in all races world-wide.

Mechanisms

Fat deposition and thrombus formation are integral parts of atherosclerosis (Fig. 3.2). This observation has influenced many attempts at modifying the pace and degree of the process either by altering dietary fat content or through use of anticoagulants. It also provides the basis for the two most popular pathogenetic hypotheses, (a) lipid infiltration and (b) platelet—fibrin deposition (encrustation

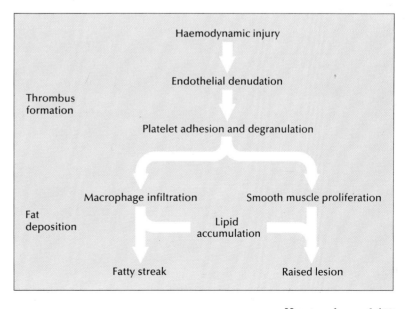

Fig. 3.2 Atherosclerosis sequence.

theory). The factor linking these is a role for smooth muscle cells which form the majority of cells in all lesions whether or not there is engulfed fat. Recent studies of all types of lesions, however, show that many are formed from monoclonal cell populations, implying that the process is more akin to neoplasia than to abnormal deposition of fat or fibrin and platelets. Studies of thrombi show a similar monoclonality and the role, particularly of platelet deposition, cannot therefore be disregarded. Mechanical factors, possibly producing focal intimal damage and including blood pressure, blood flow and sheering forces, are also implicated in the localization of some of the lesions, particularly those at points of bifurcation. However initiated or perpetuated, the process can sometimes regress, as is suggested from observations on prisoners of war and patients with wasting conditions and, more recently, angiography.

Normal vessel wall

Intima — Endothelial cells

— Internal elastic lamina

Media — Smooth muscle
— Elastic tissue

Adventitia — Connective tissue

A   Fatty streaks

Smooth muscle cells distended with fat

Intercellular (free) fat

B   Gelatinous lesion

Fibrin separated by oedema fluid

C   Raised lesion

Connective tissue cap

Debris (elastic and connective tissue)

Smooth muscle cells

Fat-filled cells

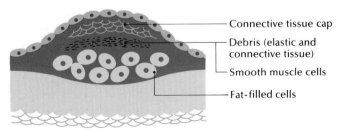

Fig. 3.3 The lesions of atherosclerosis.

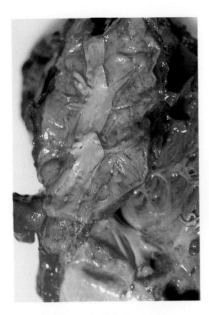 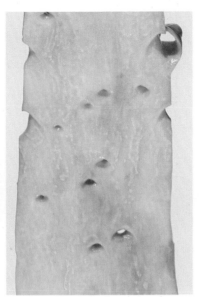 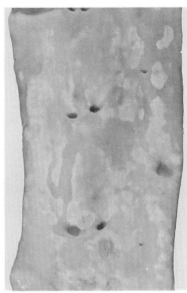

Fig. 3.4 (*Above left*) Left anterior descending coronary artery with raised yellow plaques of atherosclerosis and some fatty streaks; (*centre*) abdominal aorta of a 22-year-old male with smiilar appearances; (*above right*) uncomplicated raised lesions in the abdominal aorta.

APPEARANCES

Lesions comprising atherosclerosis are generally agreed upon although these do not necessarily represent an orderly sequence of events or have an identical pathogenesis. They are seen in arteries of all sizes including coronary arteries (Figs 3.3 and 3.4).

Fatty streaks

Glistening, tiny, oval, yellow spots frequently with a linear arrangement and most conspicuous within the aorta. These are most easily identified in children but can be found in any age group. Extracellular fat and fat within smooth muscle cells and macrophages underlie these appearances.

Gelatinous lesion

A superficial, small, greyish lesion distributed in a fashion similar to above but produced by oedema and fibrin within the endothelial tissue.

Raised lesions

These are the hallmark of the condition. They are elevated yellow to pearly white nodules most frequently found at the bifurcation of vessels. The yellow is from fat lying at the base of the lesion at the junction of endothelium and media and the white from the overlying fibrous tissue. If sufficiently large, these lesions produce significant luminal narrowing.

These lesions and particularly the raised ones can be complicated by a number of other factors (Figs 3.5 and 3.6):

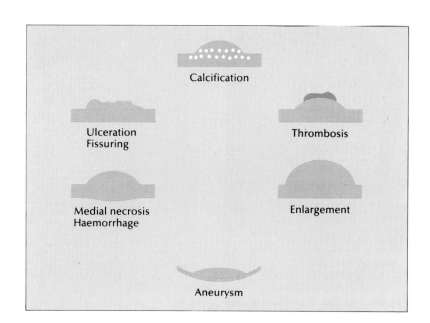

Fig. 3.5 Sequelae of atherosclerosis.

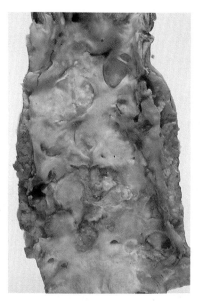 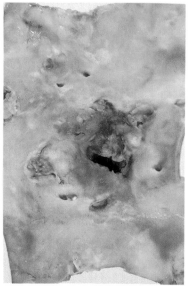 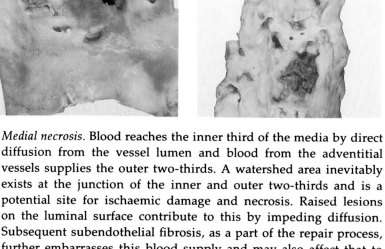

Fig. 3.6 Complications of atherosclerosis. (*Above left*) Medionecrosis: at the edge of the wall of the aorta soft greenish porridge-like material lies between the endothelial surface and the outer wall; (*centre*) ulceration with adherent thrombus; (*above right*) recent thrombus overlying atherosclerosis. The change is not uniform.

Medial necrosis. Blood reaches the inner third of the media by direct diffusion from the vessel lumen and blood from the adventitial vessels supplies the outer two-thirds. A watershed area inevitably exists at the junction of the inner and outer two-thirds and is a potential site for ischaemic damage and necrosis. Raised lesions on the luminal surface contribute to this by impeding diffusion. Subsequent subendothelial fibrosis, as a part of the repair process, further embarrasses this blood supply and may also affect that to the outer part of the media. If sufficient necrosis is present this is visible as soft, greyish-green and greasy material.

Haemorrhage. Necrosis may be sufficient to erode vessels within the wall and result in focal haemorrhage beneath the lesion. Similar

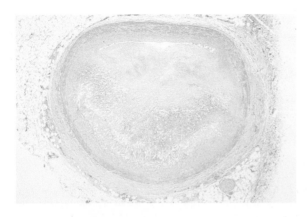 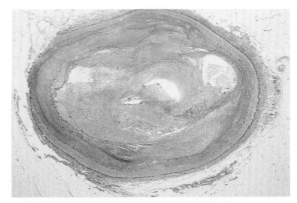

Fig. 3.7 (*Above left*) Organizing thrombus in a coronary artery superimposed upon a raised lesion. The lumen of the vessel is virtually occluded and there is fibrous replacement of much of the media; (*above right*) recanalization of the lumen of a thrombosed coronary artery. Much of the elastic tissue (stained black) is replaced by fibrous tissue (stained pink). There is haemorrhage (stained green) between the media and the fibrous tissue.

events may involve newly formed capillaries associated with the repair process with comparable results. The haemorrhage can then precipitate the raised plaque further into the vessel lumen and thereby create a focally narrowed lumen, or thrombose and split or fissure the overlying plaque.

Ulceration. This can be produced either from ulceration of the raised plaque as part of the medial necrosis or from fissuring secondary to intra-intimal thrombus.

Thrombosis. This can complicate an intact or an ulcerated lesion because the flow of blood is affected as well as the endothelium modified. Thrombosis occurs in the coronary arteries of almost half the patients dying suddenly. Embolism is a further potential but rare complication.

Calcification. Calcium deposition is attributed to the high fat content of the lesions and to necrosis but it is also a phenomenon seen with increasing age. If this occurs the affected segment loses its elasticity, becoming rigid and more prone to thrombus. The loss of elasticity is especially important in small vessels, where flow and blood pressures will be affected.

All these complications occur most frequently on the raised lesions, and so it is these that are the most important and the ones underlying the morbidity and mortality of atherosclerosis. Clearly, their effects will be greater when small calibre vessels and endarteries, like the coronary and cerebral arteries, are involved (Fig. 3.7). At autopsy luminal narrowing of two-thirds or more of one or more coronary arteries is accepted as sufficient to cause death.

Ischaemic heart disease

Cardiac ischaemia can occur with or without coronary artery atherosclerosis and with or without infarction. When infarction is present it is seen in two broad patterns, regional and diffuse (Fig. 3.8), but there are many complex and intermediate types. Virtually all infarcts are restricted to the left ventricle which, relative to the other cham-

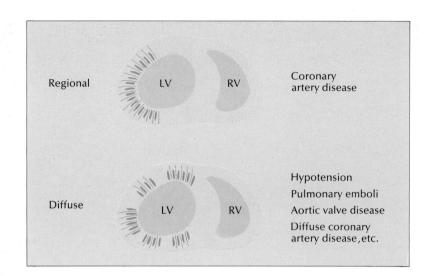

Fig. 3.8 Types of infarction.

Table 3.4 Dating of myocardial infarction

15 h	Pale oedematous myocardium
3–4 days	Macroscopic infarct
2–3 weeks	Thinning and shrinkage of myocardium
6–8 weeks	Evident scarring
3 months	White firm scarring

bers, has greater metabolic demands. Severe multivessel obstructive coronary artery disease, however, underlies ischaemic heart disease without infarction and is found in many patients with angina pectoris; these patients can therefore have a normal myocardium.

Regional infarction. This occurs only when the coronary arteries are diseased and is almost entirely confined to the left ventricle (Fig. 3.9). The site of the infarct depends upon the coronary artery that is affected and its normal areas of blood supply (Table 3.3). Collateral vessels will affect the region of infarction only if they are large enough to compensate for the diseased main vessels, a condition rarely encountered with the thrombotic occlusion that precipitates this pattern of infarction.

Thrombus superimposed upon coronary atherosclerosis is the major cause of regional infarcts even though this may not be demonstrated at autopsy. Detachment of the thrombus can occur spontaneously and from faulty post mortem technique and disappearance of thrombi from either in situ lysis or organization with incorporation into the underlying atherosclerotic lesion occurs. Moreover, any infarct will not be apparent macroscopically until 24–36 h after occlusion (Fig. 3.10) although light microscopy changes are seen earlier and ultrastructural changes preceding these. The dye Nitroblue Tetrazolium can be used to demonstrate infarction macroscopically as early as 6–8 h after occlusion but any of these times are influenced by the nutritional state of the patient, blood oxygenation, collateral vessels and their state as well as variable rates of healing. Rigid adherence to methods of dating myocardial infarcts is therefore not appropriate although systems such as those in Table 3.4 do give a broad indication of the momentum of the process.

Infarcts precipitating sudden death usually extend through the full thickness of the myocardium while others are restricted

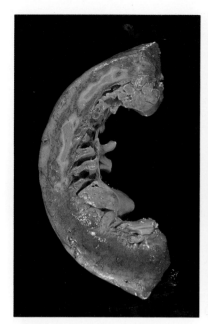 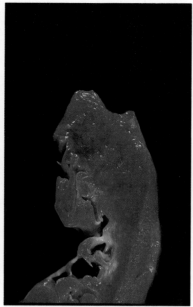 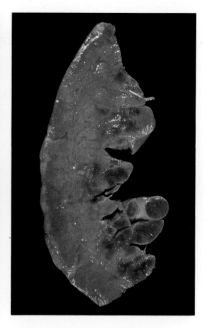

Fig. 3.9 Focal area of infarction involving the left ventricle. The yellow tissue in the centre is necrotic and much of the surrounding myocardium includes microscopic evidence of ischaemic injury.

Fig. 3.10 Early infarct of the left ventricle. There is focal haemorrhage and swelling of the myocardium but no necrotic tissue of the type seen in Fig. 3.9.

Fig. 3.11 Diffuse subendocardial infarction of the left ventricle in a patient with severe and sustained hypotension. Similar features were seen in the myocardium of the interventricular septum and free wall of the right ventricle.

to subendocardial regions and involve the inner half of the myocardium.

Diffuse myocardial infarction. This is confined to the inner zone of the left ventricle (Fig. 3.11). Extracoronary factors including hypotension, pulmonary embolism and aortic valve disease can produce this but severe obstructive atherosclerosis is the most common cause. The atherosclerosis involves all the main coronary arteries and any superimposed thrombus plays an aggravating rather than a precipitating role. The arterial disease is usually long standing with plentiful collaterals and many anastomotic vessels, so that the normal distribution territories of the main coronary vessels are no longer maintained.

Other patterns of myocardial infarction. Patterns are found that are neither solely regional nor purely diffuse and endocardial. This reflects the manner in which atherosclerosis and other events, including thrombus formation, have developed and demonstrates that the main types of infarction represent the ends of a spectrum.

APPEARANCES

These are the same for regional and diffuse infarcts (Figs 3.8–3.10). Once established, the centre of the infarcted region is yellowish

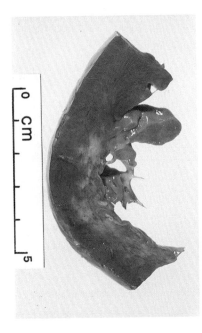

Fig. 3.12 Myocardial fibrosis in the free wall of the left ventricle.

Table 3.5 Sequelae of myocardial infarction

Sudden death
Cardiac failure
Cardiogenic shock
Arrhythmias of all types
Thrombosis and embolism

Pericarditis and effusion
Haemopericardium
Myocardial rupture
    Ventricular septal defect
    Mitral valve incompetence

Aneurysmal dilatation

with an haemorrhagic border and pale surrounding myocardium. Later, contraction occurs and the consistency is rubbery. From then on scarring by silvery white fibrous tissue develops associated with local myocardial thinning (Fig. 3.12). Other long-term changes are calcification of the scar and compensatory hypertrophy of the surving muscle.

Complications

Any type of infarct can develop single or multiple complications (Table 3.5). Clinically these are classified as early and late and functionally into those affecting either the pumping action or conduction (Fig. 3.13) but histopathologically such distinctions are not always possible.

Muscle destruction, involving a minimum of 25–40% of the myocardium, is sufficient to cause sudden death due to ventricular fibrillation, cardiac failure and cardiogenic shock. Arrhythmias of all types may stem from destruction of the conduction tissue or from transient local oedema, sympathetic overactivity or tissue anoxia and acidosis. Pericarditis is evident within 24 h in the majority of transmural infarcts and any accompanying effusion can be complicated by haemorrhage from the infarcted tissue or from the use of anticoagulants. Myocardial rupture occurs in transmural infarcts within 1–3 days post infarction, before any fibrosis has developed, but is not precipitated by hypertension, cardiac failure or exertion. Rupture takes three forms, all potentially fatal:

1 Rupture of the free wall of the left ventricle, producing a haemopericardium (Fig. 3.13).
2 Rupture of the septum leading to a ventricular septal defect.
3 Papillary muscle rupture causing mitral valve incompetence.

Aneurysmal dilatation follows a full thickness infarct but, in contrast to rupture, develops during the healing stages with thinning of the myocardium (Fig. 3.13). This may then rupture but rarely once fibrosis is established. Endocardial thrombus, with or without embolus, may be superadded to aneurysm formation but may also develop with any infarct reflecting the death of tissue, release of thromboplastins and change in cardiac function and blood flow (Fig. 3.14). Embolism develops within a two-to-three-week period following infarction and affects the brain, spleen and kidneys with lesser involvement of the gastrointestinal tract. *Dressler's syndrome* is unusual and presents 1–6 weeks after infarction. There are no specific morphological markers but it is recognized by a pericardial effusion, evidence of infarction and circulating antibodies to myocardial muscle.

Rheumatic heart disease

Rheumatic heart disease is potentially the most disabling aspect of rheumatic fever, a disease affecting the joints, the central nervous system and the skin (Fig. 3.15). Once established no treatment halts or impedes the progression of the cardiac disease which, unlike the

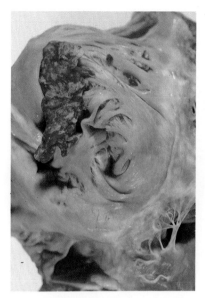
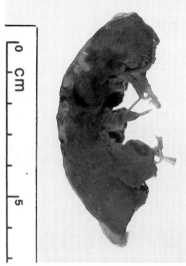
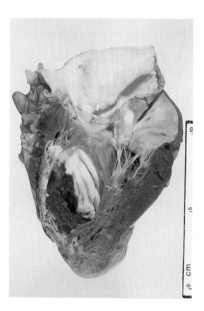

Fig. 3.13 Complications of myocardial infarction. (*Left*) Atrial thrombus. Following an infarct, atrial fibrillation and thrombus within the right atrial appendage developed; (*centre*) rupture of an infarct. Chest pain occurred two days prior to death and at autopsy there was a large haemopericardium; (*right*) aneurysm replacing much of the free wall of the left ventricle. The wall of the aneurysm is formed from pale fibrous tissue and is thinned. Thrombus has formed on the endocardial surface.

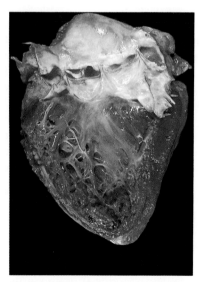

Fig. 3.14 Thrombus over an area of recent infarction. The infarct appearances resemble those in Fig. 3.9.

other aspects of rheumatic fever, rarely resolves. Rheumatic fever occurs world-wide and in all age groups but its highest incidence is among children and its highest mortality is in tropical regions. A dramatic fall in incidence has occurred within the UK since the beginning of this century due to improved social conditions, less malnutrition and antibiotic therapy. Antibiotics eradicate the upper respiratory tract infection by β-haemolytic *S. viridans* which precedes rheumatic fever and are used with symptomless carriers. The period between the streptococcal infection and rheumatic fever is 2−4 weeks and is important evidence that the disease is immunologically mediated, although exactly how is not fully established. Cross reactions between antibodies to components of the streptococcus and the patient's myocardium, joint tissues and basal nuclei in the brain provide the basis for this hypothesis but such reactions are not confined to these tissues and may be secondary phenomena arising after tissue damage. The tissue damage starts in the connective tissue of the organs involved rather than within their specialized cells.

Cardiac manifestations

The disease is a pancarditis involving all parts of the heart. Nevertheless, the valves, and particularly those on the left side, bear the brunt of the inflammation and underlie the morbidity and mortality of the disorder. The relapsing and chronic nature of the disease is represented morphologically by acute and chronic changes characterized in the acute phases by a histological marker, the Aschoff body. Although acute and chronic lesions can correlate with the clinical history, acute lesions can also be found when the disease is long standing and clinically quiescent. Acute lesions are seen in

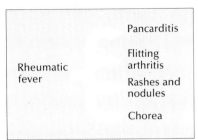

	Pancarditis
Rheumatic fever	Flitting arthritis
	Rashes and nodules
	Chorea

Fig. 3.15 Manifestation of rheumatic fever.

atrial tissue biopsied during surgery for long-standing valvular lesions and support the impression of a smouldering disorder, and explain progression despite periods of clinical remission.

Aschoff bodies (Fig. 3.16). These have a central zone of structureless eosinophilic material surrounded by a mantle of macrophages (Anitschkow cells), multinucleate cells (Aschoff cells) and variable numbers of chronic inflammatory cells. Although these bodies may be found in any part of the heart they exhibit a particular predilection for perivascular regions and, in more than half the patients, are found in the conducting tissues. Healing is associated with disappearance of these lesions and replacement by non-specific focal scarring.

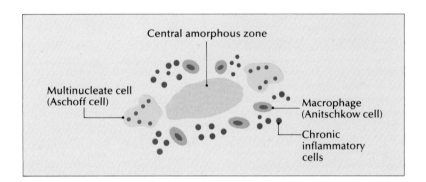

Fig. 3.16 Aschoff body.

APPEARANCES

Valves. During the acute stages these are mildly swollen and opaque and include minute growths or vegetations along their free margins. The chordae tendineae include similar features. As the disorder progresses fibrosis replaces the valve tissues, the commisures fuse and the chordae become shrunken and thickened with some fusion (Figs 3.17 and 3.18). Subsequently calcification develops giving further rigidity to the valves. At this stage the appearances are shared with any chronic inflammatory valve disorder and are not without a supportive clinical history, diagnostic of rheumatic fever. Closure of the valve is impeded with resulting incompetence and a narrowed stenotic or buttonhole orifice is ultimately produced. The altered valve surfaces and blood flow result in thrombus formation, which with organization further distorts the valves and disrupts their function.

Heart. This is enlarged and often globular, incorporating hypertrophy and dilatation, both of which are more marked with long-standing disease. The pattern of valve involvement is largely responsible for the distribution of the changes, right ventricular changes predominating with mitral involvement and left ventricular with aortic valve disease. Gross left atrial enlargement was a common feature of severe mitral stenosis but with early surgical replacement of the

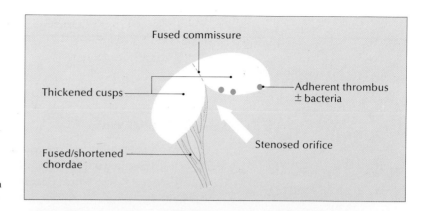

Fused commissure

Thickened cusps

Fused/shortened chordae

Adherent thrombus ± bacteria

Stenosed orifice

Fig. 3.17 Effects of rheumatic fever in the heart valve.

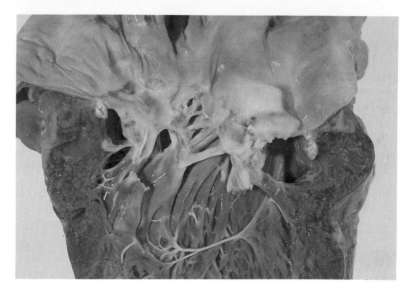

Fig. 3.18 Mitral valve with early changes of rheumatic fever. The cusps are thickened and have lost their normal translucency. There is some fusion of the cusps and the chordae are thicker than normal and shortened.

valve it is now infrequently seen. The myocardium in the early phases may include scattered foci of yellow necrosis but in long-standing examples there is only fibrosis.

Endocardium. The endocardium is spared apart from an area on the posterior wall of the left atrium (*McCallum's patch*) where, especially if there is mitral incompetence, acute changes and later fibrosis develop.

Pericardium. Either acute fibrinous inflammation with an effusion or patchy fibrosis and adhesions between the visceral and parietal pericardium are found according to the stage of the disorder.

Complications

These depend upon the valve or combination of valves involved. The altered valves are ideal sites for infection (*endocarditis*) from which emboli may break off producing further complications. Pulmonary hypertension and atrial fibrillation with atrial thrombosis and secondary embolization can occur with long-standing mitral valve disease. Heart failure is common with any pattern of valvular disease.

Miscellaneous valve disorders

Floppy mitral valve

This is a cause of mitral regurgitation and rarely, sudden death. It is being diagnosed more frequently, particularly with increasing age. There is a defect in collagen synthesis and an increased rate of collagen degeneration within the cusps and chordae tendineae. The condition can form part of Marfan's disease and Ehlers–Danlos syndrome.

APPEARANCES

The posterior cusp is primarily involved and balloons into the atrium during systole. With time the ballooned shape is maintained and the chordae tendineae become elongated and may eventually rupture. Endocarditis and calcification can also supervene.

Aortic valve sclerosis

The condition is seen only in the elderly and is categorized as degenerative, having no functional significance unless it progresses to stenosis. There is dystophic calcification of all three cusps of the aortic valve which reduces their pliability and stiffens them (Fig. 3.19). Thrombosis and subsequent organization develops on their atrial surfaces and produces further deformity.

Bicuspid aortic valve with calcific aortic stenosis

The bicuspid valve is a congenital maldevelopment and has a significant association with coarctation of the aorta. Such valves calcify prematurely in the young adult and may also be more at risk from rheumatic fever. Within surgical series these calcified bicuspid valves are the cause of aortic stenosis in at least 50% of patients but in severely distorted valves it may be difficult to distinguish the changes from severe rheumatic disease.

Endocarditis

Endocarditis is now rarely encountered by the histopathologist even though the incidence has not declined during the last thirty years. Most examples are due to bacterial infection and antibiotic therapy is clearly the major reason for the reduced mortality. Changes in the type and virulence of organisms, together with changes in the patients affected are other reasons (Table 3.6). Lancefield Group A, α-haemolytic streptococci, especially the dextran-producing members, cause the majority of infections, some following dental procedures, but virtually any organism may be associated. Within specific groups of patients certain organism predominate: *S. aureus* is common amongst intravenous drug users and *Candida* amongst patients subjected to open heart surgery (Fig. 3.20).

Table 3.6 Patterns of endocarditis

Abnormal heart valves (72% of patients)	Rheumatic and congenital	*Strep. viridans*
	Open heart surgery	*Staph. albus*
		Candida
	Degenerative	*Strep. faecalis*
	Prostheses	*Staph. pyogenes*
Normal heart valves	i.v. drug users	*Staph. aureus*
		Gram⁻ organisms
	i.t.u. patients	Staphylococci
	Immunosuppressed	Fungi
		Gram⁻ organisms
	Alcoholics	Pneumococcus
	Haemodialysis shunts	Staphylococci

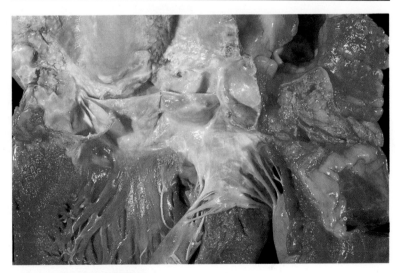

Fig. 3.19 Aortic valve sclerosis in an elderly patient. There is some thickening of the cusps combined with calcification and fusion.

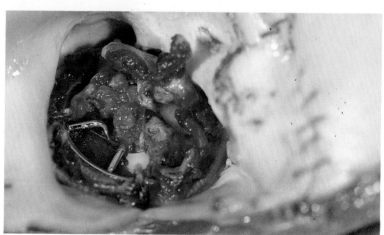

Fig. 3.20 Fungal endocarditis complicating a prosthetic aortic valve.

Despite the emphasis on micro-organisms, the condition does occur without infection and it is in this form that it is most often seen at autopsy. These patients are generally elderly and most have died from a malignancy, particularly pancreatic carcinoma.

Development

Current thinking hinges on endothelial damage as the initiating factor. Platelets and fibrin then adhere to this area giving rise to non-bacterial thrombotic endocarditis, *marantic endocarditis* (Fig. 3.21) which in lupus erythematosus is *Libman—Sacks endocarditis*. Subsequently circulating micro-organisms are trapped together with more platelets and fibrin and the vegetation thereby increases in size. Any organization will begin at the junction with the endocardium.

The evidence supporting this hypothesis is indirect since early lesions and non-fatal lesions are rarely accessible for examination but includes the following:

1 Vegetations develop on abnormal heart valves including valvular prostheses which may directly result in breaks in the endothelium and changes in the blood flow.

2 Sites of localized abnormal blood flow are involved which in turn may produce mechanical damage to the endothelium.

3 Vegetations occur on the free valve margins and on regions of endothelium subjected to regurgitant jet lesions.

4 Valve surfaces exposed to low blood pressure are affected which is where blood recoils when the valves snap shut. Additionally blood perfusion and in turn oxygenation may, in these regions, be impaired in contrast to that in the higher pressure regions.

5 The small number of lesions on the right side may equate with lower intracardiac pressures.

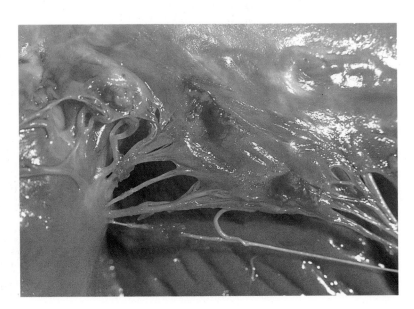

Fig. 3.21 Marantic endocarditis involving the tricuspid valve. Apart from the thrombus there are no other abnormalities to the valve.

Table 3.7 Endocarditis of single valves at autopsy

Mitral valve	86%
Aortic valve	55%
Tricuspid valve	20%
Pulmonary valve	1%

6 The predominance of *S. viridans* may either be because these organisms adhere to endothelium more easily than others or because they are more readily engulfed by endothelial cells.

APPEARANCES

The principal change is the appearance of growths or vegetations. These are found on the endothelial surface of valves and mainly involve those on the left side (Table 3.7). Lesions can occur on non-valvular surfaces, particularly those exposed to increased blood flow across a low pressure gradient (e.g., patent ductus arteriosus), and right-sided heart valves, notably amongst intravenous drug users. The vegetations lie along the lines of closure of the valve leaflets and on the low pressure surface, i.e., the atrial side of the mitral valve and the aortic surface of the aortic valve. The infecting organism can only be identified from culture of the vegetation or of the blood. The balance between the virulence of the organism and the resistance of the host are the factors determining the type of vegetation but antibiotics and the state of the valve prior to infection are also important.

Acute lesions are generally larger than more indolent and organized ones and are associated with more necrosis and ulceration (Fig. 3.22). They are also less firmly attached to the underlying endothelium than the more chronic ones. They range from millimeters to several centimetres and from small warty nodules to polypoid masses capable of destroying the valvular orifice. This allows regurgitation which may also be precipitated by perforation and prolapse of the valve cusps as well as rupture of their chordae tendineae. In well over half the examples the valve will also include evidence of rheumatic disease or a congenital disorder and in others degenerative disorders associated with calcification and ballooned valves. When otherwise normal valves are seen the combination of

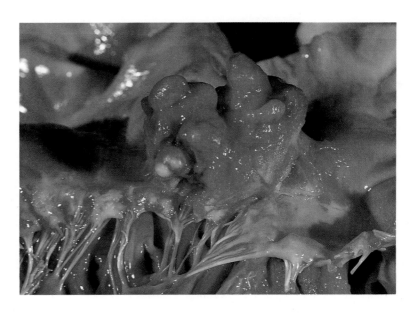

Fig. 3.22 Mitral valve with acute and chronic bacterial endocarditis. The large central vegetation is acute and friable and *S. albus* was cultured from this. In contrast the small nodular lesions to either side represent long-standing changes from which embolism is unlikely.

severe sepsis and immunosuppression is present (Table 3.6). If endocarditis is the cause of death the heart is enlarged with a flabby myocardium, sometimes including micro-abscesses and rarely infarction and pericarditis.

Complications

Cardiac failure, exacerbated by valvular regurgitation, is an important cause of death. Systemic involvement occurs in the skin, brain and kidneys (Table 3.8) with abscesses and infarcts and, in the kidneys, a proliferative glomerulonephritis. Within each site the tissue damage has been ascribed either to the micro-organisms causing the endocarditis or to immune mechanisms. Organisms have rarely been isolated and overall it is circulating immune complexes that are regarded as the basis of these complications. Nevertheless, a small number of patients do undoubtedly produce emboli from their vegetations which can lead to infarcts, especially in the spleen, lungs and skin.

Cardiomyopathy and myocarditis

These terms, although both lacking agreed definition, have been subjected to numerous subclassifications which have made assessment of their incidence extremely difficult; neither, however, are frequently seen. Cardiomyopathy is regarded as a disease of heart muscle of unknown cause or as a disease not attributable to ischaemic damage or which results from pressure and volume overload. Myocarditis has a similarly wide-ranging definition which is the presence of inflammatory cells or inflammatory processes within the heart which are combined with myocardial cell necrosis. Similar, although less extensive changes, are seen in cardiomyopathies and the two conditions therefore overlap.

Table 3.8 Complications of endocarditis

Valve	Systemic
Ulceration	**Heart**
	failure
Thrombus	**Kidney**
	glomerulonephritis
	infarction
Rupture	**Brain**
Cusps	abscesses
Chordae	infarction
Stenosis	
	Skin
	splinter haemorrhages
	subcutaneous nodules
	Other
	infarction

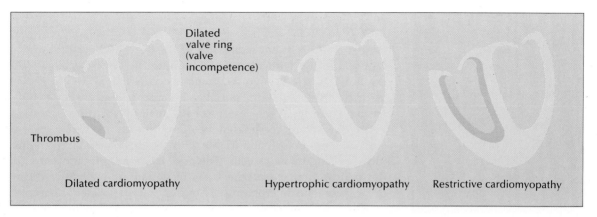

Fig. 3.23 Types of cardiomyopathy.

Three forms of cardiomyopathy are recognized and each is usually associated with an enlarged heart and patent coronary arteries (Fig. 3.23).

1 *Dilated cardiomyopathy* (formerly *congestive cardiomyopathy*). Both ventricles are hypertrophied but also dilated so that the increased thickness of their walls is partly masked. Endocardial thrombosis can develop. Since a similar condition occurs with alcoholism, this possibility must always be thoroughly investigated.

2 *Hypertrophic cardiomyopathy* (formerly *hypertrophic obstructive cardiomyopathy* and *asymmetric septal hypertrophy*). There is massive hypertrophy primarily of the left ventricle, sometimes confined to the interventricular septum, with an accompanying reduction in the size of the left ventricular chamber. Disarray of the muscle bundles and the frequent formation of whorls of muscle are pathognomonic of the condition.

3 *Restrictive cardiomyopathy* (a term encompassing *endocardial fibroelastosis* and *endomyocardial fibrosis*). There is a variable amount of fibrosis of the left ventricle which is initially confined to the endocardial regions. As a consequence the muscle is stiff and resistant to diastolic filling although systolic contraction remains normal. There is no marked increase in heart size. The condition is closely related with peripheral eosinophilia which may initiate the myocardial damage and is common in the tropics.

The term cardiomyopathy should be restricted to these three conditions and other cardiac disease with similar macroscopic findings but with a recognized cause labelled according to that cause. These latter conditions can also result in myocarditis with and without the macroscopic features of cardiomyopathy. There are nevertheless hearts with myocarditis for which no cause is found, even after exhaustive efforts to implicate viruses. These are separated into two groups:

1 those with a non-specific inflammatory infiltrate;

2 those with a granulomatous response associated with giant cells.

The first event in either of these conditions is myocardial necrosis which underlies the symptomatology and causes the inflammatory response. This occurs diffusely throughout the myocardium, evident macroscopically as small, yellow foci.

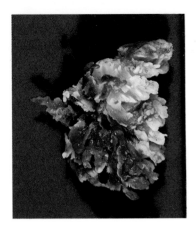

Fig. 3.24 Myxoma removed from the right atrium.

Cardiac neoplasms

Benign and malignant neoplasms of the heart and pericardium are rare (Table 3.9) with metastases forming the largest group. When the heart muscle is involved tumour occurs more often in the left ventricle than the right, possibly because of the greater mass of tissue. *Myxomas* (Fig. 3.24) form the majority of primary cardiac tumours and are considered benign although they may seed as emboli. They are soft and friable with a loose mucoid stroma which includes random small cells. The most common primary tumour of the pericardium, *mesothelioma*, is malignant and whether diffuse or localized may microscopically mimic metastatic adenocarcinoma.

The rarity of primary cardiac tumours may reflect the low turnover of myocardial cells but may also be influenced by the constant beating which may prevent tumour cells establishing themselves. This may also explain the rarity of metastatic tumours (Fig. 3.25), despite the constant perfusion of the heart with blood, which is an important pathway for tumour spread. Significantly most cardiac metastases arise from direct intrathoracic spread.

Table 3.9 Cardiac tumours

Benign	Myxoma	Most common
	Rhabdomyoma	Children. Tuberous sclerosis
Malignant	Angiosarcoma	
	Rhabdomyosarcoma	Mainly right-sided
	Metastases	Mainly from breast and lung

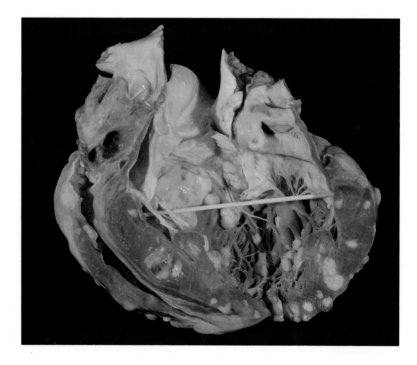

Fig. 3.25 Rare manifestation of metastatic spread. There are multiple deposits of melanoma in all parts of the heart, a few of which are pigmented. Lung and breast carcinomas also rarely involve the heart in this manner.

Table 3.10 Common congenital heart disorders

Ventral septal defect
Bicuspid aortic valve
Atrial septal defect
Patent ductus arteriosus
Fallot's tetralogy
Pulmonary stenosis
Transposition of the great vessels
Coarctation of the aorta
Hypoplastic left heart

Congenital abnormalities

The specialized muscle and conduction system of the heart are adapted to maintain a regular beat throughout life and are formed within the early weeks after conception. By this time any congenital abnormality will also be established. Most abnormalities are associated with spontaneous abortions or stillbirths but between 5–9/1000 live births will have cardiac abnormalities of which the most common are bicuspid aortic valves and a ventral septal defect (Table 3.10; Fig. 3.26). One-third of affected infants also have abnormalities in other organs but these are usually of minor significance. The best known cause of congenital heart disease is maternal rubella, but with a thorough enquiry other viruses as well as drugs and genetic factors, often in combination, are implicated.

Pericardial disorders

Many conditions affecting the heart also involve the pericardium. This can be acutely inflamed, often with fibrin formation, to produce a pericarditis of varying severity, seen most often as discrete areas of red roughening on the visceral and parietal surfaces (Fig. 3.27). In these circumstances there is focal myocardial damage but, with more widespread injury or renal failure, the change is diffuse producing substantial thickening and very conspicuous roughening.

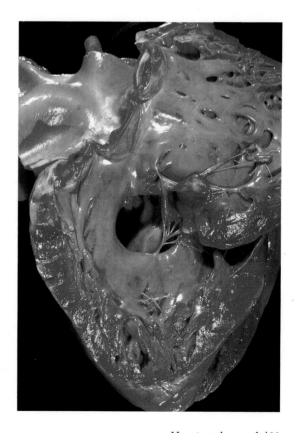

Fig. 3.26 Septal defect high in the wall of the interventricular septum.

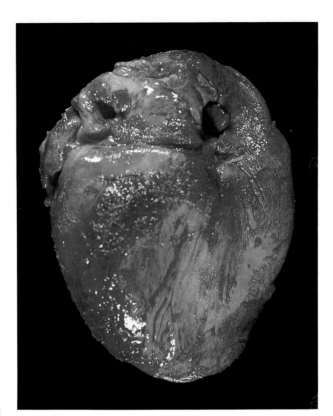

Fig. 3.27 Acute fibrinous pericarditis complicating acute renal failure. The pericardial sac included bloodstained fluid and loose adhesions bound the visceral and parietal pericardium.

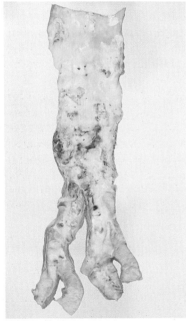

Fig. 3.28 Atherosclerosis of the abdominal aorta and both common iliac vessels. The lesions include adherent platelets and fibrin and are complicated by calcification giving the rigid appearance of the iliac vessels.

A thickened fibrotic pericardium, frequently with added calcification, is the end stage of chronic inflammation and will constrict the heart and, if unrelieved, lead to death. In most patients no cause for this *constrictive pericarditis* is found although in a few there is a history of haemorrhage into the pericardial sac and in others evidence for viral infection. Tuberculosis was formerly the principal cause for constrictive pericarditis but this is now rare.

Effusions

With either acute or chronic pericarditis an effusion, either clear, purulent or bloodstained may be found within the pericardial cavity. The volume reflects the severity or chronicity of the process as well as the amount of diseased tissue. A rapidly accumulated effusion will compress and impede the heart's action, producing cardiac tamponade, while one that collects more slowly may have no adverse effect and even escape clinical recognition. The pericardium in these conditions has had time to distend and accommodate the fluid, circumstances which do not apply for an acute effusion.

Haemorrhage into the pericardial sac (*haemopericardium*) can be associated with a fibrinous pericarditis, cardiac rupture, dissecting thoracic aneurysms, trauma including surgery, and anticoagulants and bleeding disorders. Myocardial infarction and

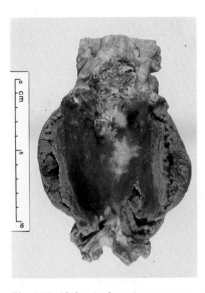

Fig. 3.29 Abdominal aortic aneurysm immediately above the bifurcation of the iliac vessels. Adherent recent thrombus lines the intimal surface and mushy, greenish atheromatous material expands and replaces the media.

dissecting thoracic aneurysms are the main causes of cardiac tamponade from acute haemopericardium and result in sudden death. That from other causes may be insidious and can clinically be unsuspected.

Aorta

Atherosclerosis

This involves the aorta and all its branches, increasing in severity with age (Fig. 3.28). Lesions are comparable to those in coronary arteries and are influenced by similar mechanisms. The changes particularly affect points of bifurcation and, in elderly patients, can cause severe calcification, ulceration, thrombosis, aneurysms and occlusion of vessels. Clinically these complications result in peripheral vascular disease, presenting as intermittent claudication, ischaemia of the skin and peripheral gangrene.

Aneurysms

Definition

An aneurysm is a localized dilatation of a vessel and is invariably due to a weakness of the media. This may be congenital as is partly the case in berry aneurysms of the circle of Willis or be caused by destruction by inflammation or degenerative changes. The natural increase in length and breadth of the aorta that occurs throughout life and continues into old age can cause confusion but this differs in that the change is diffuse rather than localized. Aortic aneurysms have different causes in different regions:

1 *Abdominal aortic aneurysms* arise from atherosclerosis (Fig. 3.29). This destroys the elastic tissue for the media and provokes necrosis. Either from these changes or because of the reactive fibrosis that follows, the media lacks the elasticity and strength of the normal wall and aneurysmal dilatation develops. These aneurysms usually lie below the origin of the renal arteries and above the bifurcation of the common iliac arteries. Both the renal vessels and the iliac vessels can be involved and this will produce local ischaemic changes.

2 *Thoracic aortic aneurysms* (Fig. 3.30) were formerly due to tertiary syphilis which provoked an endarteritis and perivasculitis of the vasa vasorum. These reactions produced ischaemia of the media with necrosis and destruction of the elastic tissue.

Most thoracic aneurysms are now related to idiopathic degeneration and necrosis of the elastic tissue and smooth muscle cells. These are also present in many aortas without aneurysms, especially in the elderly. Even so, the condition is still sometimes referred to as *cystic medionecrosis of Erdheim*. Patients are invariably hypertensive but may also have congenital disorders of connective tissue (Marfan's and Ehlers−Danlos syndromes), bicuspid aortic valves or aortic coarctation. Most aneurysms involve the ascending aorta

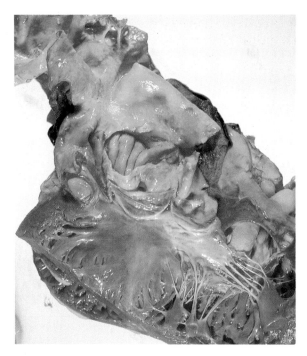

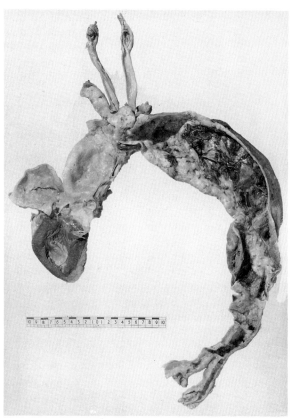

Fig. 3.30 Thoracic aortic aneurysms; (*above left*) involving rupture of the intimal surface immediately above the aortic valve; (*above right*) affecting the descending portion and complicated by thrombus.

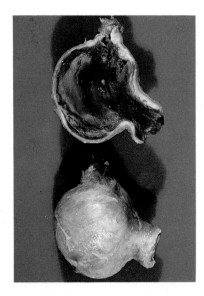

Fig. 3.31 Aneurysm of the popliteal artery following trauma. The lumen is filled with thrombus which is more organized at the periphery than the centre. The lumen is almost entirely obliterated and there were ischaemic changes in the skin of the foot and lower leg.

(Type A) where they are associated with an almost 100% mortality but others are confined to the descending aorta (Type B) and have a slightly better prognosis.

APPEARANCES

These are intimately related to the complications that have developed which are common to all aneurysms and are often all present.

Thromboembolism (Fig. 3.31). Changes in the vessel wall and blood flow make thrombosis inevitable although in thoracic aneurysms this is less common than in those in the abdominal aorta. Invariably abdominal aneurysms have a thickened wall, grossly reminiscent of an onion skin, formed from layers of organized and superimposed thrombus which gradually narrows the lumen of the aorta and impairs the blood flow. Emboli pass to the lower limbs and may precipitate gangrene.

Rupture. Any aneurysm may burst and prior to this seepage of blood may have occurred. Either event is painful and rupture is a cause of sudden death. Abdominal aneurysms rupture into the retroperitoneal tissues, particularly on the left side.

Thoracic aneurysms often rupture through the intima into the media and so create a second channel for the blood. The blood may then dissect through the degenerate media spreading along both the aorta and its branches (*dissecting aneurysm*) where it may occlude, by compression, the lumen of some of the smaller tributaries. The blood may subsequently burst from the media, either into the mediastinum and left pleural cavity or, if immediately above the aortic valve ring, into the pericardial sac, producing a haemopericardium. Rarely the dissection continues below the diaphragm and rarely the newly formed channel re-enters the aorta producing a double-barrelled aorta.

Compression of surrounding structures. Aneurysms associated with syphilis gradually erode through the sternum and vertebral column. Comparable phenomena are now rarely encountered with either thoracic or abdominal aneurysms but an abdominal aneurysm may adhere to and compress the ureters or erode through the duodenum.

Further reading

Davies, M.J. (1980). *Pathology of Cardiac Valves.* Butterworths: London and Boston.

Davies, M.J. (1984). The cardiomyopathies: a review of terminology, pathology and pathogenesis. *Histopathology* **8**, 363–93.

Hangartner, J.R.W., Marley, N.J., Whitehead, A., Thomas, A.C. and Davies, M.J. (1985). The assessment of cardiac hypertrophy at autopsy. *Histopathology* **9**, 1295–306.

Massell, B.F., Chute, C.G., Walker, A.M., Kurland. P.H. and Kurland, G.S. (1988). Penicillin and the marked decrease in morbidity and mortality from rheumatic fever in the United States. *New Eng. J. Med.* **318**, 280–5.

Mitchinson, M.J. and Ball, R.Y. (1987). Macrophages and atherogenesis. *Lancet* **ii**. 146–9.

Olsen, E.G.J. (1980). *The Pathology of the Heart.* Macmillan Press Ltd: London and Basingstoke.

Pomerance, A. and Davies, M.J. (1975) (Editors). *The Pathology of the Heart.* Blackwell Scientific Publications: Oxford and London.

Shaper, A.G. (1987). Risk factors for ischaemic heart disease. *Health Trends* **19**, 3–8.

Sleight, P. and Jones, J.V. (1983) (Editors). *Scientific Foundations of Cardiology.* Heinemann: London.

Stehbens, W.E. (1987). An appraisal of the epidemic rise of coronary heart disease and its decline. *Lancet* **i**, 606–11.

4 Lungs

The inhalation of foreign agents is the cause of most lung disease. Micro-organisms and cigarette derivatives are the main causes and less often metallic and chemical compounds and gases. Microbial infection is universally experienced but long-term effects are few and little residual damage results. This is because of the use of antibiotics and natural defence mechanisms, as well as preventative medicine and improved social conditions. Cigarette smoking in contrast damages the lungs, potentially culminating in chronic bronchitis and parenchymal destruction with emphysema and the risk of carcinoma. Among a few smokers other disorders may also be brought to light or exacerbated, for example alpha-1-antitrypsin deficiency and, in miners, coal workers' pneumoconiosis. Without cigarette smoking there would be a very substantial diminution in pulmonary pathology and a dramatic fall in mortality from lung disease.

Other important lung disorders are associated with circulation. The majority arise from disorders of the systemic circulation producing pulmonary oedema and thrombo-embolism. A smaller group centre upon pulmonary circulation and cause pulmonary hypertension.

Anatomical factors

The components of the bronchial tree are shown in Figs 4.1 and 4.2. The direct continuity of the trachea and the right main bronchus favours the trapping of large foreign bodies in the right lung but particle size and gravity are more important in the intrapulmonary distribution of smaller particles. The small size of many micro-organisms and industrial dusts permits a uniform distribution in inhaled air and within the lungs but with larger particles gravity influences the final intrapulmonary site.

Gaseous exchange only occurs in the distal components of the bronchial tree, the *acinus*, which is not identifiable macroscopically. Groups of 3–5 acini are surrounded by septae and are visible on the pleural surface of the lungs, each group forming a *secondary lobule*. The alveoli within the acinus have a lining of flattened epithelial cells (*Type I pneumocytes*) and cuboidal cells (*Type II pneumocytes*) which with their basement membrane separate the alveolar contents from the pulmonary capillaries. The elongated nature of the Type I cells gives the false impression that these

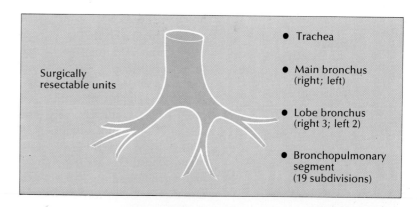

Fig. 4.1 Main conducting airways.

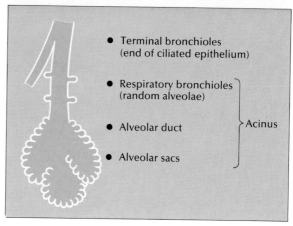

Fig. 4.2 Gaseous exchange pathways.

outnumber the Type II cells which are in fact much more common. The Type I cells are the source of surfactant, a complex of lipids and proteins, which lines the luminal surface of all alveolar cells and lowers their surface tension. Without surfactant the alveoli and lung tissue collapses and loses its elastic recoil, a state of affairs found in hyaline membrane disease of the newborn. Type II pneumocytes are also stem cells capable of forming Type I cells, a phenomenon seen in many conditions including the adult respiratory distress syndrome, where the Type I cells are irreversibly damaged.

Natural defence mechanisms

These involve:

1   The filtration of inhaled air by the nose where the largest particles are removed.

2   The cough reflex which guards the upper respiratory tract and contributes to the removal of impacted mucus plugs in the distal part of the bronchial tree.

3   The combination of the cilia lining much of the bronchial tree and the mucus secreted from the submucosal glands of the larger

bronchi and to a lesser degree from their epithelium. These mechanisms maintain the patency of the bronchial tree and remove normal and abnormal particulate matter. Without mucus the continuous upward beating of the cilia is ineffective and anything that increases viscosity of the mucus also impairs their action. Infection is the invariable consequence. Dehydration is the most common cause of increased viscosity since water is the main constituent of mucus. Congenital immotile cilia syndrome and viscid mucus in cystic fibrosis are other examples of these defects, while less complete aberrations form part of chronic bronchitis associated with cigarette smoking, where there is an excess production of abnormal mucus.

4 The serous component of glandular secretions which helps towards dissolving inhaled soluble compounds and also provides a medium for IgA secretion.

5 Lymphocytes of bronchial associated lymphoid tissue (BALT) which are found as foci in the parenchyma and in the bronchial submucosa. IgA is the main immunoglobulin produced and this may play a part in stabilizing mucus as well as in neutralizing viruses and inhibiting the direct adherence of bacteria to the mucosa.

6 Macrophages within the lumen of the alveoli (Fig. 4.3). These cells occur in a resting state as septal cells in the surrounding interstitial tissue. Once they have phagocytosed material the majority are transferred out of the bronchial tree and swallowed but a small number emigrate into the tissue around the terminal bronchioles where they enter the afferent lymphatics to the hilar lymph nodes. This exit route partly explains the localization of centrilobular emphysema and some pneumoconioses.

7 A good oxygen supply which is essential for the effectiveness of the mucociliary mechanism, alveolar epithelium and macrophage system. This is provided directly by oxygen inhaled and circulated within the rich vasculature. However, the lung apices, particularly those of the upper lobes, are relatively less well perfused because of their lower blood pressure, a direct effect of gravity. Gravity is also responsible for the relative congestion of the bases of the lungs, a factor that may underlie the localization of some types of emphysema.

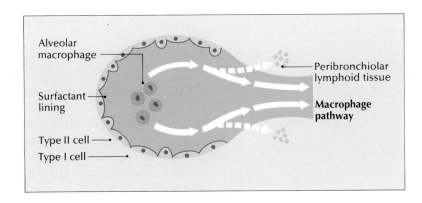

Fig. 4.3 Alveolar sac.

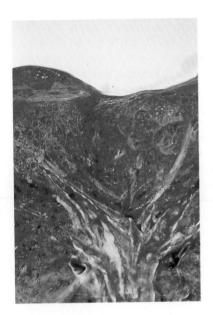

Fig. 4.4 Association of acute bronchitis with pus in the bronchial tree and pneumonia. The lung is consolidated and firm to the touch.

Inhalation disorders

Pneumonia

Terminology

Pneumonia is the term used for inflammation of the lung following microbial infection with the alveoli as the site of infection. Although most pneumonia arises from inhalation it can also develop from blood-borne infection and is then slightly more likely to involve the lower lobes. The term pneumonia is sometimes used when there is no infection and to avoid confusion it should be qualified by always naming the cause, e.g. aspiration pneumonia.

Bronchopneumonia cannot always be distinguished from pneumonia. This affects the alveoli and the bronchial tree. Distinction from pneumonia is largely academic since microbial infection starting in the alveoli or in the bronchi can spread to the other component (Fig. 4.4).

Alveolitis is used to describe allergic conditions damaging the lungs. *Pneumonitis* describes states where alveolar damage follows physical injury.

Diagnosis

Radiological support is essential clinically and the underlying micro-organism can only be recognized with laboratory help. Until a micro-organism has been isolated the clinician is faced with the possibility of a wide range of causative bacteria, viruses, fungi or protozoa.

Gram and Ziehl—Nielsen staining of sputum samples may allow the immediate recognition of some bacteria and silver staining of *Pneumocystis carinii* but for many organisms isolation on an appropriate culture medium is necessary. Potential specimens include sputum, aspirates, pleural effusions, lung biopsy tissue and blood. Where culture is inappropriate or impossible, as with some viruses, electron microscopic examination of specimens or the demonstration of a significant rise in serum antibody titre can be diagnostic. Positive allergen skin tests for tuberculosis will provide further diagnostic help.

Causative organisms

A wide range of organisms may be involved and in some patients there may be more than one type.

Bacteria. Strep. pneumoniae is the most frequent with infection by Staphylococci, often secondary to viral infections, much less common. Pneumonia from Gram negative organisms is seen in hospitalized patients and in those on long-term antibiotics or who are immunosuppressed.

Viruses. Influenza viruses are the main cause of viral pneumonia leading to a significant number of deaths in all major epidemics. Cytomegalovirus, measles and chickenpox virus are seen mostly in immunosuppressed individuals although measles pneumonia is a hazard for severely malnourished and starved children.

Fungus. Pneumonia due to these organisms is very unusual except among immunocompromised patients. In this country *Aspergillus* is the most common but *Candida* and *Acintinomycoses* species will also be found. Fungi peculiar to specific geographical areas such as histoplasmosis and blastomycosis in the USA may occur among visitors and immigrants.

Protozoa. Pneumocystis carinii pneumonia is restricted to immunocompromised patients and is a marker and a cause of mortality amongst those with the acquired immune deficiency syndrome (AIDS).

Causative factors

For a patient to develop pneumonia there is usually one or a number of ways whereby the balance between the resistance of the host and virulence of the organism is upset.

Host resistance is affected by pre-existing disease, either confined to the chest or elsewhere. Chronic obstructive airways disease, bronchiectasis and chronic congestive cardiac failure are all potential predisposing factors, as is old age, diabetes, alcoholism and immunosuppression of any type. Post-splenectomy patients are particularly prone to *Strep. pneumoniae* infections because of the loss of B-cells and lack of IgG_2 production.

Factors within the lungs increasing the likelihood of pneumonia include alterations to the mucociliary and macrophage clearance mechanisms. Temperature, humidity, alcohol and especially cigarettes all diminish the efficiency of mucociliary clearance and it is the adverse effect of cold and dryness of the air that contribute to the high incidence of pneumonia in the winter. Macrophage clearance may be decreased as part of any immunodepression but it is also influenced by the inhibitory action of some micro-organisms on chemotaxis and phagocytosis.

The specific virulence of micro-organisms is illustrated by the epithelial necrosis that the influenza virus produces in the bronchial tree, denuding it of its protective ciliated epithelium and the capsule encasing the *Strep. pneumoniae.*

APPEARANCES

Pneumonia passes through a sequence of changes reflecting the underlying and evolving inflammatory processes. These changes were described in patients with *Strep. pneumoniae* before antibiotic therapy but many are common to pneumonia from any type of micro-organism. There are nevertheless subtle differences in tissue reactions associated with certain micro-organisms but these are rarely diagnostic unless the organisms are identified (Fig. 4.5). Exceptions are the inclusion bodies of some viral pneumonias, of which the intracytoplasmic and intranuclear inclusion bodies of the cytomegalovirus are those most easily recognized; the branching hyphae and spore bodies of fungus infections (Fig. 4.6) and the closely packed cysts of *Pneumocystis carinii* pneumonia.

Following a brief phase of intense oedema the lung tissue becomes firm, congested and red and fairly sharply demarcated from the adjacent normal lung. When the pleura is involved this is dull and roughened (Fig. 4.7). This stage, from its similarity to the liver, is referred to as *red hepatization* and is rarely a stage at which death occurs. During the next four to five days there is organization and

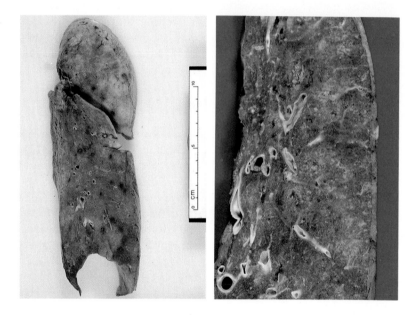

Fig. 4.5 Pneumonia due to (*left*) Gram negative cocci and (*right*) *Actinomycosis.* There are multiple scattered foci with incipient abscess formation in both lungs but the cause was only realized from culture results.

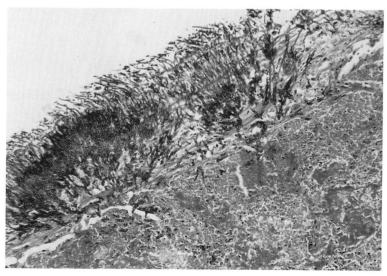

Fig. 4.6 Pneumonia arising from infection with an *Aspergillus.* The fungus is sprouting on the pleural surface but was also in the lung parenchyma.

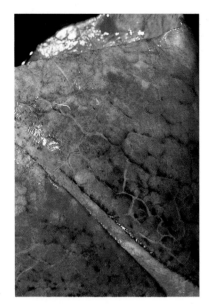

Fig. 4.7 Pleurisy overlying an area of pneumonia. There is a red and irregular deposition of fibrin which would underlie a pleural rub in the chest.

neutrophil polymorphs replace the red cells and fibrin. The lung tissue then enters the stage of *grey hepatization* and is very pale with a firm, moist and mucoid parenchyma (Fig. 4.8). The pleura is thickened and roughened and an effusion may be present which if infected is known as an *empyema*. The final stage is resolution during which macrophages ingest the necrotic debris and return the lung to normal. This sequence of events does not necessarily occur in a uniform fashion throughout the infected lung but progresses at variable rates, probably reflecting the distribution of the infecting organism.

Complications

The most serious is death. If resolution does not occur there may be an underlying bronchial carcinoma or pulmonary embolus with infarction, and fibrosis may then follow. Alternatively abscesses may supervene. Clinically the patient is often toxic and there can be septicaemic spread to any part of the body, notably the meninges and brain.

Tuberculosis in the lung

This occurs in the UK but is no longer the scourge that it was in the early part of this century. The improvement has followed from better social conditions, mass X-ray screening, milk sterilization, tuberculin testing and BCG vaccination as well as the development of appropriate antibiotics. These approaches have not been so easy to institute in the Third World where the disease still claims a high morbidity and mortality, and consequently immigrants are the main source of tuberculosis in the UK. Disease among the indigenous

Upside down

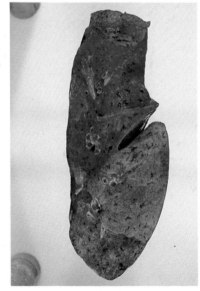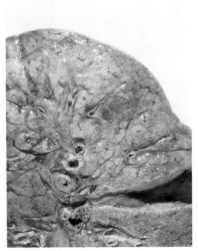

Fig. 4.8 Grey hepatization. (*Left*) Much of the upper lobe is pale and poorly aerated compared with the remaining lung; (*right*) a smaller focus in a fresh lung.

population does, nevertheless, occur, affecting those who are otherwise well, the elderly and those who are immunocompromised. Diagnosis in the latter group is realized all too often only at autopsy and atypical organisms are often found.

Organism

The bacillus is *Mycobacterium tuberculosis*, which is acid-fast in Ziehl–Nielsen preparations and is transmitted from infected individuals. Infections from *M. bovis*, where the primary host is the cow and milk the vector, are now rare. Atypical or anonymous mycobacteria can cause infection among patients with chronic bronchitis, emphysema and pneumoconioses, and especially the immunosuppressed. For diagnosis culture on specialized media and animal inoculation, each needing six to eight weeks, are necessary. Mantoux or Heaf skin tests, which rely upon a reaction to inoculated purified protein derivative (PPD) from the wall of the bacillus, can be helpful but depend upon previous exposure to the antigen.

Histological features

The histopathologist can recognize tuberculosis with certainty only if there are acid-fast bacilli. Granulomas or *tubercles* are characteristic with necrotic, amorphous, eosinophilic centres representing the fatty, or caseous cheese-like material seen macroscopically (Fig. 4.9). Surrounding the centre are macrophages, previously referred to and regarded as epithelioid cells, and Langhan's giant cells. An outer thin rim of lymphocytes surrounds the granuloma. The granulomas enlarge and fuse and ultimately their centres drop out and cavities are formed. Cavity formation is therefore another lesion highly suspect of tuberculosis. Typical granulomas can, however, be recognized without demonstrable organisms and conversely multiple organisms present in the absence of granulomas. Skin infection, *lupus vulgaris*, is an example where tubercle bacilli are rarely demonstrable and much tuberculosis in the Third World and in immunosuppressed individuals, circumstances where there are no granulomas.

Patterns of lung infection

There are two distinct patterns which may follow one another or appear as separate episodes (Fig. 4.10)

1 *Primary infection*. This is almost confined to childhood and is rarely progressive. The organisms enter via the bronchial tree to any part of the lung but most often the more peripheral subpleural air sacs. A tubercle then forms and organisms migrate via lymphatics to the hilar lymph nodes where similar granulomas develop. The focal lung infection is the *Ghon focus* and this with the involved lymph node lesions the *Ghon complex* or *primary complex*. Healing by fibrosis with scarring is the natural end result for both components

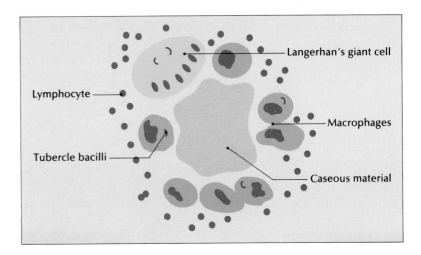

Langerhan's giant cell

Lymphocyte

Macrophages

Tubercle bacilli

Caseous material

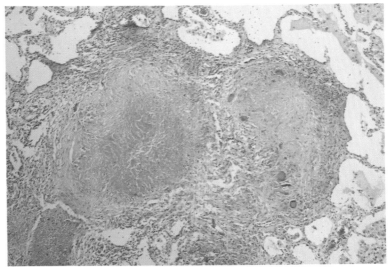

Fig. 4.9 (*Above and below*) Tubercle or tuberculous granuloma.

of the primary complex and calcification, ascribed to the affinity of calcium for fatty acids forming the wall of the bacilli, also follows. Tuberculin sensitivity is conferred on the patient and the Mantoux or Heaf test is positive.

Only a small number of those with primary infection in the UK develop more severe lung disease. Why this is so is not fully understood but an upset in the balance between the host's resistance and the organism's virulence is involved. Three forms are seen and each at any interval after the primary infection:

(a) Local expansion of the Ghon focus occurs and a cavity may appear. Erosion of bronchioles producing intrabronchial spread follows and fulminant tuberculous pneumonia accompanied by effusions and even empyema.

(b) There is progressive enlargement of the lymph node component of the primary complex. This may compress the adjacent bronchi with collapse of the lung and later secondary infection. Alternatively there may be erosion into the bronchus or trachea, intrabronchial

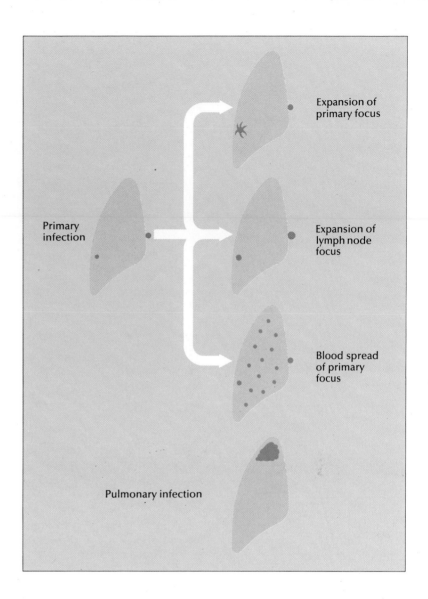

Fig. 4.10 Patterns of tuberculosis in the lungs.

spread of the tuberculosis and subsequent fulminant tuberculous pneumonia.

(c) The primary focus may be followed by *miliary tuberculosis*. Macroscopically there are pin-point granulomas within all tissues (Fig. 4.11). These, in the lungs, are recognized in chest X-rays as diffuse mottling and can be seen directly on the optic discs. Disseminated infection arises from vascular invasion spreading from the primary complex. Prior to antibiotics this was invariably fatal but solitary tuberculous lesions in adults may have arisen from subclinical miliary tuberculosis which, in the majority of sites, resolved spontaneously.

2 *Pulmonary tuberculosis.* This is unsatisfactorily named and the terms *re-infective tuberculosis, post-primary tuberculosis, secondary tuberculosis* and *adult tuberculosis* are all used. The source is either

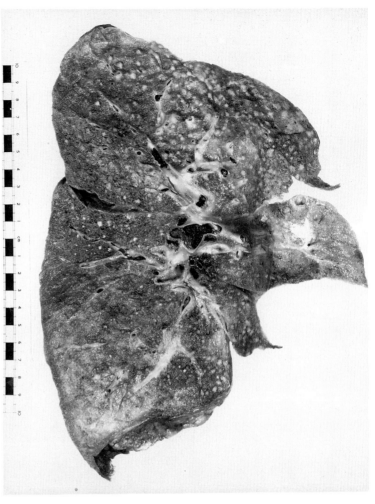

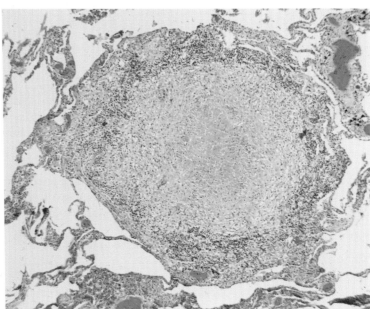

Fig. 4.11 (*Above*) Miliary
tuberculosis. Each white spot is a
granuloma and filled with
mycobacteria; (*below*) light
microscopy of a granuloma.

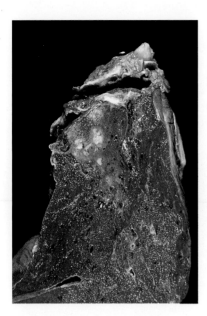

Fig. 4.12 Pulmonary tuberculosis. The apex of the upper lobe includes an early cavity with white fibrous and necrotic tissue walls. Similar features are seen in the adjacent lung.

an infected person, in which case if primary infection had occurred, the disease is truly re-infective, or from activation of organisms associated with a previous primary infection. Tuberculous bacilli can unquestionably lie dormant in tissues and even calcified tissues for many years which explains why many examples of pulmonary tuberculosis in the UK occur in elderly individuals. Whatever the sequence of infection sensitization to the bacilli may have occurred and would explain the indolent and chronic course that the disease often pursues.

APPEARANCES

Distinctive features are localization to the apices of the lungs, particularly the upper lobes, and absence of lymph node involvement (Fig. 4.12). The lesion probably starts as an isolated caseating granuloma but by the time it is recognized clinically a cavity is present. Untreated the cavity does not always enlarge but is associated with dense fibrosis within the supporting lung, calcification and pleural adhesions. Granulomas and organisms are not always so easily identified as in primary tuberculosis. Spread can occur along bronchi and pneumonia supervene but there is no haematogenous spread nor miliary tuberculosis. Vessels of varying size are nevertheless eroded since haemoptysis occurs. Should the cavity penetrate the pleural surface a pneumothorax will follow and with an enlarging cavity, effusions and empyemas.

Chronic bronchitis and emphysema

These two disorders are clinically difficult to separate and define and are referred to jointly as *chronic obstructive airways disease*. This term is unsatisfactory since it emphasizes the bronchial aspect of chronic bronchitis and detracts from the parenchymal element of emphysema. Awareness of the two separate conditions should therefore be maintained.

Chronic bronchitis involves an increase in mucus production and expectoration over observed periods. It is difficult to separate these changes from normal and timing is open to observer error, but definitions currently used are 'chronic and excessive mucus secretion in the bronchial tree' and 'cough and sputum occurring on most days for at least three months in the year, but for at least two consecutive years'.

Emphysema, in contrast, can be defined by the histopathologist provided that the lungs are inflated and morphometric techniques used. Emphysema is then recognized as permanent enlargement of a part or whole of the respiratory acinus distal to the terminal bronchiole.

Both disorders share a number of aetiological factors of which the most important is cigarette smoking. Without this habit the slow suffocation produced by these disorders could be avoided and their mortality, in England and Wales 36 000 persons per annum, dramatically decreased. Even so, cigarette smoking is not an inevitable prerequisite since the majority of smokers do not develop chronic chest disease. Why there is variation is unclear but it is consistent with different pathogenetic mechanisms both involving cigarette smoke that are believed to underlie the two conditions as well as close association of the two disorders.

Development of chronic bronchitis (Fig. 4.13)

Cigarette smoking is the most important factor and is believed to increase mucus production and to make this more viscid. Mucus originates mainly from the bronchial glands and to a smaller extent from mucous cells of the bronchial epithelium. Bronchial glands are often enlarged and may include greater numbers of mucous cells but this is not unique, since similar changes develop with age and, like those in bronchitis, later regress. Any enlargement is not uniform but patchily distributed which is why morphometric definitions of chronic bronchitis have not been universally accepted. These patchy findings make the exact role of cigarette smoke unclear, including the effect on mucus itself.

Mucus includes a greater proportion of mucin than normal and is consequently more viscid and tenacious and difficult for the cilia to clear. With stasis of mucus, infection is almost inevitable. The low level of IgA found in the lungs of those dying from chronic bronchitis may also contribute to infection, as may damage to the ciliary clearance mechanism. This can follow from both epithelial changes associated with cigarette smoking as well as direct action of smoke on the cilia. Epithelial changes range from minor degrees of dysplasia to squamous metaplasia and are associated with loss of ciliated cells.

Air pollution is an important contributor to chronic bronchitis. City dwellers have a higher incidence than those in the country and a close association exists with the coal and steel industries. Underlying these observations are common factors of low social

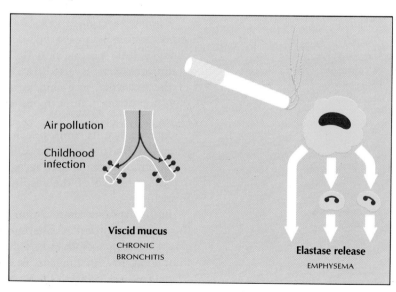

Fig. 4.13 Chronic obstructive airways disease.

class, poor living conditions and residence in the UK. A damp and often cold climate is blamed for the disorder which is still referred to as the British or English disease.

Infection *per se* is not a primary event in chronic bronchitis. This is in marked contrast to acute bronchitis, which is microbial in origin. Acute bronchitis and other respiratory infections during the first years of life, especially if the siblings have similar disorders and the parents smoke, may, however, be long-term precursors to chronic bronchitis.

Development of emphysema (Fig. 4.13)

Many factors considered for chronic bronchitis apply, including the main contributor, cigarette smoking. The effects are to destroy the lung parenchyma around the respiratory bronchioles but not to stimulate mucus secretion. Lung destruction follows an imbalance between elastase and its antagonists, allowing digestion of the extracellular matrix or stroma with permanent overdistension of the alveoli, loss of alveolar walls and development of large air spaces. Elastase is found in alveolar macrophages and neutrophil polymorphs. Increased numbers of macrophages are seen in smokers' lungs and these cells attract neutrophil polymorphs. Release of elastase initiates emphysema even with a normal complement of antagonists. However, there is no direct evidence that cigarette smoke stimulates elastase release and the possibility of a decreased antagonist role is thereby raised. A genetically determined deficiency of a potent anti-elastase, alpha-1-antitrypsin, occurs and these patients commonly develop emphysema. Furthermore, smoking diminishes the inhibitory effect of alpha-1-antitrypsin making emphysema even more likely in those with this deficiency if they also smoke. These mechanisms may also explain the intrapulmonary distribution of the most common forms of emphysema (Fig. 4.14).

Centrilobular emphysema occurs in cigarette smokers and is seen mainly in the upper zones. These are areas where the smoke collects preferentially with aggregates of macrophages surrounding respiratory bronchioles as the initial change. If elastase is released, with or without any diminution in the antagonist's role, tissue damage may follow and emphysema supervene.

Panacinar or *panlobular emphysema* occurs in the lower lobes and is found in alpha-1-antitrypsin deficiency. The natural congestion of the lower lobes involves greater numbers of neutrophil polymorphs and if elastase is released local tissue destruction may follow aided by diminution of alpha-1-antitrypsin.

APPEARANCES

Chronic bronchitis on its own is morphologically unimpressive. Mucus plugs fill some bronchi and the entrances to mucous glands and if there is superimposed infection pus will be found. In these circumstances the bronchial mucosa will be inflamed and reddened. Any bronchial gland enlargement is best appreciated in lungs

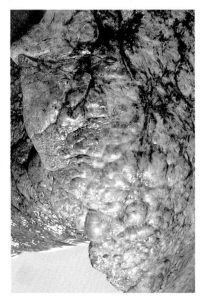

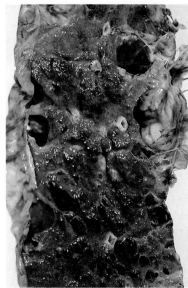

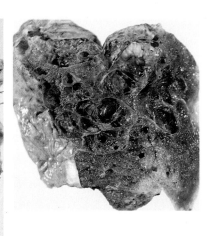

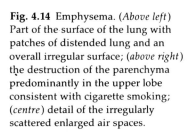

Fig. 4.14 Emphysema. (*Above left*) Part of the surface of the lung with patches of distended lung and an overall irregular surface; (*above right*) the destruction of the parenchyma predominantly in the upper lobe consistent with cigarette smoking; (*centre*) detail of the irregularly scattered enlarged air spaces.

inflated and fixed prior to examination. Within the lung parenchyma emphysema is inevitably present.

Emphysema produces apparently over-inflated lungs which are light, with a texture similar to that of wire wool saucepan cleaners (Fig. 4.14). Parenchyma spreads across the anterior mediastinum and is difficult to compress. Within the lung substance there are variably sized abnormal air spaces whose distribution can only be appreciated in sections of inflated lung. Different patterns of abnormal air spaces categorize emphysema into centrilobular and panacinar or panlobular (Fig. 4.15) but in any emphysematous lung there is almost always a mixture, contributing to the clinical difficulty in distinguishing the two types.

Other patterns of emphysema are uncommon apart from that in coal miners. Emphysema in these workers is called *focal emphysema* although distribution is not focal but similar to centrilobular emphysema. The distinctive features are coal dust around the respiratory bronchioles and absence of tissue destruction in the early stages.

Compensatory emphysema and bullous disease of the lung must be distinguished from true emphysema. *Compensatory emphysema* is a misnomer since it refers to the alveolar enlargement accompanying areas of collapsed lung, and not associated with tissue destruction. *Bullous disease of the lung* is a condition within otherwise normal lung where large subpleural air spaces or bullae occur, notably at the apices and free margins.

Complications

Respiratory failure may develop with either chronic bronchitis or emphysema and cause substantial distress. Should this become progressive cor pulmonale will develop and at any stage repeated

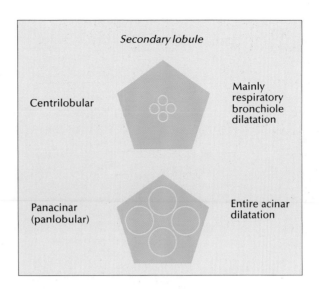

Fig. 4.15 Patterns of emphysema.

chest infection is almost inevitable. The chronic bronchitic has a greater likelihood of lung cancer than controls.

Bronchiectasis

This condition is characterized by dilatation of the bronchi. Histopathologists see only those examples where dilatation is permanent but radiologists have some evidence that affected bronchi may collapse and the dilatation revert to near normal. The condition is produced by either a destructive inflammatory disorder or a compensatory reaction to collapse of the surrounding lung and is thus not always a true inhalation disorder.

Inflammatory element. Originally this was mainly childhood viral infections, especially measles, and also acute bacterial infections, notably whooping cough. Vaccinations for measles and whooping cough, as well as the diminution of pulmonary tuberculosis and the use of antibiotics, have all radically lowered the incidence of this disorder. Today, if a child has bronchiectasis, immunodeficiency and congenital disorders of the immotile ciliary type should be looked for.

Severe damage to the bronchial epithelium results from infection with impairment of the mucociliary clearance mechanism, stasis of mucus and epithelial debris and secondary infection (Fig. 4.16). Repeated infections, some precipitated by mucus obstruction, provoke destruction of muscle and elastic tissue in the bronchial walls and subsequent dilatation.

Obstructive element. With bronchiectasis following collapse of the lung parenchyma there is also bronchial obstruction (Fig. 4.16). The

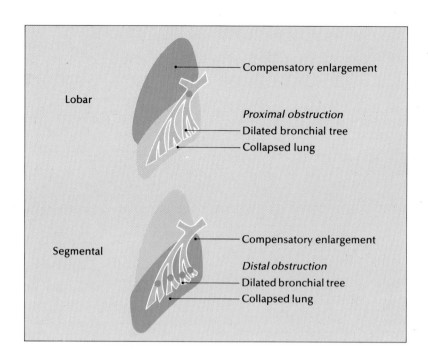

Fig. 4.16 Main patterns of bronchiectasis.

lung collapses because it is receiving insufficient air and any trapped air is then absorbed. The uninvolved lung including the bronchi undergoes compensatory enlargement which is produced by traction from the negative pressure within the chest cavity, so keeping this filled with lung tissue. Bronchial obstruction occurs either from proximal obstruction at the hilum or more distally when multiple bronchi must be affected. With distal bronchial obstruction, selected bronchi are involved but in proximal obstruction virtually all bronchi become dilated. Once obstruction is established infection and inflammation contribute to dilatation and in time render it irreversible. To provide sufficient blood for the inflammatory granulation tissue large bronchopulmonary anastomoses develop. Bronchial carcinoma is an important cause of proximal bronchial obstruction and cystic fibrosis of distal obstruction.

APPEARANCES

Bronchiectasis occurs in any part of the lungs but is most likely in the lower lobes and when unilateral is found more on the left side than the right. Gravity underlies this localization but better drainage of the right lung is also important. Dilated bronchi are obvious in the cut sections of the lung and can extend to the pleura. Two main patterns of bronchial dilatation are described (Figs 4.17 and 4.36) but mixed patterns defying precise compartmentalization frequently occur. Foul smelling pus and necrotic debris fill the involved bronchi and their walls are ulcerated and thickened. The adjacent lung is rarely normal and usually includes pneumonic and fibrotic areas as well as regions of collapse and overdistension. There is a marked vascularity associated with the many bronchopulmonary anastomoses.

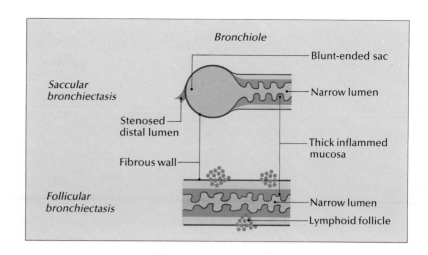

Fig. 4.17 Bronchiectasis.

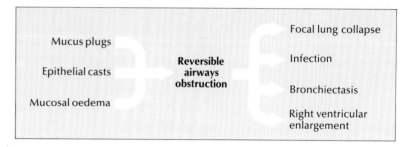

Fig. 4.18 Asthma: causes and effects.

Complications

These are largely avoidable with adequate antibiotic therapy or surgical excision of the bronchiectatic segments. Formerly lung and brain abscesses, amyloidosis, cor pulmonale and, in children, stunting of growth developed. Carcinoma is not a complication despite the frequency of focal squamous metaplasia.

Asthma

Asthma is a group of disorders predominantly due to inhalation of matter precipitating an allergic response and manifest by widespread reversible airways obstruction (Fig. 4.18). The obstruction may regress either spontaneously or in response to therapy and can be of a fairly short duration. Approximately 7% of the population in the UK is affected and death results in a constant minority.

Atopic asthma

Most asthmatics are children and they and their relatives may also suffer from eczema and hay fever. These individuals are referred to as atopic and are characterized by positive immediate Type I hypersensitivity skin tests to a number of common antigens including pollens, fungus, dust and animal extracts. These allergens combine directly with antibody, most commonly IgE but also IgG, that is on

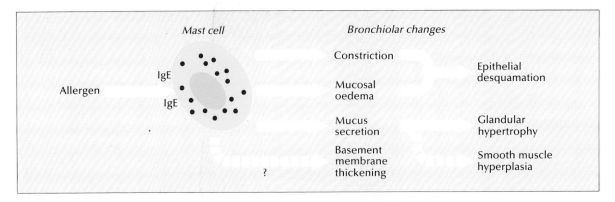

Fig. 4.19 Atopic asthma.

the surface of mast cells. Circulating levels of IgE are not always raised. Antibody—antigen reaction degranulates the mast cells and releases histamine, which precipitates bronchial constriction and mucus secretion (Fig. 4.19). The effect of the slow reacting substance and platelet-activating factor which are also released is uncertain. Eosinophilic chemotactic factor, also from mast cells, attracts eosinophil polymorphs which may liberate neutralizing enzymes to these factors including histamine. Other mechanisms including vagal inhibition, hypothalamic responses and platelets are also involved.

A positive Type I skin response does not necessarily mean that the test antigen is the cause of asthma and evidence for a direct relationship comes only from bronchial provocation tests. These involve deliberate inhalation of allergens and, if causative, the subsequent development of asthma. Some patients do not respond immediately but develop asthma hours later, a reaction shared by some responders to skin testing. These late reactions are not examples of Type I hypersensitivity and no cause for them has been found.

Non-atopic asthma

Non-atopic asthmatics are most often adults either with no recognized cause, sometimes called *cryptogenic* or *intrinsic asthma*, or those in whom the causative antigen arises in the course of their job, the disorder appearing at the end of the working day or on Monday after a free weekend. The industries concerned are many and wide-ranging, including dye, plastics and resin production as well as flour and grain products, carpentry and metal refining and plating. In some sufferers Type I hypersensitivity is involved. For many this is not so and in a small proportion there will be other aspects of the *bronchopulmonary eosinophilic syndrome*, a group of disorders with eosinophilia and infiltrates of these cells within the lung tissues.

APPEARANCES

Patients dying during an asthmatic attack have very bulky lungs, spreading from the opened thorax and across the anterior mediastinum. Most parenchyma is aerated and devoid of any destructive changes of emphysema but small areas of collapse are found on the free margins. Throughout the bronchial tree are plugs of mucus containing casts of desquamated respiratory epithelium and eosinophil polymorphs. Eosinophil polymorphs occur in large numbers in the bronchial tree and among the alveoli. Bronchial obstruction is also contributed to by mucosal oedema, smooth muscle hyperplasia and bronchial gland hypertrophy. The muscle change is probably a response to mucus plugs but is not related to spasm and glandular hypertrophy underlies excess mucin production. The pronounced basement membrane thickening that is also seen is unexplained but is not related to immune complex or antibody deposition.

Complications

These and the mortality of the disorder are largely confined to non-atopic adult asthmatics. Anoxia and less commonly focal rupture of the lung and the development of a pneumothorax are causes of death during an acute attack. Infection can arise from any asthmatic attack and in some patients precipitate asthma. Both epithelial desquamation and loss of normal ciliary clearance mechanisms as well as mucus plugging encourage infection. With repeated attacks the epithelium may fail to regenerate normally and become replaced by one devoid of cilia, making it possible for infection to arise independently and lead to bronchiectasis. The right ventricular hypertrophy, often apparent at autopsy, is the product of repeated episodes of bronchial obstruction, increases in pulmonary blood pressure and pulmonary infection.

Respiratory distress syndromes

Different patterns of respiratory distress syndromes occur in the newborn and in adults. In both age groups the clinical disorder is characterized by progressive respiratory distress, hypoxaemia and diffuse lung shadowing radiologically. Impaired functioning of Type II pneumocytes is a common factor although in the child, this is the root of the disorder but in the adult, a consequence. Inhalation is an important portal of entry for the causative agent only in some adults.

Respiratory distress syndrome in the newborn

This is a potential complication for all premature infants and especially those of multiple births, notably the second twin, and of diabetic mothers as well as infants delivered by Caesarian section. The Type II pneumocytes are immature and unable to secrete surfactant and without this the surface tension of the air sacs is too high for inflation and they remain collapsed or atelectatic. The alveolar ducts and respiratory bronchioles are unaffected and dilated and are very often lined by a band of eosinophilic material termed a hyaline membrane (Fig. 4.20). It is this hyaline membrane that has

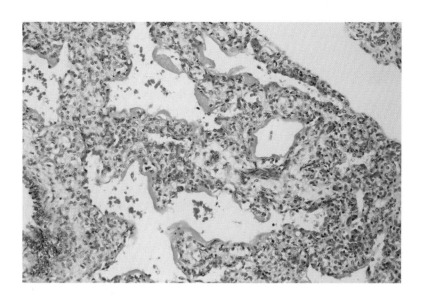

Fig. 4.20 Hyaline membranes in the lung of a premature infant dying shortly after birth.

provided the alternative name of *hyaline membrane disease of the newborn* but not all infants have these and similar linings are found in a wide variety of other disorders. They are also not evident until some hours after birth.

Formation of the hyaline membranes involves pulmonary oedema associated with a transudate as well as mechanical injury to the alveolar epithelium, each in response to the force of the respiratory effort necessary to overcome the high surface tension of the air sacs. Paradoxically the oxygen given to alleviate the symptoms may aggravate the condition by directly damaging Type II pneumocytes.

Should the infant survive over 36 h organization of the hyaline membranes and repair of the damaged epithelium occurs. Fully functional Type II pneumocytes then develop and as resolution proceeds the lungs become normally aerated.

APPEARANCES

If death occurs the lungs are airless but not collapsed. They feel solid and are often dark purple or plum coloured.

Complications

Over-assiduous attempts at ventilation may produce pneumothorax and mediastinal emphysema (air in the mediastinal tissues) as well as intraventricular haemorrhage in the brain. Focal haemorrhage is also seen in the lungs and at either site hypoxia and prematurity are further factors involved.

Adult respiratory distress syndrome

This is increasingly recognized and has multiple causes, including aspiration, inhaled toxins, shock, trauma, drugs and blood and

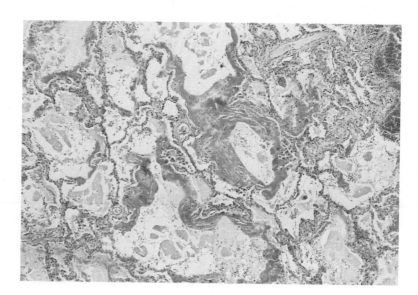

Fig. 4.21 Hyaline membranes in an adult's lungs. The patient had been in a road accident and maintained on a respirator. Other parts of the lung included areas of oedema and pneumonia, some organizing.

metabolic disorders. Most patients, in addition, have experienced oxygen therapy and artificial ventilation.

Initially there is interstitial oedema with intra-alveolar haemorrhage and congestion. The fluid leakage reflects damage to the Type I pneumocytes and separation of their intercellular junctions. These cells are especially liable to injury because they are stretched over the alveolar basement membranes and because they are unable to reduplicate. Damage may occur directly or follow from neutrophil polymorph proteases since substantial numbers of these cells are attracted in the early stages following complement activation. Further injury provokes desquamation of the Type I cells, leaving large areas of bare basement membrane through which fibrin-rich fluid passes from the capillaries into the air sacs. This fluid is part of the hyaline membranes lining the air sacs (Fig. 4.21) and is contributed to by degeneration and necrosis of capillary endothelial cells. Endothelial damage also promotes fibrin and platelet deposition in the capillaries. Endothelial cells are prone to damage for the same reasons as the Type I pneumocytes and because of their high metabolic activity but the role of this damage and its extent may not be as significant as that in Type I pneumocytes.

Course

After approximately a week reparative changes develop culminating in fibrosis by two weeks. Type II pneumocytes can divide and are the precursors of Type I cells. They replace damaged Type I cells and in doing so provide a cubical epithelium and a thicker barrier for oxygen exchange than normal. The oxygen given for the hypoxia incidentally directly damages these immature pneumocytes and a vicious circle of epithelial destruction, regeneration and further destruction is established. Proliferating fibroblasts enter the air sacs, probably via the exposed basement membrane, as well as from the interstitial tissues and cause progressive fibrosis. Damage to alveolar macrophages with the release of proteases including elastase and subsequent impaired macrophage function contribute to these processes as does vascular thrombosis.

Diffuse alveolar damage and fibrosis with death from respiratory failure is the probable end result for 60–90% of patients. Nevertheless, relentless progression is not inevitable and resolution with normal respiratory function does occur. Other survivors will have some residual fibrosis and respiratory impairment.

APPEARANCES

These reflect the progression of the disorder and any superadded infection. At first the lungs are increased in weight and are oedematous but later they are heavy and solid with plum-coloured moist pleura and tough firm-to-hard parenchyma. Both the pleura and the parenchyma usually include areas of haemorrhage. Fluid, often mucoid and bloodstained, exudes from the parenchyma and bronchial tree.

Complications

Infection and pulmonary oedema are inevitable. Liver, kidney and heart failure as well as clotting disorders and systemic infections can be anticipated either as the cause or the result and markedly increase the mortality.

Pneumoconioses

This group of disorders all arise from inhalation of dust particles which are deposited in the lungs and give rise to fibrosis (Fig. 4.22). The fibrosis must be distinguished from that arising from a wide range of agents, some producing their effects through immunological mechanisms and others through unknown means. *Farmer's lung* (Fig. 4.23) and *Byssinosis* are examples in the first category, respectively, associated with exposure to mouldy hay containing fungus and to cotton dust, while *Cryptogenic fibrosing alveolitis* is the term used for pulmonary fibrosis with no obvious cause. Nevertheless,

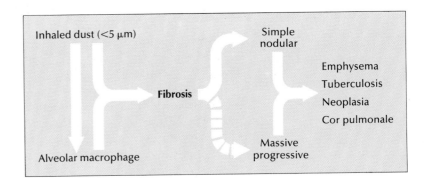

Fig. 4.22 Pneumoconiosis.

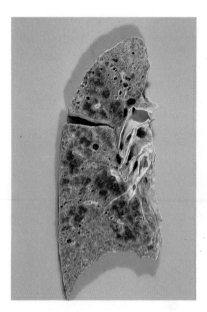

Fig. 4.23 Example of Farmer's lung.

even in this type of fibrosis the occasional presence of systemic lupus erythematosus or, more commonly, rheumatoid disease imply immunological mechanisms.

Diagnosis

The dust particles causing the fibrosis must be recognized but since these may not be evident microscopically, diagnosis leans heavily upon an occupational history and the features in the chest X-ray. The pneumoconioses are best distinguished by the causative dust but a few are referred to by the occupation involved, e.g., *silver polisher's lung*, where the putative agent is iron oxide. The dusts are both naturally occurring and those created during a wide range of industrial processes but silicon, asbestos and coal dust (Fig. 4.24) are the three most common pneumoconioses.

Mechanism of injury

Dusts provoke fibrosis because of their small size, particles < 5 μm. These reach the alveoli while larger particles are trapped and removed by the mucociliary system. A further factor seen with asbestos is the straight shape of the particles which facilitates penetration of the tissues. Individual susceptibility, duration and intensity of exposure and concentration and amount of dust inhaled are other factors influencing the development of fibrosis. The effects can be symptomatic and will be magnified when there is coincident lung disease but in many patients the disorder is only appreciated from the chest X-ray.

Dust particles reaching the alveoli are ingested by the alveolar macrophages, many of which are ultimately expectorated. A small

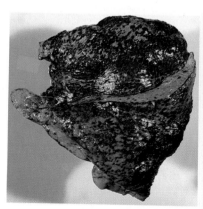

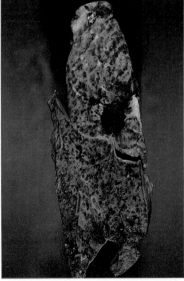

Fig. 4.24 (*left* and *right*) Coal miner's lung. The surface is almost uniformly anthracotic and within the parenchyma there is fibrosis and incipient cavity formation.

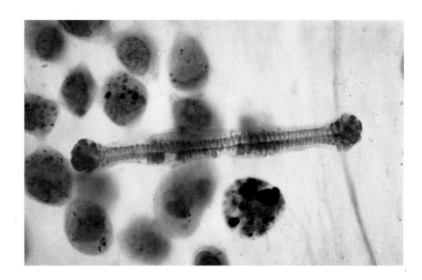

Fig. 4.25 Asbestos body in a sputum specimen.

number reach the centrilobular regions and either enter the lymphatics or accumulate in the centrilobular interstitial tissues. The dust particles are then released, following a direct action on the macrophages, and stimulate a nodular fibrosis, which with coal dust is jet black but with silica or asbestos alone has no diagnostic macroscopic features. Silica can be revealed by techniques such as micro-incineration which destroys the lung tissue, leaving the silica particles intact. Asbestosis may be associated with asbestos bodies which have a dumb-bell shape with circular ridges along the handle and are coated with haemosiderin (Fig. 4.25). These bodies are, however, found in lungs in those with no exposure to asbestos and are thus not pathognomonic.

APPEARANCES

With time and/or further exposure the nodular fibrosis may become progressive and more widespread and diffuse pulmonary fibrosis results. Even so, asbestosis affects predominantly the lower lobes and silicosis the upper. Entrapped bronchi dilate and cystic spaces form giving the lung an appearance described as *honeycomb lung*. Pleural adhesions develop sometimes in conjunction with effusions, and the patient with asbestosis may also have dense fibrous thickening of the parietal pleura, either in a uniform pattern or as scattered plaques.

Complications

Cor pulmonale, pulmonary tuberculosis and neoplasia all appear especially among the small groups of patients with the progressive forms of the disease. Cor pulmonale is common to all pneumoconioses but tuberculosis, in contrast, is seen only with silicosis and neoplasia only with asbestosis. There is no adequate explanation for this predilection but the upper lobe distribution of silicosis may influence the development of tuberculosis. Tumours related to asbestosis are carcinoma of the lung and mesothelioma of the pleura and peritoneum. Claims that some carcinomas of the gastrointestinal tract, including the stomach, and some leukaemias and myelomas are also associated are disputed.

A common misconception is that miners with coal dust pneumoconiosis have a higher incidence of pulmonary tuberculosis and lung cancer. The high incidence of these two disorders relates to their social group and cigarette consumption but not to their exposure to coal dust. Fibrotic nodules (*Caplan's nodule*) which are clinically distinct from those of coal dust pneumoconiosis appear in the lungs of some coal miners who also suffer from or subsequently develop rheumatoid arthritis. Focal emphysema and silicosis are other findings.

Circulatory disorders

Pulmonary oedema

This is a common finding at autopsy and a clinical complication to a wide spectrum of organ specific and systemic disorders. The interstitial fluid content of the lungs is increased beyond the normal 40% and oxygen exchange interfered with. The condition can develop either acutely, most dramatically so with myocardial infarction, or insidiously, and may then be associated with pleural effusions.

Mechanisms

The normal lung is protected against oedema by the counterbalancing of capillary hydrostatic pressure and plasma oncotic pressure which partly depend on the capillary wall and its integrity. Pulmonary capillary hydrostatic pressure is considerably lower than that in systemic capillaries and is greater in the lower regions of the lungs than the upper zones. Should this pressure increase, the intercellular pores of the endothelial cells and their intercellular junctions will be stretched and an easier pathway for fluid into the interstitial regions will be produced. The normal negative pressure of the interstitial tissues encourages fluid to flow in the same direction. Opposing these forces is the plasma oncotic pressure which is approximately three times that of the capillary hydrostatic pressure, and the flow of fluid and large protein molecules from the interstitial tissues via the lymphatics.

Pulmonary oedema involves damage to the capillary walls, increases in hydrostatic and interstitial tissue pressures, decreases in plasma oncotic pressure and impairment of lymphatic drainage (Fig. 4.26).

1 Capillary wall damage can be mediated by anoxia and an extremely wide range of gases, including oxygen, drugs and micro-organisms, each producing damage directly or via immune processes. Injury to endothelial cells increases the permeability of the vessel wall and releases plasma proteins into the interstitial tissues.

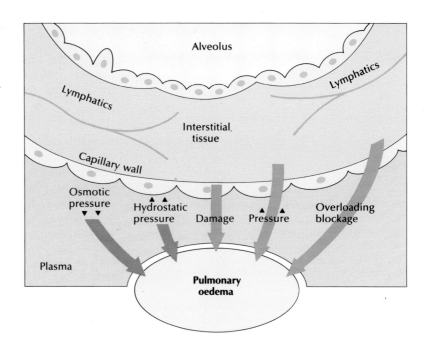

Fig. 4.26 Pulmonary oedema.

2 Any increase in hydrostatic pressure must be considerable and its effects will be greater in the lower than the upper zones, which is consistent with the frequency of oedema in these regions. Raised left atrial pressure is a key factor but an increase in pulmonary blood flow at the expense of the systemic may also be involved.

3 Increased interstitial tissue pressure is initially compensated for by an increase in lymphatic flow but once the pressure reaches zero this is insufficient and interstitial oedema follows. The resulting accumulation of protein in these regions will further increase interstitial pressure and may be the factor precipitating oedema fluid into the alveoli directly or as reflux from the terminal bronchioles.

4 Protein loss from any cause including haemodilution lowers the plasma oncotic pressure and any damage to the vessel walls exacerbates this effect. Nevertheless, if the capillary hydrostatic pressure is normal, a considerable leakage of proteins is necessary before the oncotic pressure results in pulmonary oedema.

5 Lymphatic obstruction *per se* must be widespread to produce pulmonary oedema because of the many existing anastomotic channels.

These mechanisms do not apply to all examples of pulmonary oedema. The oedema associated with intracranial disorders (*neurogenic oedema*) probably follows from a sudden rise in pulmonary capillary pressure associated with a redistribution of blood from the systemic to the pulmonary circulation. The stimulus for this may be hypothalamic and may be mediated by the sympathetic nervous system.

Oedema fluid initially collects around vessels, lymphatics and terminal bronchioles with spread later to the septal regions. As much as 500 ml fluid can be accommodated in this manner but eventually a breaking point is reached and fluid literally floods into

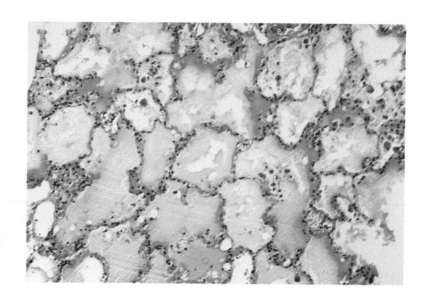

Fig. 4.27 Oedema fluid filling the air sacs. The patient had developed left ventricular failure from an acute myocardial infarct.

the alveoli (Fig. 4.27). Both the localization and alveolar flooding have no satisfactory explanation. The protein content of the fluid may impair the patient's recovery since this is only slowly cleared and if fibrinogen is present organization with fibrosis can follow.

APPEARANCES

The lungs are heavy and moist both on their pleural surfaces and within their parenchyma (Fig. 4.28). The oedema may be seen as frothy, sometimes bloodstained, fluid in the bronchial tree or flowing either naturally or following slight compression from the cut surfaces. It is also seen in the lymphatics which are conspicuous on the pleural surfaces. Such lungs hold their shape and are congested with changes often most marked in the lower lobes.

Pleural effusion

Pleural effusion is detectable fluid within one or both pleural cavities. It often accompanies cardiac failure but may also indicate pulmonary infection, malignancy (principally metastatic) and infarction as well as other conditions outside the lungs. Examination of the fluid for blood, micro-organisms and malignant cells can help to distinguish the cause.

Production

Despite the common association with cardiac failure the condition is not due to direct spread of oedema from the lungs into the pleural cavities but to an increase in systemic venous pressure and transudation through the parietal pleura. In normal circumstances fluid enters the pleural cavities and is then driven into the visceral pleural veins, and in turn the pulmonary veins, by the drop in

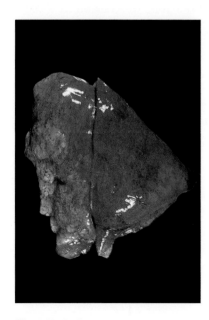

Fig. 4.28 Oedematous lung. The moistness of the surface is apparent. The lung has not been artificially inflated but holds its shape because of the fluid content. Fluid poured from the cut surfaces.

pressure gradient between the systemic and pulmonary circulations. Any protein and cells are removed by the lymphatics which drain from the parietal pleura to the mediastinal lymph nodes and from the visceral pleura to the hilar lymph nodes. Widespread obstruction to these lymphatics associated with a rise in systemic venous pressure or tumour will contribute to an effusion, as will damage to the capillary walls in the parietal pleura by increasing their permeability. Such damage may follow from increased hydrostatic pressure or inflammation.

APPEARANCES

The effusion fluid is clear and golden yellow. If there is an excessive amount of protein and fibrin, white clots form and any infection makes the fluid murky.

Pulmonary embolism and pulmonary infarction

These two conditions are intimately related although pulmonary embolism often occurs without pulmonary infarction. The most common source of pulmonary embolus is thrombus in the pelvic and calf veins but other forms (Table 4.1) are also recognized. Refined methods of investigation show that both pulmonary embolism and underlying venous thrombosis are grossly underdiagnosed and hence, in many patients, are symptomless. Lung involvement can be as pulmonary infarction and, much less commonly, as pulmonary hypertension. Pulmonary embolus, in addition, is a cause of sudden death.

Mechanisms

Venous thrombosis follows from an initial change in (a) the vessel wall, (b) the clotting mechanism and (c) the blood flow (*Virchow's triad*) which can be initiated by abdominal and pelvic surgery, immobility, cardiac infarction and failure, cancer, pregnancy, obesity and some drugs. A common denominator is often a patient of

Table 4.1 Examples of pulmonary emboli

Type	Source
Blood	Venous thrombosis
Tumour	Primary tumour
Fat/bone marrow	Long-bone, rib fractures
Amniotic fluid	Placental bed after separation
Air	Head/neck surgery; i.v. fluids; syringe-induced abortion
Foreign bodies	i.v. drug users (cotton wool fibres) i.v. medication (catheter fragments)
Parasites	Ruptured hydatid cyst; schistosomiasis

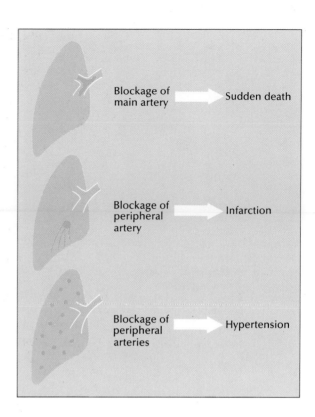

Fig. 4.29 Consequences of pulmonary embolism.

50 years or more, although no age group is exempt. Once formed the thrombus propagates along the direction of flow in the vein and may become either totally detached or parts may break off at intervals to form emboli. Iliac or femoral thrombus usually becomes totally detached, producing a large embolus, while thrombus in the deep calf veins often fragments precipitating multiple small emboli. Once emboli reach the lung one of three courses can ensue (Fig. 4.29).

1 *Massive pulmonary embolus*

A main pulmonary artery is occluded causing obstruction to over two-thirds of the pulmonary vasculature and sudden death (Fig. 4.30). Lesser degrees of vascular involvement can also cause death if there is pre-existing lung or heart disease. The obstruction of the pulmonary blood flow drops the cardiac output precipitously, the right ventricle dilating and ultimately failing. Simultaneously a reflex sympathetic response causes compensatory vasoconstriction and dramatic increase of blood flow through any uninvolved lung but, since most of the lung tissue is underperfused, the body tissues rapidly become anoxic. Inexplicably a very small number of patients survive without immediate surgical intervention, possibly because of shrinkage and fragmentation of the embolus.

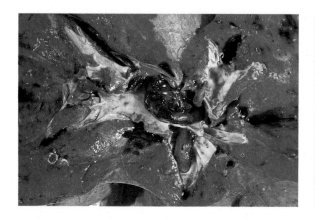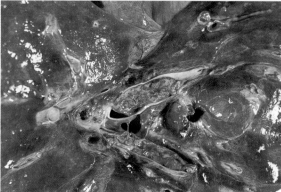

Fig. 4.30 Massive pulmonary embolus; (*above left*) very recent; the patient died suddenly; (*above right*) older in a patient who suddenly became breathless a few days prior to death.

APPEARANCES

A coiled embolus blocks either the pulmonary trunk or both main pulmonary arteries. No source for the embolus may be found but its diameter mirrors that of the iliac vessels. Neither lung is infarcted and there is no collapse. The right ventricle is dilated and sub-endocardial haemorrhage is apparent in the interventricular septum facing the right ventricular cavity.

2 *Pulmonary infarction*

This occurs if emboli reach beyond the main pulmonary arteries and become lodged in the peripheral bronchial divisions and if there are abnormalities of either the pulmonary circulation or the lung tissue. The normal lung receives a dual blood supply which includes potential anastomotic channels between the two systems as well as within each system, and which supplies oxygen in addition to that derived from the alveoli. These mechanisms effectively protect the lung from infarction and explain the frequent finding of pulmonary emboli without infarction.

Experimentally, pulmonary infarction is only produced if there is impairment to both the pulmonary venous drainage and the bronchial arterial supply. Tissue anoxia is increased by venous obstruction and any compensatory dilatation of the bronchial arteries is lessened by inherent disease or cardiac failure. The size of the region deprived of its arterial supply is also important and must be too large for direct seepage of blood from adjacent normal areas to occur and maintain tissue oxygenation. The high incidence of infarction in the lung bases where congestion is greatest supports some of these laboratory observations, as does the association with heart failure, hypotension and pre-existing lung disease, although the exact sequence of changes is disputed.

APPEARANCES

The infarct classically has a rhomboid shape with an occluded vessel (Fig. 4.31) at the apex and the base formed by the visceral

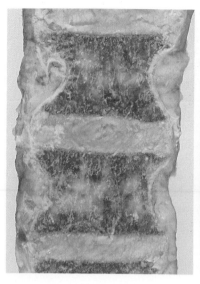 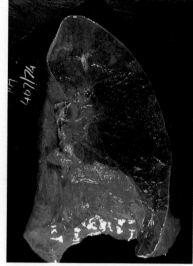 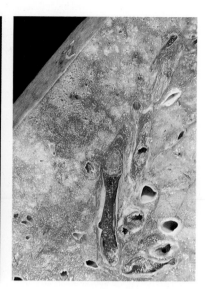

Fig. 4.31 Pulmonary infarction *Tsp 13.21*. following a pulmonary embolus. (*Above left*) Pleural appearances. The pleura is thickened and darker. (*Centre*) Parenchymal appearance from a large embolus; (*above right*) parenchymal appearance with a small peripheral embolus.

pleura. There is fibrinous pleurisy often accompanied by a blood-stained effusion and the region is firm, standing out from the surrounding tissue in the early stages and dark red. The colour is unusual since most infarcts are pale and is due to the leakage of red cells into the air sacs. The red cells can then enter the bronchial tree and give rise clinically to haemoptysis.

Complications. Most small peripheral infarcts undergo resolution but a few may leave a small fibrous scar. This is more likely with large infarcts which can also be the site of infection and abscesses encouraged by necrosis in their centres.

3 Pulmonary hypertension

This represents the most unusual complication of pulmonary embolism and arises from repeated episodes of embolism, perhaps over several years. Nevertheless, repeated showers of emboli can occur without the development of hypertension. The emboli are small, and impact in small arteries with subsequent organization, thickening of the vessel wall and loss of elasticity as well as providing a focus for thrombus formation and arteriosclerosis. Progressive involvement increases the vascular resistance and precipitates right-sided cardiac failure.

The invariable absence of a source for pulmonary emboli has led to suggestions that there is a local defect in the normal fibrinolytic system of the lung or that the initial injury is pharmacologically mediated and associated with vasoconstriction.

APPEARANCES

Thick-walled blood vessels, thrombo-embolism and arteriosclerosis are conspicuous in all parts of the lung parenchyma.

Pulmonary hypertension

An increase in pulmonary blood pressure above the normal 22/10 mm Hg represents hypertension but this is significant only if it is sustained when death from right-sided cardiac failure can follow. Transient increases in pressure occur with exercise and pregnancy as well as during fevers and with some diseases of the lungs and other organs. The conditions producing chronic pulmonary hypertension involve primary disorders of either the heart, the lungs or both and a convenient, although not all-embracing, classification recognizes passive congestion of the lungs, increased blood flow through the lungs and obstructive lesions within the pulmonary vasculature as the most common underlying mechanisms (Table 4.2).

Mechanisms

The important factor, whatever the cause, is the slow progression of the disorder which allows the pulmonary vasculature to accommodate. Nevertheless, pulmonary hypertension, as seen with some congenital heart disorders, can manifest itself early in the life of a child. Once the compensatory reactions of the lung's vasculature are overstretched, changes appear with the end effect of a fairly rigid, inelastic vasculature and a much reduced cross-sectional area. The role of spasm and the release of vasoconstrictor substances, although attractive in the early phases, remains unproven.

APPEARANCES

Grossly, the lumen of vessels is narrowed and the vasculature prominent and rigid. When hypertension is associated with congestion these features are confined to the lower lobes but with other causes distribution is more uniform. There is arteriosclerosis in the main pulmonary arteries and more significantly their smaller branches. The heart has a hypertrophied right ventricle, an association known as cor pulmonale.

Table 4.2 Mechanisms involved in pulmonary hypertension

Passive congestion (left atrial hypertension)	Mitral stenosis Chronic left ventricular failure Left atrial myxoma
Increased blood flow	Large left-to-right shunts e.g., ventral septal defects
Arterial obstruction	Chronic lung diseases Thromboembolic disease
Other	Kyphoscoliosis Chronic hypoxia from living at high altitude or chronic lung disease Cirrhosis

Lesions within the pulmonary vessels can only be fully appreciated microscopically where they affect the muscular branches and include intimal thickening by either cellular proliferation or fibrosis and medial hypertrophy. These both produce some luminal narrowing which is masked initially by generalized, and later by localized, dilatation. Complex plexiform lesions involving endothelial cells and platelet−fibrin deposits can then develop and when there is sudden severe hypertension fibrinoid necrosis is an end result. These lesions all overlap but not all appear in all examples of pulmonary hypertension and none is uniformly distributed, either within affected vessels or throughout the lung.

Vessels in pulmonary hypertension associated with congenital heart disease are graded such that Grade 1 includes only medial hypertrophy and Grade 6 the entire range of changes. Use of this system has demonstrated that early lesions, whatever the cause, are reversible and hence at this time the disease is curable if the cause can be corrected.

Cor pulmonale

This is defined as hypertrophy of the right ventricle arising from disease affecting the function and/or the structure of the lungs except where the pulmonary changes arise from disease primarily affecting the left side of the heart (WHO 1961). Increase in size in the right ventricle has no precise correlation with the duration of pulmonary disorder or the degree of associated hypertension and anoxia but the end result is right-sided cardiac failure.

Recognition rests on accurate assessment of the size of the right ventricle and of the associated pulmonary disorder. Virtually any diffuse lung condition involving either the parenchyma and/or the vasculature may be present as well as structural deformities to the thoracic cage and disorders of the control of respiration, of which the most common is cerebrovascular disease. The lung disorder causes pulmonary hypertension which if sustained produces compensatory right-sided cardiac hypertrophy and, if unrelieved, right-sided cardiac failure.

Lung tumours

Carcinoma

Lung cancer is the major cause of death from cancer in the Western Hemisphere and has relentlessly increased in incidence since the last World War. Both the high mortality and increasing incidence are particularly apparent within the UK where, as in other countries, males are mainly affected. Approximately 40% of all male cancer deaths in England and Wales are from lung cancer. The tumour is directly related to the number of cigarettes smoked but surprisingly the risk decreases if the habit is dropped for several years. The disease is therefore largely preventable. Nevertheless, industrial and occupational factors are involved as well as environmental

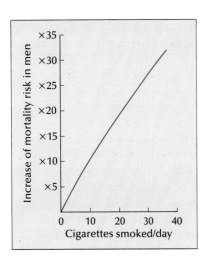

Fig. 4.32 Cigarette smoking and lung cancer mortality. Adapted from *Smoking and health now: a report of the Royal College of Physicians* (1971).

pollution, particularly within large cities. Experimentally, efforts to identify the cause of lung cancer, including those centring around cigarette smoke, have failed to produce tumours exactly identical with those in man.

Cigarette smoking and lung cancer

The relationship is based upon the following observations:
1 A linear relationship exists between the number of cigarettes smoked and the mortality risk from lung cancer (Fig. 4.32).
2 Variations in cigarette smoking that either increase the amount of smoke or its duration in the respiratory tract also increase the risk of cancer. These include smoking from an early age, inhalation of smoke, keeping the cigarette in the mouth between puffs, a large number of puffs, smoking to the butt, not using a filter and relighting extinguished cigarettes.
3 The cigarette smoking/lung cancer relationship has been substantiated in retrospective and, more importantly, in prospective studies in all continents and many countries.
4 If cigarette smoking is stopped the mortality risk declines and, after abstinence for 10 years, becomes equivalent to that for non-smokers.
5 Lung cancer patients have an increased incidence of other cigarette smoking related conditions such as chronic bronchitis and ischaemic heart disease, as well as the bronchial epithelial changes found in smokers with no lung cancer.
6 The rising incidence of lung cancer in women correlates with their increased cigarette smoking and the decline amongst men, particularly in the higher social groups, with men dropping the habit.

Although similar observations apply to pipe and cigar smoking the risk of cancer is less. The common factor is the smoke and its products which include polycyclic aromatic hydrocarbons which are *tumour initiators*, (substances capable of starting a malignant process) and phenols and fatty acids, *tumour promoters*, (substances able to complete but not initiate carcinogenesis). These products produce skin cancers experimentally but the amounts necessary are in marked excess of those experienced by the cigarette smoker and the skin tumours are histologically, unlike human lung cancers. Direct evidence between cigarette smoke and lung cancer is therefore lacking. Only one in eight heavy smokers in fact develop lung cancer. It is suggested that these patients have an inherited tendency to develop lung cancer which smoking unmasks. Supporting evidence includes the similarity of the physical and mental make-up of the patients and the occurrence of the disease amongst family members and twins.

Occupational factors and lung cancer

Exposure to some dusts and chemicals which are often contaminated by radiation carries a risk. Among these are uranium, chromate, arsenic, nickel and haematite as well as coal gas, tar and asbestos. Cigarette smoking may have a synergistic effect in these patients.

Atmospheric pollution and lung cancer

Any relationship is unclear but lung cancer is more common in all large cities than in rural areas. Within cities there is both industrial and vehicle exhaust pollution producing carcinogenic promoters and initiators as well as traces of radioactive substances.

Diagnosis

This is made from tissues obtained by transbronchial and pleural biopsy, autopsy examination and cytological examination of sputum or bronchial brushings.

There are a number of lung cancers but a few common patterns, all including a heterogeneity of cells but with one type predominating. The common patterns are:

1 Squamous cell carcinoma which forms approximately half of all lung cancers and is that particularly associated with cigarette smoking. Squamous metaplasia and dysplastic changes (Fig. 4.33) like those in some chronic bronchitis and cigarette smokers infer that these conditions precede the carcinoma.

2 Oat-cell or small anaplastic cell carcinomas (Fig. 4.34) include cytoplasmic dense core granules at electron microscopy associated with polypeptide secretion and ectopic hormone production. They arise from similar cells within the bronchial epithelium.

3 Adenocarcinomas (Fig. 4.35) may arise from the bronchial mucous glands and cause confusion with metastatic tumour, notably from the gastrointestinal tract. They are also difficult to distinguish from primary tumours of the alveolar and bronchiolar epithelium

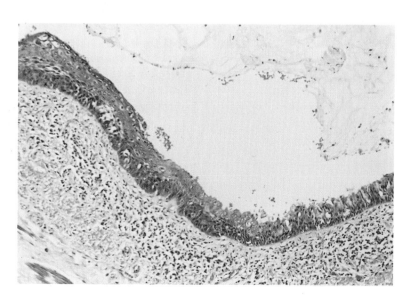

Fig. 4.33 Bronchial epithelium with a spectrum of changes from normal (on the right side), through squamous metaplasia to dysplastic (on the left side). The patient was a heavy smoker.

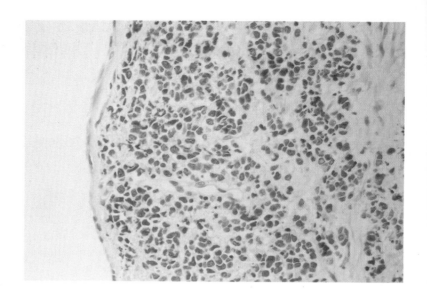

Fig. 4.34 Oat-cell or small anaplastic cell carcinoma of the lung.

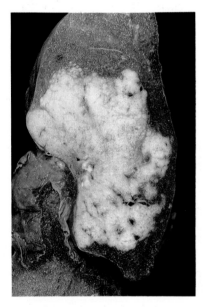

Fig. 4.35 Lung carcinoma. The histology was that of an adenocarcinoma. The appearances infer an origin from the hilum and hence a primary lung tumour.

which are seen more often in women and may then relate to cigarette smoking.

4 Large cell anaplastic carcinomas.

APPEARANCES

Grey-white tumour surrounds a bronchus which is usually at the hilum of the lung (Fig. 4.36). The right lung is involved more than the left and the upper lobe bronchi more than the lower. The carcinoma may vary in size from a small warty excrescence to a massive tumour when necrosis and haemorrhage are common features, and spread into the lungs and along the involved bronchus almost invariable. The affected bronchus is frequently obstructed and the distal lung collapsed with bronchiectatic changes and foci of pneumonia. Primary lung tumours do occur away from the hilum, some associated with scars and long-standing cavities (Fig. 4.37) but such tumours must, even though single, be considered as metastatic until proved otherwise. Failure to find an alternative primary lesion or the histological appearances provide the clues to a primary origin.

Spread

This is directly into the lung, mediastinum and pericardium. Blood-borne metastases go especially to the liver, adrenals, brain and skeleton and lymphatic metastases to lymph nodes, mainly those at the hilum. With extensive lymphatic permeation, the lymphatics in the pleura and the parenchyma are conspicuous, a condition known as *lymphangitis carcinomatosis*. In these circumstances and after direct infiltration of the lung and pleura there may be a bloodstained pleural effusion containing malignant cells.

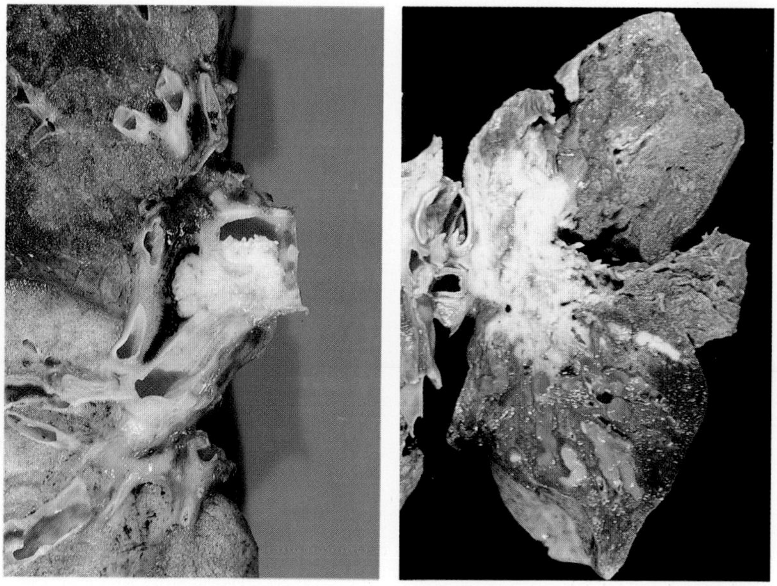

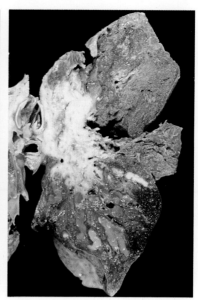

Fig. 4.36 Lung carcinoma. (*Above left*) Small tumour involving the main bronchus. The lower part of the involved lobe shows grey consolidation reflecting obstruction and infection; (*above right*) a large tumour infiltrating into the lung parenchyma and producing bronchiectasis in the lower lobe. The dilated bronchi are filled with mucus.

Systemic effects

Lung cancer more than any other is associated with systemic effects unrelated to the presence of metastases (Table 4.3). Most of these are not unique to lung cancer and their frequency with lung cancer mirrors the common occurrence of this tumour. Some are the result of ectopic hormone production but the majority are largely unexplained. Those due to ectopic hormones are not confined to the oat-cell pattern.

Mesothelioma

This affects the pleura and is related to exposure to asbestos, particularly the crocidolite type. However, the tumour is not confined to those workers such as laggers who are immediately exposed to the fibres, but may also affect those more distantly involved such as relatives or secretaries within the contaminated regions. A long

Fig. 4.37 Lung carcinoma associated with a cavity. *Ignore*

Table 4.3 Systemic effects of lung cancer

Weight loss (6.4 kg)
Clubbing; hypertrophic osteoarthropathy
Neuromyopathies including myasthenia gravis and cerebellar degeneration
Psychotic disturbances
Migrating thrombophlebitis; marantic thrombi
Anaemia; polycythemia; red cell aplasia
Ectopic hormone production: ACTH, ADH, parathormone, calcitonin, prolactin, HCG and serotonin (carcinoid syndrome)
Non-metastatic hypercalcaemia
Scleroderma; acanthosis nigracans

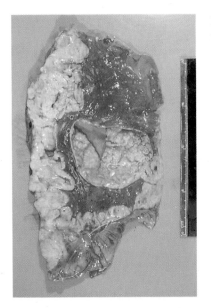

Fig. 4.38 Mesothelioma of the pleura. Inevitably, because of its origin, the tumour encases the lung.

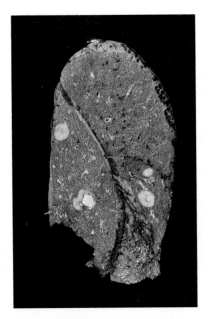

Fig. 4.39 Metastatic osteosarcoma. There are several round and discrete nodules of tumour, each of comparable size.

latent period of up to even 40 years separates exposure and the recognition of mesothelioma. The combination of indirect exposure, the widespread use of asbestos during the preceding decades, the prolonged latent period and an increasing incidence of mesothelioma are causes for anxiety that there will be an explosive epidemic of this tumour.

APPEARANCES

The tumour develops from mesothelial cells and most frequently arises from either the pleura or the peritoneum. Spread along the parietal and visceral pleura replaces this with tough white tissue which will eventualy completely encompass the lung (Fig. 4.38). Although one lung is generally affected bilateral involvement is seen and in the underlying lung there is not necessarily any evidence of asbestosis. The pericardium can be similarly replaced, encapsulating and restricting the heart, and infiltration through the diaphragm also occurs.

Death from the 'frozen' chest contents usually results before metastatic spread but blood-borne metastases, notably to the liver, brain and lung, occur occasionally.

Miscellaneous tumours

Secondary tumours

Metastatic tumour is probably the most common malignancy found within the chest by the general physician and surgeon. Tumours reach the lungs via the blood and their immense vascularity presumably plays some role in ensuring that some malignant cells then settle and proliferate.

The feature distinguishing metastatic tumour from primary lung cancer is the multiplicity of most metastatic tumours.

The deposits appear in two distinct patterns although mixed varieties also occur: (a) multiple, round, white nodules of several centimetres diameter scattered throughout the lung parenchyma and referred to as cannon ball secondaries (Fig. 4.39); (b) diffuse small deposits are found within the parenchyma which are more easily appreciated by touch or the gritty sensation experienced when they are cut into.

Other tumours

There is an extremely wide range of benign and other malignant tumours including those developing from the bronchial epithelium, the connective tissue, especially nerve, and the pulmonary lymphoid tissue. Some of these tumours straddle the line between benign and malignant but few of them produce symptoms or signs diagnostic of their origin or likely behaviour.

Further reading

Dunnill, M.S. (1987). *Pulmonary Pathology* (2nd Edition). Churchill Livingstone: London and New York.

Harris, P. and Heath, D. (1977). *The Human Pulmonary Circulation* (2nd Edition). Churchill Livingstone: London and New York.

Hasleton, P.S. (1983). Adult respiratory distress syndrome — a review. *Histopathology* 7, 307–32.

Lancet (1988). What causes oedema? *Lancet* i, 1028–30.

Scadding, J.G., Cumming, G. and Thurlbeck, W.M. (1981). *Scientific Foundations of Respiratory Medicine*. William Heinmann Medical Books Ltd: London.

Spencer, H. (1985) *Pathology of the Lung* (4th Edition). Pergamon Press: Oxford and New York.

5 Alimentary tract

Peptic ulceration and gastritis

Malabsorption
Coeliac disease

Inflammatory bowel disease
Microbial infection
Idiopathic inflammation

Diverticular disease

Miscellaneous conditions related to systemic disorders
Vascular disease
Radiation
Immunodeficiency

Tumours
At risk groups
Malignant precursors
Epidemiology
Non-epithelial tumours

Tumour appearances
Benign tumours
Malignant tumours

Symptoms referable to the alimentary tract are the most common reason for patients of all ages presenting to doctors. Many symptoms, even without investigative procedures, are often clearly related to disease elsewhere and some may never be associated with organic disease. Those arising from the gastrointestinal tract are often not diagnostic of a particular disorder although it is sometimes possible to distinguish between disease of the *upper gastrointestinal tract* (oesophagus, stomach and small intestine) and that of the *lower gastrointestinal tract* (appendix, caecum, colon and rectum). Upper tract disease can result in the vomiting of fresh blood (haematemesis) or passing altered blood per rectum (melaena, Fig. 5.1) while the passage of fresh blood implicates lower gastrointestinal tract disorders. Indigestion or abdominal pain and many other symptoms are even less specific, which is why gastroenterologists place considerable reliance upon investigative procedures for diagnosis. The ease with which endoscopy of all parts of the gastrointestinal tract can be performed makes this an especially attractive tool: gross appearances are visible and biopsy is possible. Endoscopy and biopsy now largely replace the former dependance upon X-ray changes and analysis of gut secretions and products but may, in their turn, be superseded by measurements of gut polypeptides. These hormones are numerous (Table 5.1) and form part of a complex system encompassing the gastrointestinal tract, pancreas and

Table 5.1 Hormones in gastrointestinal tract

Cholecystokin (CCK)	Duodenum; jejunum
Gastric inhibiting polypeptide (GP)	Duodenum; jejunum
Gastrin	Stomach; duodenum
Glucagon	Small and large intestine
Motilin	Duodenum; jejunum
Neurotensin	Stomach
ACTH-like peptide	Stomach
Somatostatin	Stomach; duodenum; jejunum
Secretin	Duodenum; jejunum
Substance P	Small intestine
Serotonin	Stomach; small and large bowel
Vasoactive intestinal polypeptide (VIP)	Stomach; duodenum
Pancreatic polypeptide	Duodenum
Encephalin	Stomach; duodenum
Thyrotropin releasing hormone	Small intestine
Bombesin	Small and large intestine

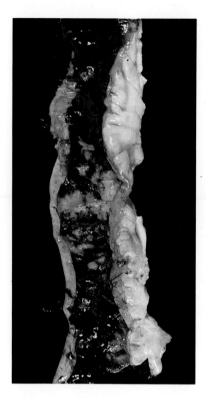

Fig. 5.1 Altered blood filling the colon and associated with bleeding oesophageal varices.

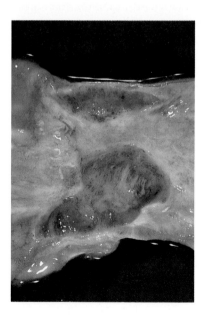

Fig. 5.2 Benign chronic ulceration of the lower third of the oesophagus following gastric reflux. The ulcer is shallow and the walls sloping to the floor.

brain. They affect the normal functions of the gastrointestinal tract and are altered in disease processes either as a primary phenomenon or as a secondary response.

Normal function

The alimentary tract provides access to the body for food and water. These, like all ingested materials, are processed, then part or wholly absorbed and any waste and unwanted products excreted. The bowel is adapted for these functions by:

1   Varied secretions occurring at different levels.
2   A constant high epithelial cell turnover and potential for repair.
3   The motility and blood supply.
4   The large surface area contributed to by the length and folding of the mucosa.
5   The substantial lymphoid population and traffic within the mucosa.

Many of these properties also protect the body from the entry of noxious substances including ingested antigens and microorganisms. They can also be affected by local or systemic disease with any subsequent changes causing further alimentary tract disorders.

Peptic ulceration and gastritis

These are closely allied inflammatory conditions, often unsuspected and not always the basis of the patient's complaints. Their diagnosis rests largely upon histological findings. Peptic ulceration cannot always be distinguished from malignant ulceration without biopsy. Gastritis can be evident histologically but not appreciated endoscopically although acute erosions, a variable part of gastritis, will be seen. Peptic ulceration also occurs within the ectopic gastric mucosa found in Meckel's diverticulum, in the jejunum as part of the Zollinger—Ellison syndrome and in the lower third of the oesophagus if there is gastric reflux (Fig. 5.2) or hiatus hernia. The *Zollinger—Ellison syndrome* involves severe, often multiple, ulceration of the upper tract, hypersecretion of gastric acid and a pancreatic endocrine tumour.

Causes

These are unknown although in both conditions there are well recognized precipitating factors, some of which are shared but all of which are experienced without ulceration or gastritis (Table 5.2).

1   Changes in the normal defence mechanisms of the stomach may be important. These maintain a delicate balance between destruction of the mucosa and its preservation. Hydrochloric acid of the gastric juice, formed by the parietal cells, and pepsin from the oxyntic cells are factors that promote mucosal destruction whilst mucus and bicarbonate secretion counterbalance these. Mucus forms a physical barrier and also acts as a buffer. This action is facilitated by its constant replacement which in turn depends upon the integrity

Table 5.2 Factors associated with peptic ulceration and gastritis

	Ulcer	Gastritis
Common factors		
Cigarette smoking	√	√
Coffee	√	√
Alcohol	√	√
Aspirin		√
Blood group	O	A
Uncommon factors		
Irradiation		√
Chronic obstructive airways disease	√	
Chronic renal failure	√	√
Gastrin-secreting tumour	√	
Cirrhosis	√	√
Burns, shock, head injury		√

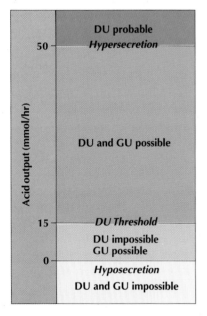

Fig. 5.3 Gastric acidity and ulceration (DU = duodenal ulcer, GU = gastric ulcer).

and reduplication potential of the mucosa. The buffering is also contributed to by the bicarbonate secreted from the fundal and pyloric glands. Alcohol inhibits the synthesis and secretion of mucus and is hence invariably associated with gastritis.

2 Increasing acidity correlates well with the potential for ulcers developing (Fig. 5.3).

3 Excess gastrin secretion. This hormone stimulates hydrochloric acid release and is inhibited when the antral mucosa is exposed to a low pH. Both the absence of ulceration with achlorhydria and the increased incidence with excessive gastrin secretion, as in the Zollinger–Ellison syndrome, are in keeping with these observations.

4 Other factors in some patients include changes in patterns of gastric emptying and reflux of duodenal juices. Gastritis is almost invariable following a partial gastrectomy or gastrojejunostomy and duodenal reflux is demonstrable in many patients with gastric ulcers.

5 The presence of end arteries and stretching of the mucosa over the muscle folds, particularly within the antral regions, may help to localize the disorder.

None of these explanations accounts for acute and chronic patterns, the potential for spontaneous healing, the circulating parietal cell antibodies found with some forms of gastritis or the localization of ulceration or gastritis. Ulcers can occur in any part of the stomach but most are confined to the antrum and along the lesser curvature, an area which naturally with age becomes lined by antral mucosa. Gastritis is also found in the antrum but in its acute forms and when advanced (gastric atrophy) the entire stomach is affected.

APPEARANCE OF PEPTIC ULCERS

Ulcers, either acute or chronic, are most often single and most are less than 2 cm diameter. Multiple ulcers occur in slightly over 5% of patients, more so with the acute than the chronic forms. In the duodenum opposing ulcers on the anterior and posterior walls are

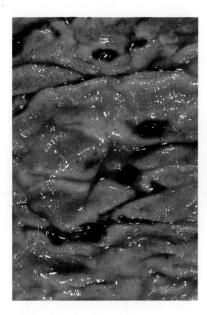

Fig. 5.4 Multiple acute ulcers in the stomach in a patient with long-standing renal failure.

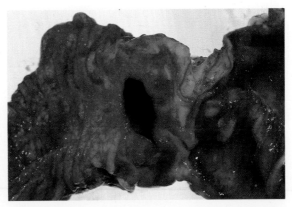

Fig. 5.5 Chronic ulcer in the first part of the duodenum. This was associated with a large haemorrhage from a vessel in the floor.

called *kissing ulcers*. Large ulcers raise the possibility of malignancy but large benign ones are seen, especially on the lesser curvature, and may deform the stomach to an hour-glass shape. Acute ulcers (Fig. 5.4) are round with reddened bases including fibropurulent material and flattened atrophic mucosa, often the site of gastritis. The edges are characteristically straight in contrast to the raised and rolled or overhanging edges of the malignant ulcer. A vessel may be seen at the base. If the ulcer is chronic there is fibrosis which deforms the shape, produces a scar and impedes re-epithelialization (Fig. 5.5).

Complications

These are bleeding, perforation, fibrosis and possibly malignant change.

Bleeding and perforation invariably lead to hospitalization and can be fatal, especially in the elderly. As a result there may be a biased view of their frequency. Haemorrhage is the more common of the two and is either chronic, producing anaemia and occurring from erosion of the granulation tissue in the ulcer bed, or is more spectacular with erosion of a vessel and acute blood loss. Perforation is usually equally dramatic, especially with acute ulcers on the anterior or free wall of the stomach or duodenum when peritonitis results. If, however, adhesions have developed between the stomach or duodenum and an adjacent viscus, perforation can be confined and an abscess form.

Fibrosis causes adhesions, scarring of the ulcer (Fig. 5.6) and, if sufficiently chronic, deformity of the organ. In the body of the stomach an hour-glass shape results while in the pyloric region, pyloric stenosis. Rarely the viscus may be deformed by adhesions and an acquired or traction diverticulum develop.

Malignancy, even in the most chronic ulcers, is surprisingly rare. It is estimated that only 1% of ulcers terminate in carcinoma. Its appearance is recognized from biopsies from the edge of the ulcer and can be missed if only the fibropurulent floor is biopsied.

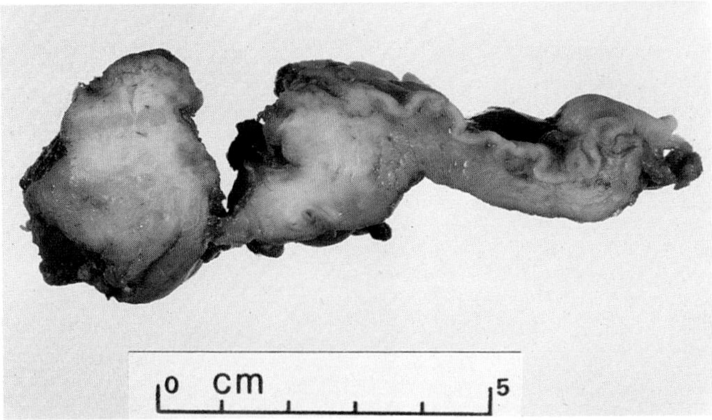

Fig. 5.6 Chronic ulcer in the antrum of the stomach. The fibrosis affects the entire thickness of the wall and contributed to the lack of healing.

APPEARANCE OF GASTRITIS

Gastritis is ultimately a histological diagnosis even if it follows infections (Table 5.3).

1   Acute forms are characterized by petechial haemorrhages, oedema and multiple small greyish erosions throughout the mucosa (Fig. 5.7). Microscopically the acute inflammatory reaction is accompanied by some epithelial necrosis and may be confined either to the superficial parts of the mucosa or extend through its full thickness. Resolution or blood and fluid loss producing shock and death may result.

2   Chronic gastritis may pass unrecognized at endoscopy. There are several histological subtypes, probably part of a single disorder and not clinically distinguishable. Chronic inflammatory cells are found in the mucosa and when there are also neutrophil polymorphs the condition is regarded as active rather than quiescent. If the changes are confined to the superficial zone of the mucosa its overall thickness is normal (Fig. 5.8) but when the deeper layer is affected the mucosa is thin. The terms chronic superficial and chronic atrophic gastritis describe these two conditions but in practice their distinction is not always clear-cut. The former can either undergo resolution or proceed to the chronic atrophic form and persist for many years. The atrophic form has to be distinguished from gastric atrophy, the final end-point, which affects the entire stomach mucosa, rather than foci, and has a less marked inflammatory cell

Table 5.3 Classification of gastritis

Type		Course	Distribution	Site
Acute haemorrhagic		Resolution Death	Focal	Entire stomach
Chronic gastritis Subtypes				
Ch superficial	active quiescent	Resolution Ch atrophic	Focal	Antrum >body
Ch atropic	active quiescent	Persists (years)	Focal	Antrum >body
Gastric atrophy		Lifelong	Diffuse	Entire stomach

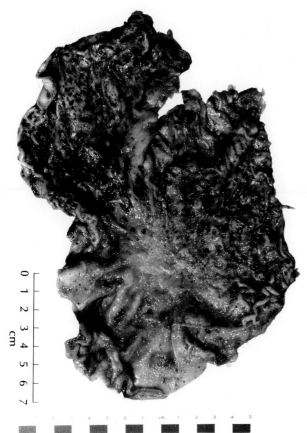

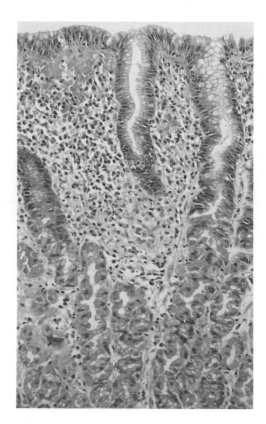

Fig. 5.8 Chronic superficial gastritis with a band of chronic inflammatory cells beneath the surface epithelium in the body of the stomach.

Fig. 5.7 Acute gastritis complicating leukaemia. Most of the stomach mucosa is involved by small erosions.

response. Gastric atrophy is related to circulating parietal cell antibodies and often pernicious anaemia and is the only form of gastritis which is a precursor of gastric carcinoma.

3 There are other histological variants in gastritis of which the most important is *intestinal metaplasia* (Fig. 5.9). In this condition foci of mucosa assume histological, histochemical and ultrastructural features of small intestinal mucosa. The change is common adjacent to peptic ulcers and seen with gastritis. It does not progress to carcinoma but may be related since 50% of gastric cancers have a histological pattern similar to small intestinal mucosa. Intestinal metaplasia is also common among high risk groups for gastric carcinoma. Other subtypes of gastritis are granulomatous, cystic, follicular and regenerative or hyperplastic and while these can occur in isolation they generally accompany the main forms.

Malabsorption

As the term implies, absorption is impaired and therefore malnutrition can be anticipated. The extent of this will reflect the cause of

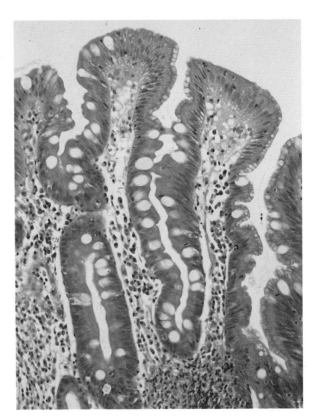

Fig. 5.9 Biopsy from the body of the stomach in which the epithelium has the features of small intestinal epithelium. The change is *intestinal metaplasia* and it contrasts with the epithelium in Fig. 5.8.

which there are many, varying in different age groups. Malnutrition can be due to disorders of the gastrointestinal tract, pancreas, biliary tract or liver and also from abnormal dietary habits. Operative procedures short-circuiting parts of the bowel as well as bowel resections are other important causes. The effects are numerous and the patient may present with a variety of complaints, some not immediately relevant to malabsorption. Investigations, including endoscopy and biopsy, may be the only means of accurately identifying the underlying cause (Table 5.4).

Coeliac disease

This persistent familial disorder of the small intestine is an important cause of malabsorption at any age. Gluten within the diet causes flattening and even loss of the villi (*villous atrophy*) recognizable endoscopically and under the dissecting microscope (Fig. 5.10). Increased numbers of T-cells within epithelium and plasma cells within the mucosa are other features (Fig. 5.11). Functional and structural changes are correctable with strict adherence to a gluten-free diet but the harmful constituent of gluten has not been identified, nor has the mechanism of injury. Since many patients have autoimmune disorders including thyroid disease and diabetes mellitus, and also small intestinal lymphoma develops, immune mechanisms have been postulated. The familial incidence and the association with HLA B8 and DRW3 support this idea as may the close association with dermatitis herpetiformis.

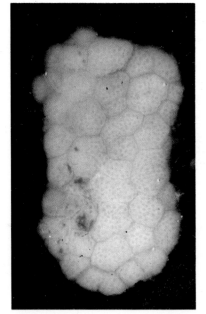

Fig. 5.10 Flattened mucosa of coeliac disease as seen under the dissecting microscope.

Table 5.4 Examples of disorders provoking malabsorption and their principal biopsy appearances

Coeliac disease	Loss/flattened villi
Tropical sprue	Loss/flattened villi
Amyloid	Intercellular deposits
Whipple's disease	Foamy cells
Hypogammaglobulinaemia	Absent plasma cells; *Giardia lamblia*
Lymphoma	Tumour cells
AIDS	Loss/flattened villi; micro-organisms
Pancreatic disease	Pancreatitis; tumour; mucoviscidosis
Liver disease	Hepatitis; obstruction, etc.

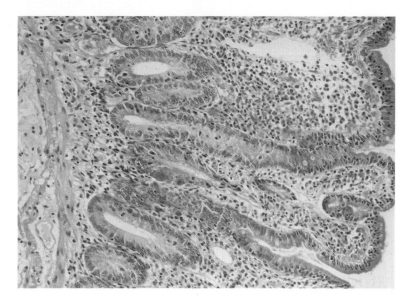

Fig. 5.11 Coeliac disease: the villi of the small intestine are short and flat. The number of lymphocytes is increased and some have infiltrated the epithelium. The crypts are large and prominent.

Dermatitis herpetiformis

This is a blistering disorder of the skin in which local IgA deposits are seen, sometimes with other immunoglobulins and complement. No specific circulating antibodies, as is the case also in coeliac disease, are recognized and, like coeliac disease, there is no clear understanding of the role of immune responses. The disorder can be controlled with gluten restriction and all patients will have some of the histological changes of coeliac disease.

Complications

The most important is malabsorption but lymphoma and, less frequently, carcinoma in the small intestine also occur. Carcinoma may also develop in the oesophagus and pharynx. A small spleen is found but this has not been associated with any specific symptomatology or laboratory finding.

Inflammatory bowel disease

This term refers to any bowel disorder with a significant inflammatory response but in practice it is confined to disorders within the small and large intestine and does not embrace oesophagitis, gastritis or appendicitis. The intestinal disorders fall into two main groups, firstly those following a variety of microbial infections, X-ray therapy and some drugs and second those for which no cause has been identified, namely Crohn's disease and ulcerative colitis. Since tissue responses in both groups are similar, distinguishing the infective disorders rests upon identifying the causative organism. This may mean stool examination and culture, often on more than one occasion, and may be aided by serology. Rarely the histopathologist may recognize organisms such as *Mycobacterium tuberculosis*, *Candida*, *Giardia* and *Amoeba*. Identifying an organism within the bowel by whatever means does not, however, mean that organism is always harmful or even the cause of the patient's symptoms. *Giardia*, *Cryptosporidiosis*, *Spirochetosis* and *Campylobacter* are all organisms whose pathogenicity is, in some patients, a matter of dispute.

Both microbial and non-microbial inflammatory bowel disorders have important local and systemic effects which can arise from temporary or permanent functional changes within the mucosa. Infection by *Vibrio cholera* produces an immediate massive outpouring of fluid faeces (rice water stools) which, if the patient survives, ceases and leaves no long-term effect. Crohn's disease, which leads to epithelial destruction and fistula formation, can result in lasting malnutrition arising from malabsorption. As part of any of these changes, alterations in the normal gut flora can arise and further embarrass the gut's function. The bacterial overgrowth can be contributed to by any form of therapy, but especially antibiotics, as well as by stagnation of bowel contents. Toxic dilatation of the gut and blind loops of bowel bypassed after fistula formation are important causes of bowel stasis. The effects on the mucosa are to alter its absorptive capacity and its immune responses, so allowing easy access of potentially harmful toxins, drugs and other materials. If there is long-standing inflammation with lasting structural changes the condition may progress to malignancy. This is seen particularly in those forms of ulcerative colitis producing little bowel disturbance and persisting for twenty years or so.

Microbial infection

Micro-organisms of all types can infect the small and large bowel. It is nevertheless possible to generalize about those most commonly found in each part and sometimes to recognize the pathogen, either directly or from the morphological changes it produces.

Viral infections

These are an exception in that the organisms are rarely identified and their histopathological effects even less often biopsied.

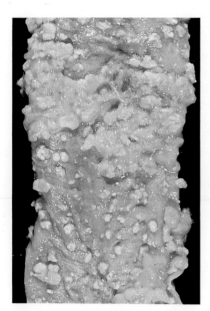

Fig. 5.12 Pseudomembranous colitis. A yellow membrane of slough partly covers the inflamed mucosa.

Bacterial infections

Most bacteria infect the small intestine. The *Salmonella* target on its lymphoid tissue, especially that in the terminal ileum, producing longitudinal raised mucosal ulcers with black sloughing necrotic bases. Septicaemia follows and locally perforation and haemorrhage may occur. *Staphylococci* are associated with necrotizing entero-colitis in neonates, when they may either cause ischaemia or become established on an ischaemic gut, a dilemma often difficult to un-ravel. Similarly post-operative infection in any age group is often the sequelae of antibiotic therapy and alteration of the normal bowel flora.

Shigella and some *Clostridia* predominantly infect the large bo-wel. *Shigella* is the main cause of bacillary dysentery in Europe and its spread is largely due to the house fly. *Clostridia* form part of the normal flora of both the small and the large intestine and are only harmful when the mucosa is damaged or ischaemic. An example, confined to the colon, is *pseudomembranous colitis* (Fig. 5.12). Focal areas of mucosa or the entire mucosa are covered by partly adherent and partly sloughing yellow mucus, the pseudomembrane, and there are inflammatory changes within the underlying mucosa, the colitis. The organism responsible is *C. difficile* and many patients will have received antibiotics.

Mycobacteria and most *Clostridia* are bacteria which exhibit no preference for either the small or the large bowel. *Mycobacteria* can be recognized either in Ziehl—Nielsen preparations or indirectly from caseating granulomas. Macroscopically there are transverse mucosal ulcers within the intestine which, if multiple, are especially suggestive. Most examples arise from swallowed bovine bacilli but a few are from open pulmonary tuberculosis. When *M. bovis* is the cause, a Ghon focus forms in the draining mesenteric lymph nodes. In Britain today such infection is uncommon, largely because of the screening of cattle and the pasteurization of milk, but also because of the improved recognition and treatment of tuberculosis. Tu-berculosis within the gastrointestinal tract is now either part of a miliary disorder or from atypical mycobacteria in patients with compromised immune responses.

Fungal and protozoal infections

Among the common fungal infections *Candida* predominates in the small intestine and *Actinomycosis* within the large intestine. A similar distribution is shared by *Giardia* and *Amoebae*. All of these organ-isms are potentially recognizable within the tissues, so providing a precise cause for the bowel inflammation.

Idiopathic inflammation

These disorders are Crohn's disease and ulcerative colitis. At one time Crohn's disease was regarded as confined to the small intestine and ulcerative colitis as a disorder of the large intestine. It is now accepted that Crohn's disease also involves the large intestine and that the division between the two is not always clear. All age groups are affected with a peak incidence at 30 years and an equal sex incidence in Crohn's disease but a slightly higher incidence among women for ulcerative colitis. Although there is a world-wide distribution, those in the Western hemisphere are most affected and Asian Jews in particular. Crohn's disease has undergone a true and inexplicable increase during the last twenty years but ulcerative colitis remains static. The symptomatology of both conditions is broadly similar with periods of remission and relapse and histo-pathology plays a role in separating the two disorders, particularly when only the colon is involved (Table 5.5). Distinguishing the conditions is important because of differences in prognosis and treatment.

Cause

The cause of both disorders is unknown. Although micro-organisms may play a part, neither condition is primarily infective since there is no clear case clustering and neither disease is transmissible. The occurrence of granulomas in Crohn's disease has stimulated nu-merous investigations for a role for mycobacteria, other bacteria and viruses but none have shown evidence that organisms produce the disease. Lysosomes, food allergy, collagen abnormalities and psychosomatic factors have also been studied but for none of them is there a clear pathogenetic role.

There is a family history in about 30% of patients with Crohn's disease. Ankylosing spondylitis, a disorder closely related to HLA B27 hepatotype, is more common than expected among these pa-tients but they are unusual in that they are not HLA B27 positive. Other vague evidence for a genetic factor is the high incidence among Asian Jews.

Research, at present, is directed towards an immune cause. Reasons for this include the clinical response to steroids and immu-nosuppressive drugs, the presence of circulating colonic epithelial antibodies and immune complexes as well as changes in the ratio of immunoglobulins (B-cell distribution) within the mucosa. How-

Table 5.5 Distinguishing features of ulcerative colitis and Crohn's disease in the large bowel

	Ulcerative colitis	Crohn's disease
Inflammation	Mucosal	Transmural
Granulomas	None	50−70%
Fissures	None	Pathognomonic
Distribution	Continuous	Segmental
Fistulae	Iatrogenic	10%
Polyps	Occur	Uncommon
Carcinoma	20X expected	3−5X expected

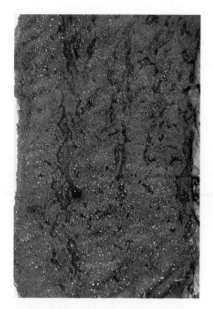

Fig. 5.13 Part of the wall of a colon with acute ulcerative colitis. There is ulceration and severe acute inflammation, shown by the hyperaemia.

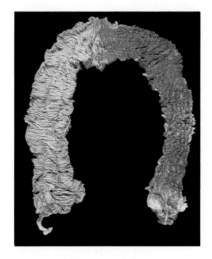

Fig. 5.14 Colectomy specimen for ulcerative colitis. There is a sharp cut-off between the acutely involved rectal, sigmoid and left colon areas and the less affected proximal part.

Fig. 5.15 Contrast between colon involvement in Crohn's disease and ulcerative colitis.

ever, none of these observations are specific and they may be secondary responses. The systemic effects of either condition, which include autoimmune disorders, particularly liver disease, are more positive reasons for an immune basis even though these are seen in only a small proportion of patients.

APPEARANCES

Ulcerative colitis

As the name implies this is an ulcerative condition (Fig. 5.13). It is associated with variable destruction of the mucosa and relative sparing of other parts of the intestinal wall. The disease starts in the rectum and spreads to the adjacent mucosa in a continuous pattern (Fig. 5.14). There is thus no normal mucosa within affected areas. The most severe changes are in the distal parts, although the rectum may seem relatively normal because of the use of topical steroids. In acute disease the inflamed bowel may be hugely dilated with a thin wall and filled with blood, mucus and loose faeces. Ulcers and polyps secondary to the inflammation and granulation tissue (*pseudo-polyps*) replace the mucosa. Following chronic disease the colon is usually shorter than normal with a very smooth mucosa. Slightly nodular areas may, on histology, reveal a dysplastic epithelium and sometimes adenocarcinoma. The tumour can be multifocal and has a bad prognosis.

Crohn's disease

In the small intestine Crohn's disease is fairly readily recognized but in the large intestine distinction from ulcerative colitis can be extremely difficult and may even be impossible (Fig. 5.15). This is

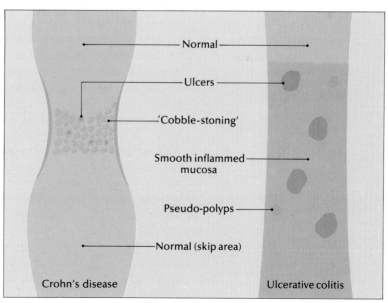

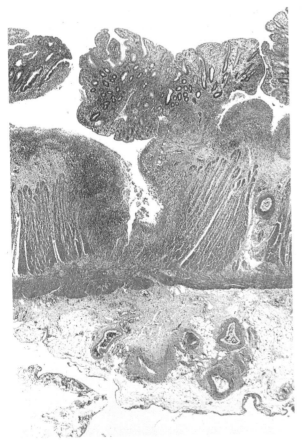 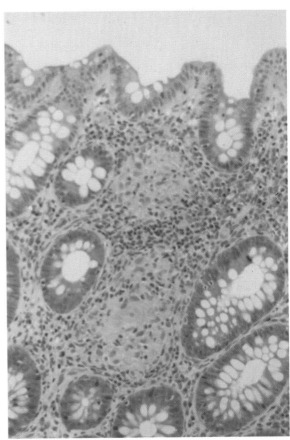

Fig. 5.16 Crohn's disease of the colon; (*above left*) transmural inflammation and fissuring and (*above right*) granulomas.

particularly so if only the morphological features are considered (Table 5.5). The disorder is not confined to the mucosa but involves the entire bowel wall. The two hallmarks are transmural inflammation and fissures spreading through the wall (Fig. 5.16). Granulomas are also seen in half to one-third of specimens. Fissures can result in fistula formation between loops of bowel and between bowel and adjacent organs including the bladder and skin. The most helpful macroscopic feature is the separation of areas of abnormal bowel by areas of normal bowel (*skip areas*) (Fig. 5.17). The abnormal areas are segmental and include thickened and shortened bowel wall with a characteristic cobble-stone pattern to the mucosa. This reflects oedema in the submucosa trapped in zones by the tissues anchoring the epithelium and is thus a feature of any condition associated with submucosal oedema. Discrete mucosal ulceration (*aphthous ulcers*) and possibly pseudo-polyps are other features. Dysplastic changes and malignancy are not common complications, although carcinoma can supervene in both the involved small and large intestine. Inflammation of other parts of the alimentary tract including the mouth and anus occurs and produces similar histological changes. Arthropathy, eye and skin disorders are important systemic complications.

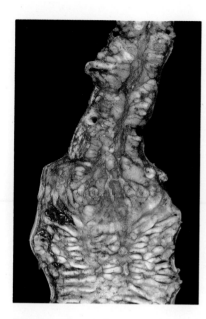

Fig. 5.17 Narrowed segment of bowel involved by Crohn's disease adjacent to a non-involved (skip) area. A cobble-stone pattern is seen in the Crohn's area.

Table 5.6 Sites of diverticula formation

Pharynx	Killion's dehiscence
Oesophagus	Below Killion's dehiscence Opposite tracheal bifurcation Supra-diaphragmatic
Stomach	Posteriorly at the cardia Secondary to ulcer and gall bladder disease
Duodenum	Intraluminal Vessel entry points Secondary to ulceration
Small intestine	Ileum — antimesenteric border (Meckel's) Jejunum — mesenteric border (multiple)
Colon	Sigmoid: between mesenteric and antimesenteric borders

Diverticular disease

Diverticula occur in various sites within the gastrointestinal tract (Table 5.6) and may be congenital or acquired. They can be further sub-divided into either true, when the diverticulum includes all layers of the gut wall, or false, when only the mucosal coat and possibly muscularis mucosa are involved (Fig. 5.18). True diverticula arise from traction on the wall outside the gut, while in false diverticula propulsion from within is the precipitating event. Either type may be single or multiple. The more diverticula, the greater the opportunity there is for inflammation, possibly involving perforation, haemorrhage and obstruction of the affected area. An important factor in these events is the size of the diverticulum and especially the circumference of its orifice. Wide-mouthed diverticula are less prone to complications since material is less likely to become entrapped. True diverticula are also exposed to fewer complications since their complete wall with an intact muscle coat can expel the contents.

The diverticula most often encountered are Meckel's diverticulum in the small intestine and multiple diverticula in the pelvic and especially sigmoid colon.

Meckel's diverticulum

This is a true diverticulum found on the antimesenteric border of the ileum and is the residue of the vitelline duct. An unusual feature is the occurrence of gastric, duodenal or colonic mucosa as well as heterotopic pancreatic tissue in the wall. Inflammation can develop as well as peptic ulceration and obstruction. The latter arises from either intussusception or persistence of a fibrous band uniting the diverticulum and the umbilicus.

Colonic diverticula

When not inflamed these are referred to as diverticulosis and when inflamed as diverticulitis or diverticular disease. The disorder

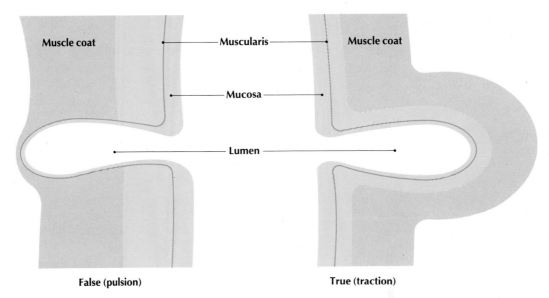

False (pulsion) True (traction)

Fig. 5.18 Types of diverticula.

increases in incidence with age, although it can occur in any age group, including children. The cause remains unknown but current ideas embrace age, vascular sites and increased intraluminal pressure. A role for either bile salts or polypeptide hormones is unsubstantiated.

1 The decline in the mechanical strength of tissues with age may be important but obviously affects the entire colon. It is not restricted to the sigmoid part where 95% of diverticular disease occurs. Senile atrophy may nonetheless underlie the few examples of diffuse disease.

2 Diverticula develop at the sites of vascular entry to the bowel (Fig. 5.19). These may be points of weakness in the circular muscle coat but if the large bowel is distended under pressure with water or air, rupture occurs through the taenia and not at these sites.

3 Intraluminal pressure increases when the bowel is active and is higher in colons with diverticular disease than in those without. The increased bulk of circular muscle in diverticulosis may underlie increased intraluminal pressure but the resting intraluminal pressures in normal and diseased bowel are similar. The muscle hypertrophy is not the result of absent ganglia, analogous to Hirschsprung's disease in children, since ganglia are present and there is also no compensatory enlargement of nerve bundles (Fig. 5.20). The muscle bulk may be to counteract the sphincter action of the rectum and it may be this that localizes the disorder.

Stool mass might influence the initiation and progression of the disorder. The disease is found predominantly in the Western hemisphere and is rare in Africa and the Orient. A major difference between these populations is in their diet, and especially the fibre content. Fibre binds water and thereby increases the stool mass. This is allied with increased transit times and increased intraluminal

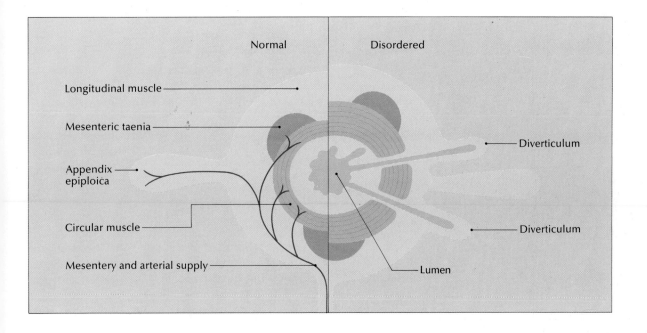

Normal

Disordered

Longitudinal muscle

Mesenteric taenia

Appendix epiploica

Circular muscle

Mesentery and arterial supply

Diverticulum

Diverticulum

Lumen

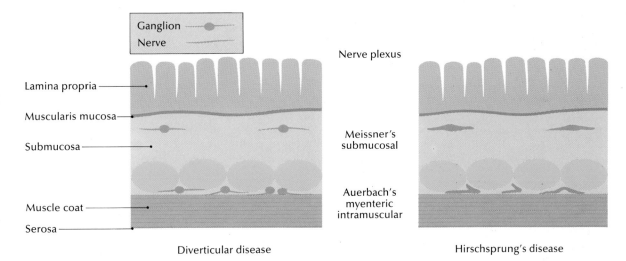

Ganglion

Nerve

Nerve plexus

Lamina propria

Muscularis mucosa

Submucosa

Meissner's submucosal

Auerbach's myenteric intramuscular

Muscle coat

Serosa

Diverticular disease

Hirschsprung's disease

Fig. 5.20 Diverticular disease and
Hirschsprung's disease.

pressures as well as lower bacterial counts than occur in controls on
low fibre diets. Such diets are consumed in the West where the
main fibre source is fruit and vegetables and most is removed by
milling flour. Similar diets produce diverticular disease in rats and
rabbits but human vegetarians eating very high fibre diets suffer
from diverticular disease. The apparent influence of fibre may be
false, since life expectancy in Africa and the Orient is shorter than
in the West and most sufferers from diverticular disease are elderly.
Diet may be more important in alleviating symptoms and lessening
complications than in the pathogenesis of the disorder.

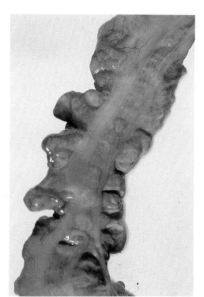

Fig. 5.21 Diverticular disease of the sigmoid colon.

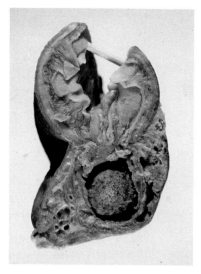

Fig. 5.22 Faecolith trapped within a diverticulum.

Diverticular disease is mostly restricted to the sigmoid colon. Two and less often three rows of diverticula are seen between the mesenteric and antimesenteric borders of a thickened segment of bowel (Fig. 5.21). This contrasts with the disorder in the small bowel where diverticula occur on the mesenteric border. On the mucosal surface mouths of varying circumference lead into the diverticula where there is often entrapped faeces (Fig. 5.22). Diffuse diverticular disease and a solitary caecal diverticulum are unusual manifestations of the disorder.

Complications

Most subjects are unaware of their diverticular disease and will never recognize any related symptoms or experience any complications. Inflammation is the most frequent complication and the basis for most others. Inflammation in response to entrapped bacteria may remain confined to the diverticulum (diverticulitis) or lead to perforation with either a localized paracolic abscess or widespread peritonitis. Fistula between adjacent viscera including the bowel, bladder and vagina; obstruction from substantial oedema or more often adhesions; and haemorrhage are further consequences. Haemorrhage can be massive if a large vessel is eroded, or slight, but chronic when related to granulation tissue. Carcinoma does not supervene.

Miscellaneous conditions related to systemic disorders

Just as gastrointestinal ailments affect the rest of the body, so disorders elsewhere can produce changes within the gastrointestinal tract. These may either be localized or widely dispersed. Peptic ulceration, although usually found in isolation, is a complication of numerous conditions including chronic kidney, liver and lung disease as well as a range of endocrine disorders. Fibrocystic disease or mucoviscidosis (Fig. 5.23), vascular disease, systemic amyloid and immunodeficiency are all examples of systemic disorders with the potential for widespread alimentary tract changes and diabetes mellitus, connective tissue disorders and radiation, conditions capable of inducing local or generalized changes.

Vascular disease

The principal vascular disorders of atherosclerosis, vasculitis and thrombo-embolism can all adversely affect the alimentary tract and produce ischaemic bowel disease. Their effects depend upon the size and number of vessels involved, the extent of this involvement and the rapidity with which it occurs, closely associated with the presence and state of collateral vessels. The right-angle take-off of the coeliac axis and its wide lumen are believed responsible for its immunity relative to the other major mesenteric vessels from

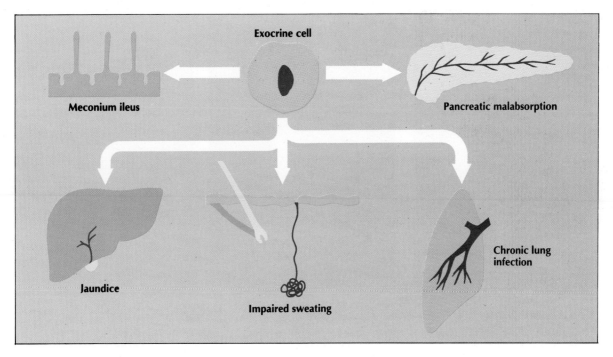

Fig. 5.23 Fibrocystic disease/ mucoviscidosis: the spectrum of the disorder.

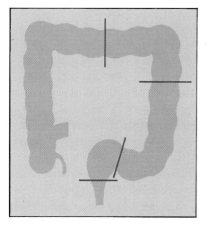

Fig. 5.24 The colon: watershed areas.

thrombo-embolism; in contrast the angled origin of the superior mesenteric artery predisposes it to atherosclerosis and thrombo-embolism. Similar complications can develop in the inferior mesenteric artery which has a very small lumen, but the abundant collaterals invariably protect the tissues supplied. If the cross-section of two of these large vessels is reduced below two-thirds ischaemic bowel disease follows. The localization depends on the vessels affected and if watershed areas are involved. These areas lie at the junction of major blood vessels and depend upon adequate oxygenation from perfusion rather than directly from a major vessel. The splenic flexure and the junction of the sigmoid colon and rectum are areas within this category and consequently are common sites of ischaemic bowel disease (Fig. 5.24).

Apart from the vascular supply, impaired perfusion from other causes as well as oxygenation of the blood also contribute to ischaemia. Cardiac failure, arrhythmias and shock, especially when combined with fluid/blood loss, are the most important reasons for impaired perfusion. These conditions are frequently seen with ischaemic bowel disease and may be aggravated by anaemia and increased blood viscosity, invariably superimposed upon an impaired vascular supply.

APPEARANCES

Ischaemic injury can be manifested in a variety of forms, some of which are curable and others generally fatal. A volvulus (Fig. 5.25), intussusception and hernia can each produce ischaemia by torsion

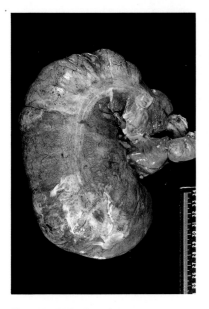 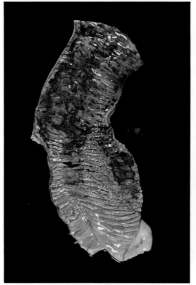 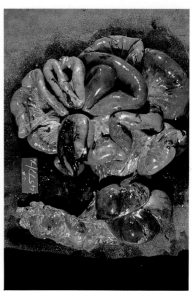

Fig. 5.25 Volvulus of the caecum in which the ischaemic damage has produced necrosis of the wall manifest by the purple discoloration and peritonitis.

Fig. 5.26 Part of an ischaemic colon showing the sharp demarcation between the area receiving an adequate blood supply and that with an impaired supply.

Fig. 5.27 Massive small bowel ischaemia following mesenteric artery thrombosis.

and occlusion of the blood supply which, in the hernia, is predominantly arterial and in the intussusception, venous. Uncomplicated recovery occurs if the torsion is quickly corrected but a stricture from the subsequent fibrosis may result when this is delayed. The affect on bowel function will depend upon the site involved. Malabsorption is a potential result if the small intestine is affected and alteration of bowel habit when the disorder is in the large bowel.

Small areas of focal ischaemia from small vessel disease cause ulceration. When the disease is restricted to single vessels this may be silent or produce blood loss; with multiple involvement, complications are more likely.

Ischaemic colitis and massive ischaemia of the major part of the small intestine are both conditions that are difficult to treat. Ischaemic colitis is a phenomenon of the watershed areas and a post-operative complication of surgery for abdominal aneurysms (Fig. 5.26). It is confined to the left side of the colon and is macroscopically similar to other types of colitis. Since the mucosa is the main site of injury and the muscle is less affected, massive fluid loss invariably results and perforation is uncommon. Epithelial repair can follow within four to five days but only if the crypts survive. Without re-epithelialization, granulation tissue and impaired function persist and strictures invariably follow.

Massive small bowel ischaemia commonly follows mesenteric artery thrombosis (Fig. 5.27) but embolism from atrial fibrillation and a paradoxical embolus via a patent foramen ovale are other causes. Shock and fluid loss can be fatal and, when recovery follows resection, severe malabsorption is inevitable.

Radiation

This can cause ischaemic damage similar to that outlined above. The sites most affected are the sigmoid colon, the rectum and the terminal ileum, reflecting the use of this therapy in cervical and bladder tumours. The techniques used and the amount of radiation received influence the development of ischaemia but previous pelvic surgery, diabetes mellitus and atherosclerosis are also important.

APPEARANCES

An immediate acute inflammatory reaction can occur which usually resolves. Of more consequence is the appearance of ischaemic lesions months and years after treatment. These are associated with occlusive vascular changes in the wall of the gut and necrosis, ulceration and strictures. The symptoms vary with the site of the involved bowel.

Immunodeficiency

This is manifest in the alimentary tract which, especially in adults, may be where presenting symptoms occur. Infections of all types occur. Giardiasis is especially related to IgA deficiency and candidiasis to some T-cell disorders and secondary immunodeficiency states. Multiple and repeated infections are characteristic and are an important part of the acquired immunodeficiency syndrome. Malabsorption can arise as a secondary phenomenon but also as an unrelated and incompletely understood condition. Protein loss from infection and steatorrhoea contribute, as does the development of lymphoma and amyloid. Subtotal villous atrophy, nodular lymphoid hyperplasia and gastritis are the histological findings. These all differ from those in other conditions in the paucity of plasma cells. Gastritis, although resulting in pernicious anaemia, is without antibodies.

Tumours

Benign and malignant tumours are found throughout the gastrointestinal tract with a greater incidence of malignant than benign tumours. The malignant tumours contribute significantly to patient morbidity but their mortality is largely dependent upon the stage at diagnosis. A carcinoma confined to the gastric mucosa has an 80–95% 5-year prognosis, while for one that has spread beyond the mucosa, the 5-year prognosis is reduced to less than 30%. Similar figures can be quoted for oesophageal and colonic cancers (Fig. 5.28). For many of these patients, therefore, a near normal life span is possible if adequate screening methods for early tumours can be found. These in turn may also lead to tumour prevention.

'At risk' groups

In practice screening for cancer depends upon the recognition of 'at risk' populations, groups and families. Certain provinces of China

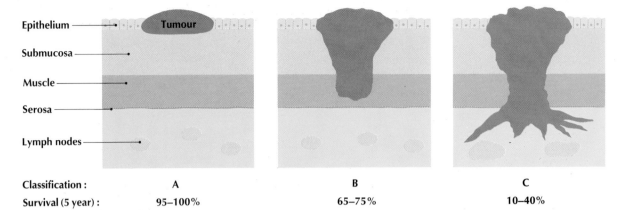

Epithelium			
Submucosa			
Muscle			
Serosa			
Lymph nodes			

| Classification : | A | B | C |
| Survival (5 year) : | 95–100% | 65–75% | 10–40% |

Fig. 5.28 Duke's classification of colonic carcinoma.

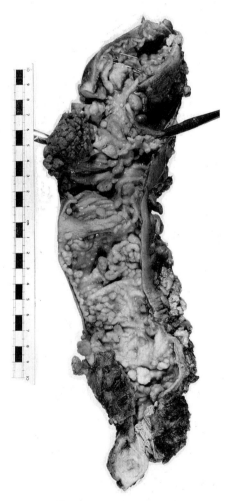

Fig. 5.29 Carcinoma of the colon (top) and benign tubulovillous adenomas: their presence raises the possibility that an adenoma was the precursor to the carcinoma.

show a high incidence of oesophageal cancer, and by cytological screening using swallowed balloons this has been diagnosed at an early stage and the mortality reduced. Similarly, with the knowledge that coeliac disease can be complicated by lymphoma and ulcerative colitis by carcinoma, careful monitoring of these patients may reduce the effects of these tumours. An analogous approach is used among the relatives of patients with familial polyposis to avoid the development of colonic carcinoma.

Malignant precursors

The histopathologist aids in screening programmes by either diagnosing potentially malignant changes or by recognizing established premalignant conditions.

Potential malignant changes include some hyperplastic and metaplastic conditions, particularly if accompanied by dysplastic changes, dysplasia itself and early carcinoma. The latter may be confined to the epithelium (*carcinoma in situ*) or to the mucosa (*intramucosal cancer*), depending on the viscus involved.

Premalignant conditions vary with the part of the gastrointestinal tract affected and include a large number of conditions with differing malignant potential (Table 5.7). Pernicious anaemia and its associated gastric atrophy carries a risk of malignancy three to four times that expected and similar figures apply to those ulcer patients with some form of gastrectomy or drainage procedure. Disorders resulting in partial oesophageal obstruction are possible precursors of malignancy while benign polyps in the colon, especially when large (>5 cm) and multiple (>5) are similarly implicated (Fig. 5.29).

The drawback to monitoring any of these conditions is that long latent periods are involved. The ulcerative colitic who develops carcinoma has generally had the disease for between 10 and 20 years and a similar time interval elapses between gastric surgery and the appearance of gastric cancer. Circulating tumour markers would provide a simple method for detecting the development of malignancy, but at present there are none specific for early gut tumours. Those that occur are neither specific for malignancy nor

Table 5.7 Potential pre-malignant conditions

Oesophagus	Hiatus hernia
	Diverticulum
	Achalasia
	Stenosis
	Chronic inflammation
Stomach	Gastric atrophy (pernicious anaemia)
	Post-gastric surgery
	Gastric polyps (Ménétrièr's disease)
	Gastric ulcer
Small intestine	Coeliac disease
	Crohn's disease
	Familial polyposis
Large intestine	Ulcerative colitis
	Villous adenoma
	Multiple polyps
	Previous colonic carcinoma

for any part of the gastrointestinal tract. Carcino-embryonic antigen (CEA) can be useful in the recognition of metastases if a rise in the serum levels occurred with the initial tumour. In these circumstances a further rise results when metastases appear. Unfortunately, CEA may appear with inflammatory conditions and also with disorders outside the gut.

Epidemiology

Few causes of malignancy within the gut are known and none apply to all patients or explain the focal nature of the condition.

Diet

This has been considered the most important potential source of carcinogens since this includes natural foods, additives, colorizers, preservatives, products of storage, cooking and digestion as well as unintentional contaminants, pesticides and industrial pollutants. The carcinogen(s) may not necessarily exist *per se* in the diet but appear after ingestion, either because promoters are present or because there is *in vivo* formation of carcinogens from non-carcinogenic substances. Micro-organisms, either as part of the normal flora or as abnormal flora, may affect any of these processes. Changes in transport produced via the diet by affecting contact between the bowel contents and the wall as well as the concentration and speed of transit of the contents are other potential factors. In practice, despite intensive studies it has proved impossible to pin-point any dietary component as the cause of a particular alimentary tract tumour.

Experimentally, tumours can be induced but only in selected species and in restricted parts of the alimentary tract. Relative to human consumption, massive doses of the potential carcinogen are generally required. The tumours are confined mainly to the liver and small intestine and often depend upon the absence or presence of micro-organisms but the common clinical malignancy, colorectal cancer, is rarely produced. The interpretation of the experimental results is that in sites of high cell turnover the small intestine, carcinogens or intermediate products have a greater chance of affecting DNA transformation and producing malignancy. A similar explanation may apply to colorectal carcinomas in man. In these sites of low cell turnover, the slow transit times that exist may allow greater exposure of mucosa to possible carcinogens formed during transit and dependent on bowel flora.

Bile and Clostridia

The carcinogen, 20-methylcholanthrene, is formed from deoxycholic acid, a component of bile, in the presence of *Clostridia* and an anaerobic environment. *Clostridia* species are carried by many of the European populations who also suffer from colonic carcinoma but they are rarely found within African populations, an area with a low incidence of colonic cancer. These observations imply that this mechanism of *in vivo* carcinogenesis may be important in colonic cancer.

Nitrosamines

These carcinogens arise from ingested nitrates that have been converted by bacteria via nitrites to nitrosamines. Bacteria do not usually occur in the stomach except after surgery. This sequence may thus contribute to the incidence of gastric carcinoma following operations in this site.

Other factors

Genetic and geographical factors are important. It must also be realized that tumour incidence changes spontaneously, as the reduction in gastric cancer during the last twenty years illustrates.

Non-epithelial tumours

Few of the considerations discussed apply to non-epithelial tumours. The most common connective tissue tumour is the generally benign leiomyoma which has no obvious cause. Lymphomas, which form a substantial group of malignant tumours, should always raise the question of an impaired or abnormal immune system. Some primary immunodeficiency states, particularly, can be associated with primary small intestinal lymphomas and there is also a relationship between these and coeliac disease.

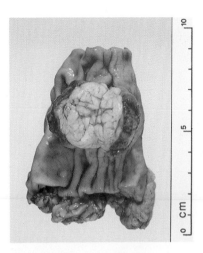

Fig. 5.30 Lipoma of the stomach wall.

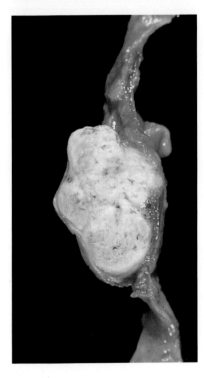

Fig. 5.31 Leiomyoma of the stomach.

Tumour appearances

Benign tumours

These include epithelial, connective tissue and lymphoid types (Fig. 5.30). The distinction from malignant tumours is often apparent from their small size and can usually be confirmed by microscopy.

1 *Leiomyomas* are found in all parts of the alimentary tract with the highest incidence in the oesophagus and stomach (Fig. 5.31). They may be asymptomatic or associated with bleeding or obstruction. Their size and microscopic features are not absolute indicators of their future behaviour since some are malignant. Those most likely to metastasize are large and include frequent and often bizarre mitotic forms and invade locally.

2 *Epithelial polyps or adenomas* particularly if large, numerous or villous, can also be associated with malignancy and distinction must therefore be made between the tubular, tubulovillous and villous patterns (Fig. 5.32). These occur especially within the large bowel with or without symptoms.

3 *Regenerative or inflammatory pseudo-polyps and hyperplastic polyps* are most often found in the large bowel and are not malignant. They can be confused in the rectum with the solitary rectal ulcer. This is a benign condition possibly due to local ischaemia and/or prolapse and clinically mistaken for carcinoma.

Malignant tumours

1 *Epithelial*

These form the majority of malignancies throughout the alimentary tract. The large bowel is the most common site and the small bowel the least. Gastric and oesophageal carcinoma carry the worst prognoses overall but, at any site, tumours in younger patients behave more aggressively and have a worse prognosis. Carcinomas of the oesophagus and anal canal are squamous but those in other parts are adenocarcinomas. Adenocarcinomas develop in the oesophagus when there is metaplastic gastric mucosa or when the epithelium in the lower third is columnar (*Barrett's oesophagus*). The epithelial changes follow from persistent gastro-oesophageal reflux. Spread of gastric cancers into the oesophagus will mimic oesophageal adenocarcinomas. Basal cell carcinoma and, more unusually, malignant melanomas can be found at the anal canal.

APPEARANCES

The tumours have a variety of macroscopic appearances which affect the timing and manner of their presentation.

(a) Infiltrative tumours tend to deform and narrow the gut and

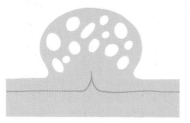
Tubular

Incidence : 80–90%

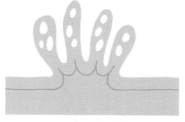
Tubulo-villous

10–15%

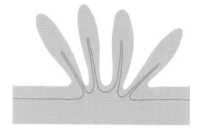
Villous

3–5%

Fig. 5.32 Adenomatous polyps.

Fig. 5.33 Infiltrative carcinoma of (*left*) stomach and (*right*) oesophagus.

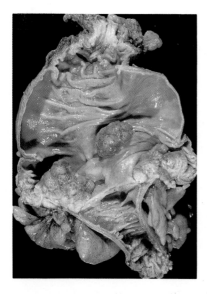

Fig. 5.34 Polypoid carcinoma of the colon. There is some dilatation of the bowel above the tumour due to obstruction.

thereby lead to obstruction at an early stage. The narrowed area may produce a localized annular constriction or affect a large part of the viscus, in the stomach producing the rigid *'leather bottle stomach'* (Fig. 5.33).

(b) Alternatively the tumour develops as a localized mass, often fungating and sometimes polypoid (Fig. 5.34). A variety of symptoms can then occur including intermittent obstruction, intussusception or persistent mild haemorrhage with the gradual development of an iron deficiency anaemia. The patient in these circumstances presents late often with established metastases.

(c) Between these extremes is the ulcerative tumour leading to acute or chronic haemorrhage or perforation (Fig. 5.35).

Any of these patterns may be superimposed (Fig. 5.36) upon another and all are found in any part of the alimentary tract. Multiple primary tumours occur most uncommonly except when cancer complicates ulcerative colitis and occurs in the small intestine. Tumours may, histologically, vary from highly differentiated adenocarcinomas, with or without marked mucus production, to undifferentiated anaplastic tumours hardly recognizable as adenocarcinomas. A well known variant is the *signet ring type* (Fig. 5.37). The

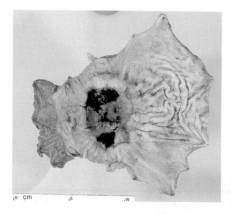
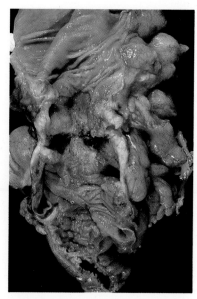

Fig. 5.35 Ulcerative carcinomas of (*left*) stomach and (*right*) rectum.

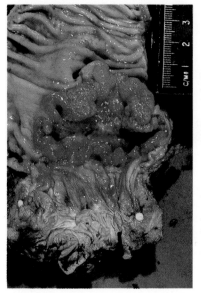

Fig. 5.36 Carcinoma of the rectum that is ulcerative and infiltrative.

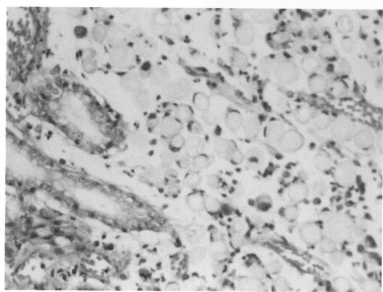

Fig. 5.37 Adenocarcinoma of the stomach with typical signet ring cells. The nucleus is displaced by intracytoplasmic mucus which swells the cell.

tumour cells include intracytoplasmic mucin which deforms the nucleus so that the cell is comparable to a signet ring. Such cells are seen lying individually or in infiltrating strands and this microscopic pattern underlies many of the infiltrative types of carcinoma.

Spread. The tumours spread directly through the bowel wall to contiguous structures and to more distant sites by vascular, lymphatic and intraperitoneal routes. The portal drainage provides an additional route for venous spread and probably contributes to the high incidence of liver metastases accompanying many carcinomas of the gastrointestinal tract. The substantial lymphatic drainage of the stomach virtually ensures lymph node spread in most gastric carcinomas. Spread to the ovaries, especially from gastric cancers, can result in bilateral metastases or *Krukenberg tumours*. Transcoelomic spread is often advocated as the route for these metastases but it is probable that this too is an example of lymphatic spread. Tumour can be seen in the ovaries within lymphatic channels and there is rarely tumour on the surface of the ovaries.

Other pathways for tumour spread, although rare, involve direct implantation either from biopsy needles or following surgical intervention. Tumour at surgical resection lines and within laparotomy scars are the consequences.

No organ is exempt from metastases but the liver, lungs and lymph nodes are those most involved. The histopathologist examining a biopsy of such a metastasis is rarely able to localize the primary site with confidence, since similar appearances occur with tumour from any cuboidal or columnar epithelium. Primary growths within the breast, lung, pancreas and ovary are all tumours that can mimic adenocarcinomas from any part of the alimentary tract.

2 *Non-epithelial tumours*

Lymphomas differ from carcinomas in that they are often multiple and, in their early phases, confined to the submucosa. They complicate coeliac disease in the small intestine, occasionally ulcerative colitis in the large bowel, but usually have no recognized precursor in the stomach or large bowel. The majority are non-Hodgkin's lymphomas with many B-cell types and some T-cell types. The view that they are mostly histiocytic is no longer tenable although a proportion fail to exhibit either B- or T-cell markers.

Malignant connective tissue tumours are all exceedingly rare apart from the leiomyosarcomas. These are often impossible to recognize until metastases have formed.

Further reading

Jass, J.R., Love, S.B. and Northover, J.M.A. (1987). A new prognostic classification of rectal cancer. *Lancet* i, 1303–6.

Lewin, K.J. (1986). The endocrine cells of the gastrointestinal tract: the normal endocrine cells and their hyperplasias. Part 1. In: *Pathology Annual*. Volume 21. Ed. by S.C. Sommers, P.P. Rosen and R.E. Fechner. Appleton Century-Crofts, Norwalk Connecticut.

Morson, B.C. and Dawson, I.M.P. (1989). *Gastrointestinal Pathology* (3rd Edition). Blackwell Scientific Publications: Oxford and London.

Whitehead, R. (1985). Mucosal biopsy of the gastrointestinal tract (3rd Edition). W.B. Saunders Co. Ltd.: London.

6 Liver

The liver synthesizes, detoxicates and excretes a wide range of substances and also acts as an endocrine and exocrine gland. The failure to develop an effective artificial liver illustrates both the complexity and the multiplicity of these functions, all performed by each individual liver cell. The liver cells form 80–90% of the organ's cell population and are arranged as lobules with central veins and peripheral portal tracts. Functionally this lobular pattern is false since perfusion with dyes demonstrates cell groupings or acini which are centred on portal tracts. Attempts to describe liver disease in terms of acinar rather than lobular architecture have not found universal acceptance, and in practice lobular structure is that most easily recognized and used by most histopathologists. Liver cell disease is diagnosed from clinical and biochemical findings but any abnormalities. are not necessarily in proportion to the severity of the liver cell involvement and can be mild or absent even with substantial liver injury.

Cholestasis

The most common functional abnormality observed by the patient is jaundice. This is invariably due to the bile accumulation within the liver (*cholestasis*) (Fig. 6.1), although numerous mechanisms are involved. Bile stasis can precede clinical jaundice and if severe will

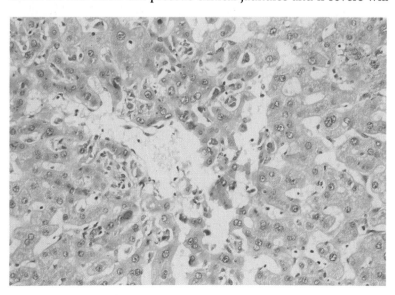

Fig. 6.1 Cholestasis: the greenish-yellow pigment around the central vein is bile. The patient was receiving numerous drugs and was jaundiced.

itself cause liver cell damage and so exacerbate the underlying disorder. The most common cause is obstruction to the extrahepatic biliary tree by calculi, tumour or strictures, but there are many others in which injury is often confined to the liver cell (Table 6.1). Disorders of the biliary tract may initially induce changes in the micro-organelles, in particular the endoplasmic reticulum, but later the reduction in bile flow is contributed to by the inflammatory response and fibrosis in the portal tracts. It is these events, particularly, that make it difficult to distinguish between intra- and extrahepatic biliary tract obstruction in liver biopsies. The mechanisms producing cholestasis unrelated with biliary obstruction are, like those of normal bile excretion from liver cells, not completely understood.

APPEARANCES

Affected livers in long-standing examples are enlarged and dark green and may have progressed to cirrhosis. Cirrhosis following extrahepatic biliary obstruction is referred to as *secondary biliary cirrhosis*.

Regeneration

The variance between clinical observation and liver cell damage is to some extent due to the immense regenerative capacity of the liver. This response also underlies the importance of liver biopsy in diagnosis, the liver's regenerative and reserve capacity initially masking many disorders. This facility is surprising given the complex functions of each cell, but is possible because of the uniformity and structural simplicity of liver cells.

Table 6.1 Important causes of cholestasis

	Site of obstruction
Common	
Calculi	
Tumour	Extrahepatic biliary tree
Stricture	
Drugs	
Alcohol	Hepatocellular
Viral hepatitis	
Cirrhosis	Hepatocellular and
Congestive cardiac failure	intrahepatic biliary tree
Idiopathic	
Uncommon	
Mucoviscidosis/cystic fibrosis	
Alpha-1-antitrypsin deficiency	
Pregnancy	
Primary biliary cirrhosis	
Biliary atresia	

Each cell is polygonal and includes the micro-organelles found in all epithelial cells with no specialized types present. The mitochondria which provide oxidative energy for many of the cells' functions are, however, numerous and frequently abnormal in shape. They may contain crystalline structures in some congenital and acquired liver disorders. Abundant glycogen and endoplasmic reticulum in each cell further reflects the liver's metabolic activity.

Regeneration, involving hyperplasia and hypertrophy, follows the removal of 10% or more of the liver and can restore the liver to its original size and architecture. This response is an integral part of any disease involving liver cell necrosis and is most obvious in cirrhosis, where it is aberrant in that the normal anatomy is not restored.

Vascular disorders

The liver's vascular supply is arterial as well as venous, the portal system, with drainage via the hepatic veins. The liver cells are in receipt of a quarter of the cardiac output, although this can be dramatically increased in the face of some physiological demands. Four-fifths of this blood supply is provided by the low pressure portal system and only one-fifth by the hepatic artery. The latter is the main source of oxygen and the portal system of nutrition. Nevertheless, alterations in the balance of supply occur and there is a temporary adaptive facility available when one or other supply is compromised. Cirrhosis and venous outflow obstruction (*Budd–Chiari syndrome*) are causes of persistent changes in the portal blood flow, with consequent portal hypertension, while systemic hypotension and disseminated intravascular coagulation can affect the arterial supply (Fig. 6.2). Intrahepatic portocaval anastomoses found in cirrhosis affect both arterial and portal supplies. Results of vascular impairment are degeneration and necrosis which in the liver are

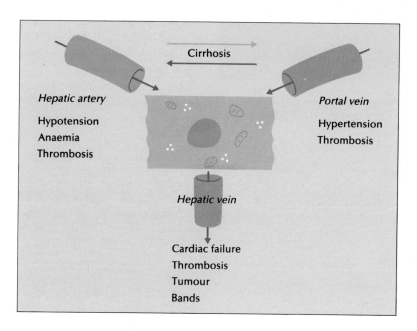

Fig. 6.2 Factors impairing the liver's blood supply.

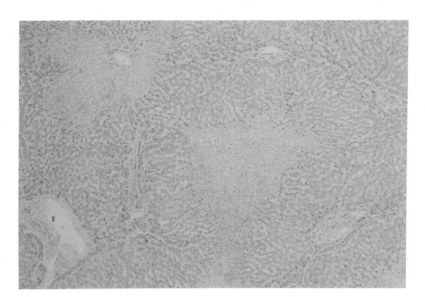

Fig. 6.3 Severe venous congestion. Liver cells in the centre of the lobules are necrotic and the sinusoids distended with blood.

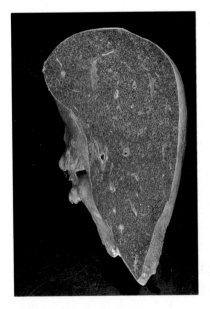

Fig. 6.4 Nutmeg liver, the consequence of long-standing cardiac failure.

particularly likely because of the immense metabolic activity of each cell and are most severe with hepatic artery involvement. Cells particularly at risk are those furthest from the portal tracts and nearest the central veins. Hence, in venous congestion from cardiac failure degenerative changes appear first in the perivenular cells, and if the process progresses these will become necrotic with those nearer the portal regions undergoing degeneration (Fig. 6.3).

APPEARANCES OF VENOUS CONGESTION

Congestion of the sinusoids contributes to enlargement and a macroscopic appearance analogous to that of a nutmeg and characteristic of cardiac failure (Fig. 6.4).

Although liver cell necrosis is theoretically easily precipitated, infarction of the liver is a fairly rare event. The double blood supply protects against this and, to produce infarction, both blood supplies must be compromised either by vessel wall disease such as polyarteritis nodosa or by hypotension. Apparent infarcts (*infarcts of Zahn*) are seen when the portal vein is occluded and when there is systemic hypotension sufficient to reduce the portal blood flow.

APPEARANCES OF ZAHN INFARCTS

Affected areas are subcapsular and formed from dilated sinusoids filled with blood (Fig. 6.5). The dilatation is secondary to atrophy and shrinkage of the liver cells but liver cell necrosis is not a feature.

Immune responses

Specialized cells are present in the liver but in much smaller numbers than the hepatocytes. These include endothelial cells lining

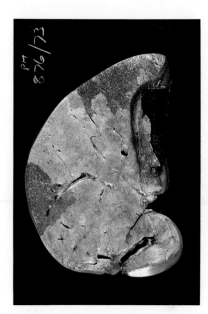

Fig. 6.5 Infarcts of Zahn. These are the two peripheral dark areas involving the capsule. The patient had acute pancreatitis and was hypotensive.

sinusoids and Ito cells, or lipocytes, in the space of Dissë. *Ito cells are the storage organs for vitamin A* and synthesize the liver's collagen. Also lining the sinusoids are *Kupffer cells*, or macrophages. These form 15% of the total cell population of the liver and provide the largest aggregate of these cells in the body. They are phagocytic but unlike other macrophages are unable to process antigen for antibody responses. Kupffer cells are bathed directly both in the portal blood which is rich in antigens from the gut and in antibody-rich blood from the spleen. It is suggested that their function is to sieve out harmful substances from entering the systemic circulation. The increased incidence of systemic infections seen with many liver disorders supports this concept. The immunological defence of the liver is further contributed to by lymphocytes migrating to and from the parenchyma and more notably the portal tracts, as well as local synthesis of complement by macrophages (Fig. 6.6).

Hypergammaglobulinaemia, circulating autoantibodies and hypocomplementaemia are part of many liver disorders and clearly indicate immune reactions, as does the local influx of lymphocytes seen with these disorders. Immunoglobulin changes are explicable in terms of altered T-cell function with release of B-cells. Complement consumption develops either from decreased synthesis or increased utilization associated with immune complex formation. Underlying all of these processes could be defective antigen filtering by the Kupffer cells as a consequence of liver disorder or secondary to intrahepatic vascular shunting. Intrahepatic shunts, as occur in cirrhosis, reduce the numbers of exposed Kupffer cells as well as impair their saturation with antigen. Antigen may then enter and persist in the liver so provoking local immune damage or inducing autoantibody injury but only if there is also a defect in T-cell function.

The disorders particularly related to immune injury are primary biliary cirrhosis and some forms of chronic active hepatitis unrelated to Hepatitis B virus infection. *Primary biliary cirrhosis is only a*

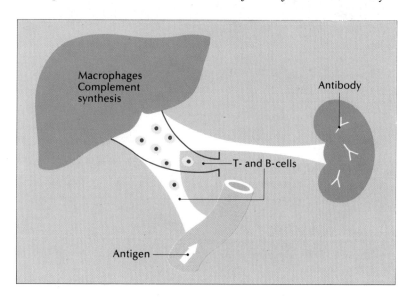

Fig. 6.6 Immunity and the liver.

cirrhosis terminally and can exist for many years before this stage is reached. The target tissue in primary biliary cirrhosis is the biliary epithelium while that in *chronic active hepatitis* is the periportal hepatic cells. It is because both disorders centre upon the portal tracts that distinction between them histologically can be very difficult. Both diseases predominate in women and are invariably associated with autoimmune disorders in other tissues. Primary biliary cirrhosis is characterized by a 90% frequency of antimitochondrial antibodies as opposed to the 20% frequency in chronic active hepatitis. A reversed frequency pattern is seen for antibody to smooth muscle between the two disorders. Chronic active hepatitis patients have an HLA B8 DRW3 phenotype, but none has emerged for primary biliary cirrhosis.

Involvement in systemic disorders

A consequence of the double blood supply and multiple functions of the liver is that it will be involved in many systemic disorders, infectious and non-infectious.

1 Infectious: miliary tuberculosis is one of the common causes of hepatic granulomas, particularly when the immune system is compromised. Amoebic abscesses (Fig. 6.7), hydatid cysts and malaria are infections which, although more common outside the UK, are occasionally encountered in immigrants and inveterate travellers. Disseminated viral infections, notably in the immunosuppressed and neonate, affect the liver as, potentially, does any severe microbial infection.

2 Non-infectious: disorders involving the blood components will have sequelae within the liver. Any severe anaemia contributes to a fatty liver, while lymphomas and leukaemias can result in hepatic deposits and platelets and coagulation disorders in thrombosis and intrahepatic haemorrhage. In all these there may be iron deposition (*haemosiderosis*) (Fig. 6.8), often aggravated by treatment with iron-containing compounds and foci of haemopoietic cells. The changes

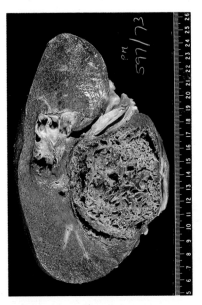

Fig. 6.7 Amoebic abscess.

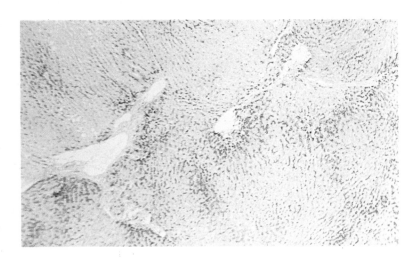

Fig. 6.8 Haemosiderosis. Iron is stained blue. The patient had chronic renal failure and had received regular blood transfusions.

of viral hepatitis may also be present, particularly if multiple transfusions have been given or, as in haemophiliacs, clotting factor concentrates received.

The close proximity of the heart and liver ensures that any impairment of blood flow, especially from cardiac failure, produces perivenular congestion and potentially a nutmeg liver. Polyarteritis nodosa, systemic lupus erythematosus and rheumatoid arthritis all have expression in the liver and amyloid as part of systemic deposition is also seen. In sarcoidosis, granulomas are found in the majority of patients with widespread disease.

Other disorders produce no diagnostic changes but are associated either with non-specific liver changes such as fatty change or mild hepatitis, and, less often, with more distinctive but not unique changes. Sclerosing cholangitis found with a few examples of inflammatory bowel disorders and the rare cholestases associated with pregnancy provide such examples.

Systemic effects of liver disease

The diversity of the liver's function means that any impairment may potentially modify that of other organs. In practice this is commonly found with widespread acute and chronic liver disease but not with minor degrees of liver cell damage.

Portal hypertension and associated varices and splenomegaly are the features most often looked for by the physician. Gall-stones, peptic ulceration, gastritis, pancreatitis and diabetes mellitus are also all described, most consistently with alcohol-related liver disease. Renal failure or the hepatorenal syndrome can be the terminal event with changes within the kidneys ranging from none to tubular necrosis, including bile deposition in the tubules and glomerulonephritis. Vasoconstriction of intrarenal arteries and circulating endotoxins contribute to renal failure as does intravascular coagulation, complement activation and hypotension. Hyperdynamic circulation characterizes many types of chronic liver disease including alcohol-related, and is exacerbated by anaemia and intrapulmonary shunting of blood as well as by a reduced peripheral resistance. The cardiomyopathy of alcoholic liver disease can precipitate cardiac failure but ischaemic heart disease is less common than in other patients. In the lungs pulmonary oedema is common and in those with alpha-1-antitrypsin deficiency this can be complicated by pre-existing emphysema. Pulmonary infection is facilitated by congestion, oedema and emphysema but defective Kupffer cell function, depressed immune responses and reduced chest expansion induced by ascites also play a role. Testicular atrophy and gynaecomastia of chronic liver dysfunction may follow either from the metabolic impairment produced by the liver cell injury or from that similarly produced in the pituitary and hypothalamus. Encephalopathy of liver failure is also imprecisely understood. Thyroiditis, like gastritis, may form part of a diffuse disorder of autoimmunity and hence is seen in those liver diseases particularly associated with abnormal immune responses.

Table 6.2 Viruses and hepatitis

Most common
- Hepatitis A virus (HAV)
- Hepatitis B virus (HBV)

Others
- Non A, Non B hepatitis virus
- Hepatitis delta virus
- Cytomegalovirus
- Epstein—Barr virus
- Herpes simplex virus
- Yellow fever virus
- Adenoviruses
- Coxsackie B
- Enteroviruses

Hepatitis

This term describes the inflammatory response in the liver to a very wide range of stimuli. These include infective agents, especially viruses (Table 6.2), as well as poisons, gases, drugs, alcohol and a range of systemic and infective disorders (Table 6.3). Nevertheless, the most common causes world-wide are the different hepatitis viruses, such that the term has become synonymous with this form of infection. Recognition ultimately relies upon histology although it may be suspected with varying degrees of confidence from clinical, biochemical and serological findings. With non-viral causes in many patients no aetiological agent is found. Clinically the disorder ranges from asymptomatic patients with subclinical inflammation to those with slowly or rapidly progressive liver failure. Similarly, prognosis varies between rapid death and a normal life span. Between these extremes are chronically ill patients with constant or relapsing but progressive liver disease which, in some, will form cirrhosis.

Acute hepatitis is a disorder of less than six months' duration. If symptoms or asymptomatic liver changes persist beyond this period the disorder falls into the chronic category (Table 6.4).

Chronic hepatitis is particularly associated with hepatitis virus infection and three morphological subclassifications exist, although there are overlapping and merging patterns (Table 6.5).

1 *Chronic persistent hepatitis.* This is characterized by a predominance of inflammatory changes within the portal tracts, absence or minimal amount of fibrosis and no change in the liver architecture. The disorder can only be recognized from a liver biopsy and the

Table 6.3 Non-viral causes of hepatitis

Systemic disorders	Some drug groups
Disseminated infections	Psychotropic
Connective tissue disorders	Antituberculous
Inflammatory bowel diseases	Antibiotics
	Analgesics
	Anaesthetics
	Hypotensives
	Antimetabolites
	Immunosuppressants

Table 6.4 Acute HBV hepatitis

Course	Liver
Full recovery (90%)	No virus Spotty necrosis
Chronic hepatitis (10%)	Virus Piecemeal and bridging necrosis
Fulminant fatal hepatitis (1%)	No virus Widespread necrosis

most essential feature is that microscopic changes remain static for long periods in serial biopsies.

2 *Chronic active hepatitis.* As the name implies, the inflammation is aggressive with a marked tendency to progress to cirrhosis and clinically there is liver impairment. There is fibrosis and architectural distortion and, characteristically, *piecemeal necrosis.* This term describes liver cell destruction at the interface of the liver parenchyma and the connective tissue either within portal tracts or at the edges of cirrhotic nodules. Non-viral causes are important (Table 6.6).

3 *Chronic lobular hepatitis.* This is an acute hepatitis lasting for more than six months. Inflammation and liver cell necrosis is randomized within the lobules and any portal tract changes are minor as in chronic persistent hepatitis.

The division of hepatitis into acute and chronic forms is, nevertheless, not as clear-cut as it might appear. The disorder may remain unrecognized for some time prior to diagnosis and may persist asymptomatically. Relapses and exposure to other hepatotoxic agents are further causes of confusion, as is coexisting cirrhosis. Morphological divisions according to the site of injury within the acinus and their focal or diffuse distribution throughout the liver are sometimes helpful in indentifying the cause but are rarely, without clinical information, diagnostic. Histology does, however,

Table 6.5 Chronic hepatitis

Types	Course	Liver
Chronic persistent	Static Resolution Few progress	Virus diffusely Portal inflammation
Chronic active	Variable Progressing to cirrhosis and liver failure	Virus focally Portal inflammation Piecemeal necrosis Fibrosis
Chronic lobular	Not progressive	No virus Spotty necrosis

Table 6.6 Non-viral causes of chronic active hepatitis

	Liver cell markers
Unknown (lupoid or HBs Ag negative)	None
Drugs methyldopa some laxatives isoniazid paracetamol	None
Wilson's disease	Copper and Mallory bodies
Alpha-1-antitrypsin deficiency	Specific intracytoplasmic globules
Alcohol-related liver disease	Mallory bodies
Primary biliary cirrhosis	Copper and Mallory bodies

distinguish the condition from *granulomatous hepatitis* which most often arises from sarcoidosis or tuberculosis.

Hepatitis virus infection

There are three groups of hepatitis viruses: Hepatitis A (HAV), Hepatitis B (HBV) and the Non A, Non B group (Table 6.7). HAV has a uniform distribution world-wide and by adulthood most populations are immune but have experienced few symptoms. HBV has a more variable distribution pattern but is the most important cause clinically of hepatitis. The impact and distribution of Non A-Non B is less easily defined but this virus is the principal source of post-transfusion hepatitis.

B virus hepatitis

Patients' infection is from carriers, most commonly via blood and blood products but transmission is also possible via saliva, semen, vaginal discharges, breast milk and serous exudates. Infected and unsterilized needles and syringes are important vectors as are occasionally communally shared razors, toothbrushes and scissors. Although close contact is important recipients of blood transfusions including haemophiliacs, those on dialysis or given organ transplants, medical personnel of all types, institutionalized groups, intravenous drug addicts, male homosexuals and any immunodeficient patient are also at risk.

Serological diagnosis

Recognition of the actively infected patient and distinction from a carrier depends upon the types of circulating viral antigens and antibodies. The virus forms three types of antigen to which antibodies appear (Fig. 6.9). The central core of the virus provides the c antigen (HBcAg) and the outer coat, or surface, the s antigen (HBsAg).

Table 6.7 Hepatitis viruses

	HBV	HAV	Non A, Non B
Type	DNA	RNA	3 types
Size	42 nm	27 nm	Unknown
Antibodies	HBs Ab HBc Ab HBe Ab	HAV Ab	None
Source	Blood Body fluids Liver	Faeces Serum Bile Liver	Blood Coagulation factors Water
Incubation period (days)	50−80	15−40	18−89

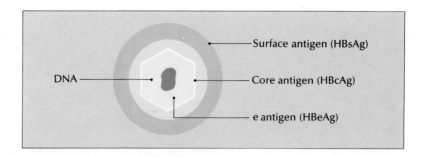

Fig. 6.9 Hepatitis B virus.

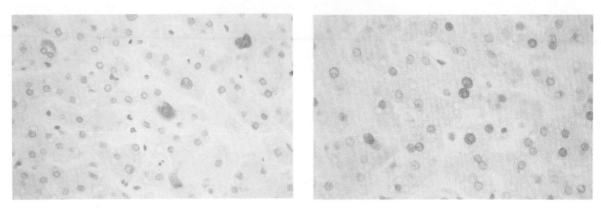

Fig. 6.10 Hepatitis B virus antigen; (*above left*) the surface antigen is labelled brown with an antibody and is dispersed throughout the cytoplasm; (*above right*) the core antibody, similarly labelled, is restricted mainly to the nucleus.

Circulating HBsAg characterizes the hepatitis B carrier. The third antigen, e (HBeAg), is a proteolytic breakdown product of the core antigen and appears before clinical symptoms. All antigens and their antibodies occur in the serum but the virus can also be demonstrated within liver cells by electron microscopy and by specific peroxidase or fluorescent labelled antibodies (Fig. 6.10).

Histological effects and course

Infected cells can be swollen with a finely granular cytoplasm containing vast amounts of excess surface antigens (*ground glass cells*) (Fig. 6.11). This antigen is also seen on the cell membrane but the core antigen (HBcAg) is virtually confined to the nucleus. The presence or absence of these antigens in liver cells and the distribution of infected cells has been used to subdivide acute hepatitis and predict transition to the chronic form of the disease. Full recovery can be anticipated among those patients whose biopsies include virtually no antigen of either type. Persistence of HBcAg, especially in a focal pattern, can be associated with progression but generalized HBcAg occurs in many asymptomatic carriers, some with chronic persistent hepatitis, and also immunocompromised patients. Other indices of recovery are the absence of piecemeal necrosis, lack of necrosis linking portal tracts and central veins (*bridging necrosis*) and small numbers of plasma cells. Elderly patients, particularly women, are most likely to progress. In 10% of patients chronic hepatitis appears and in less than 1% massive necrosis, which in over two-thirds leads rapidly to death.

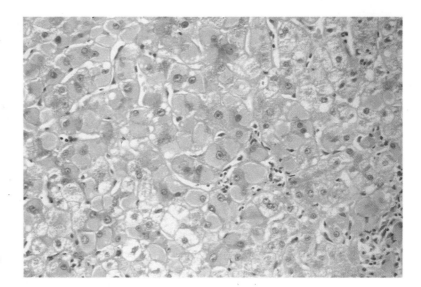

Fig. 6.11 Ground glass cells. These liver cells are packed with Hepatitis B surface antigen.

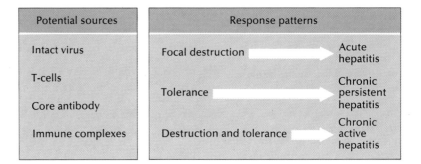

Potential sources	Response patterns	
Intact virus	Focal destruction →	Acute hepatitis
T-cells	Tolerance →	Chronic persistent hepatitis
Core antibody		
Immune complexes	Destruction and tolerance →	Chronic active hepatitis

Fig. 6.12 Liver cell injury with Hepatitis B virus.

Mechanism of injury

The reasons for the variable course and different patterns of liver reaction are not fully understood (Fig. 6.12). The virus does not directly damage the liver cells and is not the sole cause of their destruction. In marked destruction, as in acute hepatitis, there is no virus demonstrable while, in carriers and chronic persistent hepatitis with little cell necrosis, the virus is widespread. Chronic active hepatitis, however, is characterized by foci of liver cells containing virus and progressive liver cell necrosis.

It is suggested that liver cell destruction of acute and chronic active hepatitis is primarily the effect of immune injury. This is mediated by T-cells and arises from antibody to core antigen on the surface of the liver cells. This antigen in chronic persistent hepatitis and carriers, in contrast, provokes a more substantial humoral reaction which blocks the core antigen and thereby the cytotoxic T-cell response. The surface antigen is protective and, like HBe antigen, has no part in the liver the cell destruction.

The concept of combined viral and immune damage is incomplete, largely because agreement on cellular responses has not been reached and also because the role of HBc antigen has not been documented.

Immune complexes also occur and are an alternative mechanism of injury in some carriers and in patients with chronic persistent hepatitis, especially the immunocompromised and those on maintenance dialysis. Kupffer cells may further affect progressive disease by contributing to immune complex formation. They may either fail to inactivate antigen or serve as sources for viral division, but both of these possibilities remain to be evaluated.

APPEARANCES

The liver in acute hepatitis is rarely seen macroscopically. This is mainly because the patient recovers, but also because autopsy examination is generally avoided. At laparotomy the liver is of normal size and reddened but, if there is cholestasis, it will be green to yellow. Within the parenchyma no changes may be evident but in some livers there are discrete, scattered, pin-point, yellow foci of necrosis. When there has been an uncomplicated recovery there is no trace of any abnormality grossly. The small group of patients dying with fulminant acute hepatitis have a small bright yellow liver which is strikingly soft, sometimes to the extent that it collapses on a firm surface.

Patients who have proceeded to chronic hepatitis have an enlarged liver. This has an irregular surface and fairly tough parenchyma, varying with the degree of fibrosis. Cirrhosis and hepatocellular carcinoma develop in a small minority of these patients. Others, in whom hepatitis virus cannot be found, will have evidence of multisystem disease, postulated as immune, including thyroid, joint, intestinal tract and kidney disorders.

Alcohol related disorders

Improved standards of living and associated affluence have led to an increase in alcohol consumption among all social classes. A four-fold increase has occurred within the UK during the last 20 years. All groups of society are affected, although certain occupations more so than others, reflecting the availability of alcohol and peer and social pressures. Brewers, barmen, sailors, printers, sales and business men and doctors are those particularly at risk.

Liver injury

The most important site of tissue injury of alcohol is undoubtedly the liver. Even so, the mechanisms by which this arises remain obscure, as do the reasons for some patients being affected and others not. The proof of an association between liver disease and alcohol is therefore circumstantial and epidemiological. Animal models have been unsatisfactory, largely because a different pattern of disease is produced, although among a small number of baboons the changes closely mimic those in man. A sustained intake of alcohol over several months or years in the order of a minimum of 2-3 pints of beer or 4-5 measures of spirit daily, is more likely to

Table 6.8 Disorders associated with Mallory bodies

Commonly
  Alcohol abuse
  Wilson's disease
  Indian infantile cirrhosis
  Primary biliary cirrhosis

Uncommonly
  Long-standing biliary obstruction
  Intestinal bypass surgery
  Diabetes mellitus
  Drugs

produce lasting liver injury than random binges, although in women, possibly because of their smaller body mass, the periods and amounts are both less. There is no firm evidence for any genetic influence; the high incidence of alcohol-related liver disease among family members reflects shared social and behavioural patterns.

Mallory bodies are common to all forms of injury and are considered almost the hallmark of alcohol-related liver disease, although they occur in other conditions involving liver cell injury (Table 6.8). They are fibrillar bodies discernible by the light microscope as variably shaped and sized eosinophilic masses similar to hyaline (Fig. 6.13). They reflect an aberration of intermediate filament synthesis. These filaments provide the micro-scaffolding of liver cells and are normally dispersed and not closely aggregated, as occurs in Mallory bodies. Mallory bodies often herald cell death and may, by acting as an antigenic focus, play a role in perpetuating injury initiated by alcohol, a hypothesis contradicted by the lack of progression of liver injury in the majority of patients. They are concentrated in the perivenular regions and around the periphery of cirrhotic nodules and disappear within six to eight weeks of alcohol abstention.

Alcohol-related liver injury is manifest in four ways. Combinations occur but progression from one form to another has neither been clearly documented nor is inevitable.

Fatty liver

The development of a fatty liver probably involves mechanisms other than those producing hepatitis and cirrhosis. Nevertheless, it is present with the other manifestations of alcohol-induced liver damage and it is the most common and often only finding in liver biopsies from alcoholic patients. The fat is seen usually as large cytoplasmic globules within hepatocytes and less often as diffusely dispersed small globules (Fig. 6.14), although the reason for this difference is unknown.

Fatty liver (*steatosis*) arises from an imbalance between the natural constant deposition and removal of fat within the liver. Removal of fat depends upon a number of enzyme pathways including those in the Kreb's cycle. Alcohol depresses these pathways and so slows the removal of fat. The alcohol is degraded to acetaldehyde and acetate and produces, as a by-product, reduced nicotinamide adenine dinucleotide (NADH) which blocks all similar pathways, including those involved in fat metabolism. Since 70–80% of ingested alcohol is metabolized in the liver, particularly the perivenular regions, the site and the degree of steatosis partly reflects the quantity of alcohol ingested. Formerly, malnutrition and the subsequent mobilization of body fat to the liver was believed to be the cause of a fatty liver. Current evidence all indicates that the alcoholic is not severely malnourished and that similar changes cannot be produced by abnormal diets unless alcohol is also present.

Many of the enzymes affected are synthesized within the mitochondria and this may explain the frequency of bizarre and large

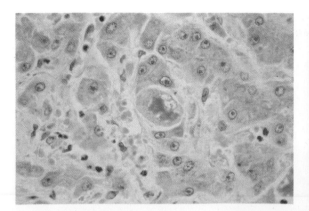

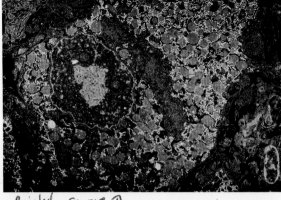

Printed as -ve ↑

Fig. 6.13 Mallory body; (*above left*) hyaline-like material fills much of the cytoplasm of the liver cell; (*above right*) ultrastructural features including the fibrillar pattern. The patient drank heavily and had cirrhosis.

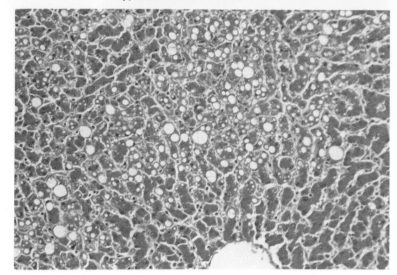

Fig. 6.14 Fatty globules within many liver cells in a biopsy from a patient who was drinking heavily. In this example there are large and small globules.

mitochondria in hepatic cells in alcohol-related liver disease (Fig. 6.15). Any aberration of mitochondrial function would affect the synthetic and secretory functions of the cells, structurally reflected by an increase in the endoplasmic reticulum. This may be a metabolic hyperplasia to compensate for the basic injury to mitochondria, or a response to their inadequate function.

APPEARANCES

Fatty change is seen principally in biopsies taken either to investigate minor derangements of liver function, liver enlargement, or as a part of the investigation of other disorders. At laparotomy or autopsy the liver is enlarged, sometimes massively, and pale (Fig. 6.16). The parenchyma is soft and bulges and fat droplets lie along the cutting knife's surface. Cholestasis, probably secondary to direct compression of the bile canaliculi by the fat-filled liver cells, is unusual but results in yellow-green bile staining. If there is hepatitis and/or cirrhosis, these will dominate the appearances and liver enlargement may not be evident. Neither portal hypertension nor the stigmata of liver failure are common complications of a purely fatty liver.

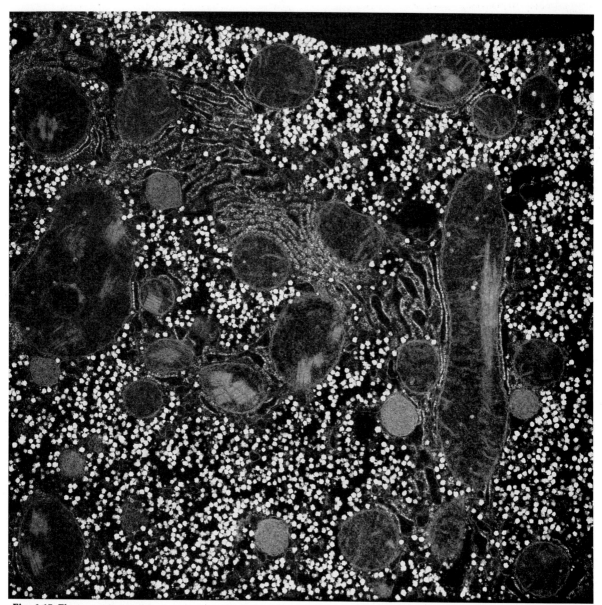

Fig. 6.15 Electron microscopy features of part of the cytoplasm of a liver cell. The mitochondria at the cell membrane border are of normal size while others are enlarged and include a variety of shapes. Many mitochondria also include crystalline inclusion bodies. All these changes occur in association with alcohol injury to the liver.

Hepatitis

This, like fatty change, is found histologically more commonly than is clinically suspected and can revert, structurally and functionally, to normal. Distinction from other causes of hepatitis in the absence of a history of alcohol abuse relies principally on finding Mallory bodies. The hepatitis which follows long periods of alcohol abuse includes changes ranging from focal to extensive necrosis, the latter rapidly resulting in death in over 10% of patients. This poor prognosis can be contributed to by continued drinking, a laparotomy for suspected extrahepatic biliary obstruction, cirrhosis and involvement of the perivenular hepatocytes associated with hyalinization (*central sclerosing hyaline necrosis*).

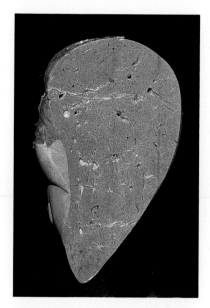

Fig. 6.16 Fatty liver. The liver weighed 2300 g (normal < 1800) and had a greasy parenchyma. The patient was a known alcoholic and had died from an inhalation pneumonia following a bout of drinking.

Hepatitis may follow direct injury to the liver cells from alcohol but the presence of T-cells also suggests an immune reaction. Further evidence for this comes from circulating lymphocytes cytotoxic to liver cells, reduction of peripheral T-cells and, in women especially, increased incidence of non-organ-specific antibodies such as those to smooth muscle. Damage to Kupffer cells with loss of the normal protective antigen filter is one possible way that this sensitization arises. Alternatively, an autoimmune response to proteins released from the damaged hepatocytes, and in particular the Mallory bodies, may be important, especially in perpetuating the injury.

APPEARANCES

These vary from a normal liver to one with scattered pin-point yellow spots, to a deeply jaundiced yellow organ which may or may not harbour cirrhosis. When the involvement is slight there may be no symptoms but generally, although not invariably, more wide-spread liver cell necrosis results in symptoms from cholestasis, liver failure and portal hypertension.

Cirrhosis

This disorder, although popularly believed to be the inevitable consequence of alcohol abuse, develops in less than one-third of heavy drinkers. A high association with HLA B8 implies a genetic predisposition. The time period required varies but is generally between 15 to 20 years and the minimum amount of alcohol in the region of 50 g daily. Abstinence improves survival such that two-thirds of patients survive, but does not lead to regression in the cirrhosis. Even so, a third of patients survive five years with continued drinking.

Direct injury to the liver cells and perpetuation of this by immune destruction, similar to that in alcohol-related hepatitis, are thought to be the essential mechanisms. Additionally there is active fibro-genesis and the vascular architectural changes common to all forms of cirrhosis. These result in a self-perpetuating pattern of changes which will be exacerbated by any further damage to liver cells such as by drugs, viral infection, blood loss and alcohol.

APPEARANCES

These grossly are similar to those of other causes of cirrhosis (Fig. 6.17). The parenchyma, however, particularly in wine drinkers, has a markedly brownish discoloration due to iron deposition.

Complications

Systemic effects of liver failure and portal hypertension usually accompany alcohol induced cirrhosis. Pulmonary infection is common terminally, often reflecting the life style of some individuals but also the hypoproteinaemia and depressed immune responses.

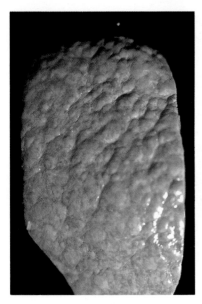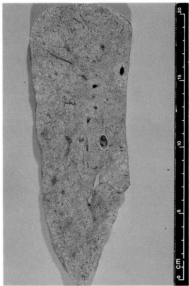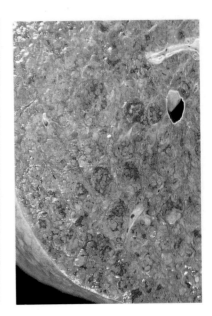

Fig. 6.17 Cirrhosis associated with alcohol; (*above left*) nodular capsular appearance; (*centre*) uniform replacement by nodules and (*above right*) close-up of the nodules.

Alcohol-related diseases, in particular pancreatitis and cardiomyopathy, may also be found at autopsy. Atherosclerosis, however, may not be as severe or diffuse as expected for the patient's age and sex, but why this is so is not apparent.

Liver cell carcinoma

This does not differ from hepatocellular carcinoma of non-alcoholics. It appears only after the cirrhosis is fully developed and then only in 5–15% of these patients. The progression to neoplasia from regenerative liver nodules is clearly a possibility.

Cirrhosis

Cirrhosis is the final, although not inevitable, result of numerous hepatic disorders and as such represents end-stage organ disease. The initiating factors and incidence vary among different populations according to their social habits and their exposure to hepatotoxic agents (Fig. 6.18). Alcohol-related cirrhosis is common in the Western world whereas Hepatitis B virus-associated liver disease is a more common basis among the developing countries. In its early stages there may be no clinical or biochemical derangement, but with time liver failure, portal hypertension and their complications appear. Death at this stage may be delayed, even for years, if the cause of the cirrhosis, particularly alcohol, can be removed, so arresting the progression of the disorder. *Latent* or *compensated cirrhosis* thus occurs. No cirrhosis, however, is reversible and claims for this are unsubstantiated.

The lesion is diffuse fibrosis with parenchymal nodules and loss of the normal liver architecture. Implicit is necrosis and regeneration of liver cells, although these may not be evident and do not

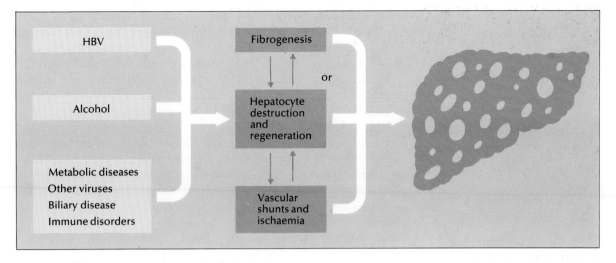

Fig. 6.18 Cirrhosis.

occur either in direct proportion to one another or in immediate sequence. The architectural distortion affects the liver's vasculature with the development of direct shunts between the portal and systemic systems and consequent ischaemia. This in turn aggravates hepatocyte damage and encourages the self-perpetuating nature of the disorder. Haemorrhage, infection and other hepatotoxic agents will have similar effects.

Classification

Morphological classifications have not been entirely successful. That most commonly used is between *micronodular* and *macronodular cirrhosis*, the distinction depending upon the presence of nodules of predominantly less or more than 3 mm diameter, respectively. Unfortunately, cirrhosis with nodules of widely differing diameters is also encountered and nodular variation is part of the evolving spectrum of the disorder. Further, no pattern is specific to any one cause and consequently the classification gives no precise diagnostic information. In addition, macronodular cirrhosis, especially, can be very difficult to recognize in needle biopsy specimens.

Development

1 For cirrhosis to develop, liver cell necrosis must be initiated and, importantly, perpetuated. A patient with alcohol-related hepatitis who stops alcohol abuse and liver cell injury may not develop cirrhosis but for those who continue to drink there is a much greater likelihood of cirrhosis appearing. Once cirrhosis is established withdrawing the cause will not reverse its self-perpetuating nature.

Hepatocyte necrosis stimulates liver cell regeneration although exactly how is unknown. Regeneration does not necessarily proceed at the same pace as the liver cell necrosis. This is particularly evident in early stages of alcohol-related cirrhosis where little regeneration is apparent in contrast to later stages where this is dominant. The regeneration in cirrhosis is imperfect, in that normal liver cell parenchymal appearances are not produced.

2　Fibrous tissue in the liver includes Type I and Type III collagen. Type III collagen initially appears after hepatic injury and is later replaced by Type I collagen. The proportions of each are probably similar in the normal and the cirrhotic liver, although the quantity in the cirrhotic liver is obviously greater. Collagen can be synthesized by a wide range of cells including fibroblasts, macrophages and smooth muscle cells, but within the liver perisinusoidal Ito cells are probably also important. Active fibrogenesis is the main cause of the fibrosis in cirrhosis. Cell death may also provide a stimulus, as may the release of lymphokines associated with the chronic inflammatory cell infiltrate. Collapse of the liver framework from cell loss is a further, although small, contributor to the diffuse fibrosis.

3　Vascular pathways form in the fibrosis that eventually links the portal tracts and terminal hepatic veins. This provides direct contact between the portal and venous outflow systems and thereby deprives the hepatocytes of portal blood perfusion. These shunts can divert as much as 80% of portal blood from the liver cells and indirectly result in the disgorging of toxins, metabolites and antigens directly into the systemic circulation which must partly contribute to the infections experienced by cirrhotics. Similar direct channels form between the hepatic arteries and the terminal hepatic veins with the important result that oxygen supply to the liver cells is reduced. The combined effect of these vascular alterations is to deprive the liver cells of their nutrition and oxygenation and so contribute to degeneration and necrosis. The effective functional liver cell mass is thus less than the anatomical cell mass, an effect further aggravated by any hepatotoxic agent. Added embarrassment to the normal blood flow comes from collapse and compression of the liver sinusoids and larger venous channels secondary to liver cell loss, increasing fibrosis and expanding regenerating nodules. The principal extrahepatic effect of these vascular alterations is portal hypertension with varices and splenic enlargement.

APPEARANCES

Nodularity of the liver is the basis of the diagnosis macroscopically (Fig. 6.19). Each nodule is brownish but this may be altered by any fat accumulation, jaundice or excessive iron. Each nodule is surrounded by silver-grey bands of fibrous tissue (Fig. 6.20).

The early stages associated with some causes are marked by uniformly small nodules (up to 3 mm in diameter) (micronodular cirrhosis). At this stage destruction is the dominant process and the liver is smaller than normal. As regeneration gathers pace a macronodular pattern develops with loss of the uniformity of the nodules, their enlargement and an increase in liver size. Close examination can reveal the altered relationships of the portal and terminal hepatic vein regions and foci of necrosis and haemorrhage. Later, when

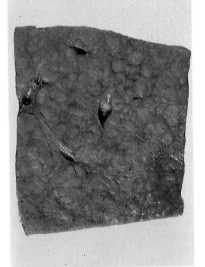

Fig. 6.19 Cirrhosis in a haemophiliac, probably due to Non A, Non B hepatitis virus.

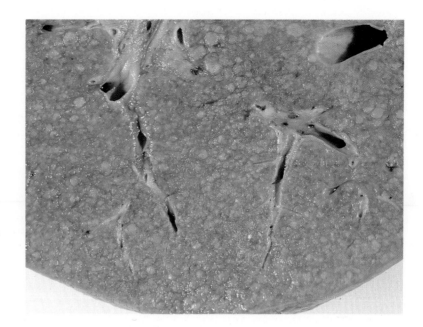

Fig. 6.20 Cirrhosis following a past history of Hepatitis B virus infection. The patient was deeply jaundiced and this is the cause of the green staining in the liver. The variably sized pale yellow to white nodules are liver and the intervening tissue fibrosis.

fibrosis predominates, the liver becomes smaller and is then referred to as a *'hob-nail'* liver with bulging regenerative nodules separated by broad bands of scar tissue. An associated liver cell carcinoma may be obvious because of the size of the tumour and difference in colour and texture. However, in some livers the tumour is indistinguishable from the cirrhosis and is only appreciated after light microscopy.

Complications

Gastrointestinal haemorrhage is a common cause of death among cirrhotics and may arise from ruptured oesophageal or gastric varices and also from peptic ulcers and gastritis. The oesophageal varices (Fig. 6.21) are a result of portal hypertension and can accompany varices in gastric submucosa, mesenteric veins, abdominal wall and haemorrhoidal venous plexus, all of which are more apparent at laparotomy than autopsy. Splenomegaly accompanies these findings. When death is due to liver failure, haemorrhage can be more widespread and is then influenced by defective coagulation from the impaired hepatic synthesis of clotting factors. Ascites is the result of portal hypertension and defective liver cell function. These alter the flow of lymph, protein synthesis and electrolytic balance, all of which can be, in addition, adversely affected by diet and diuretic therapy. Infection, primarily from defective Kupffer cell filtration and function and depressed immune responses, is another common complication. Septicaemias without a primary source of infection are well recognized as is infection in the lungs, influenced by ascites and impaired chest movements. Renal failure develops and is manifest by enlarged and often pale or jaundiced kidneys — the renal features of the hepatorenal syndrome.

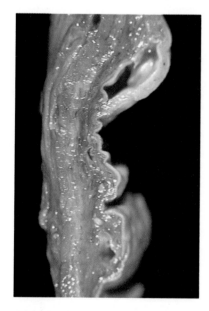

Fig. 6.21 Oesophageal varices: the spaces in the wall below the luminal surface are the varices.

Tumours

Benign and malignant primary liver tumours are rare in the UK (Table 6.9). Metastatic tumour, in contrast, is common. World-wide, however, liver cell carcinoma is one of the most common cancers. The frequency and distribution closely relate to that of the Hepatitis B virus and there is a strikingly high incidence in men. Cavernous haemangiomas are the most common benign tumours.

Table 6.9 Common liver tumours

Benign	Malignant
Liver cell adenoma	Liver cell carcinoma
Bile duct adenoma	Cholangiocarcinoma
Haemangioma	
	Angiosarcoma
	Hepatoblastoma

Metastatic tumours

Any primary tumour can metastasize to the liver. This is mainly via the portal and systemic vasculature but a lymphatic route is occasionally involved. Hepatic metastases occur in at least a third of disseminated tumours and lymph node metastases are also invariably found. Lung, breast and large bowel carcinomas are the most common primary sources. In many patients the metastases are symptomless but in others there is liver enlargement and mildly impaired liver function. The patient's prognosis once metastases are recognized is between 12–18 months although metastatic carcinoid, diagnosed from the carcinoid syndrome, does not hold such a poor outlook.

APPEARANCES

The liver can vary in size from normal to grossly enlarged and the tumour from a few scattered nodules to virtual replacement of the entire organ. The tumour is seen on the surface as well as within the substance and occurs as rounded, often umbilicated, masses of varying size (Fig. 6.22). Haemorrhage and necrosis complicate the larger nodules which also coalesce.

Liver cell carcinoma

This tumour is distributed throughout the world but especially in the Far East and Africa. It is associated with a number of factors but most particularly the Hepatitis B virus and cirrhosis (Table 6.10). The rise in alcoholic cirrhosis in Britain has been paralleled by an increase in incidence. The frequency in men is 3–9 times that of women. The age range is 30–40 years in the Far East in contrast to of 50–60 years in the West. The 5-year prognosis is nil with the majority of patients dying within 6 months from diagnosis.

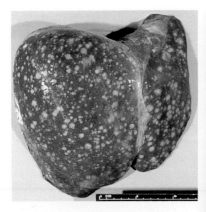

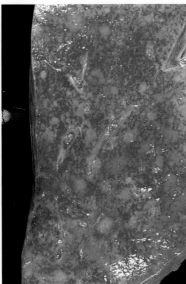

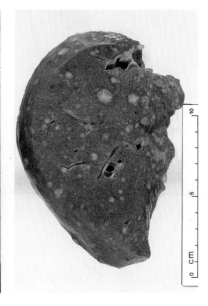

Fig. 6.22 Metastatic tumour in the liver from a primary; (*above left*) in the colon; (*centre*) in the breast and (*above right*) in the lung. These appearances are not specific for these primary tumours but demonstrate the variable appearances and involvement that can occur with any metastatic tumour.

1 Hepatitis B virus: evidence relating this virus and liver cell carcinoma stems from a wide range of studies and is believed to indicate a 90% association in some countries. An implication is that mass Hepatitis B virus vaccination allied with improved hygiene and health measures could, within 20 years, largely eradicate liver cell carcinoma. The relationship depends on the following.

(a) Geographical distribution of the tumour mirrors that of Hepatitis B virus infection, although not all populations are equally involved. The Chinese in Malaysia, an area with a high rate of Hepatitis B virus infection, have considerably more liver cell cancer than Malays and Indians, as do Chinese in the USA, a region of relatively low Hepatitis B virus prevalence.

(b) Patients with liver cell carcinoma have a higher incidence of all markers of the virus in their serum and in their liver cells than controls. The viral antigens can usually only be demonstrated in non-neoplastic cells.

Table 6.10 Patterns of liver cell carcinoma

Population	UK, USA	Sub-Sahara, Far East
Age (years)	60−80	40−50
Sex	>Male	≫Female
Cirrhosis	Macronodular	Macro- and micronodular
Main cause	Cirrhosis and alcohol	Chronic HBV Aflatoxin
Clinical presentation	Cirrhosis	Tumour
Alpha-fetoprotein	++	+++
Course	Fulminant	Rapid

(c) Integrated Hepatitis B virus DNA has been demonstrated within the nuclei of some liver cell tumours. In these there is also always integrated viral DNA in non-tumour liver cells.

(d) Patients with cirrhosis and chronic active hepatitis, both of which are linked with Hepatitis B virus infection, are at increased risk for liver cell carcinoma.

(e) Prospective studies of HBs Ag carriers, most notably in Taiwan, indicated a risk of liver cell carcinoma 340 times that of the non-carrier, a figure substantially higher than that relating cigarettes and lung cancer. Similar studies from Japan showed a significantly high incidence of liver cell cancer amongst HBs Ag positive cirrhotics and, from Senegal and Korea, that HBs Ag carriers were more common among the mothers of such patients than controls.

(f) A tumour cell line has been cultured which secretes HBsAg and has only integrated viral DNA in the nucleus.

(g) Woodchucks, ground squirrels and Chinese domestic ducks all spontaneously develop liver cell cancer and all suffer infection from viruses synonymous to the Hepatitis B virus. Incorporation of viral DNA from the Woodchuck virus has been demonstrated within the tumour cells and within liver cells prior to the appearance of the carcinoma.

All these observations clearly implicate Hepatitis B virus in some if not most liver cell carcinomas. Integration of the virus into the hepatocyte genome is the key event preceding the carcinoma. It is thus suggested that this will eventually occur close to a cellular oncogene, so impairing the normal growth mechanisms and thereby allowing the emergence of less mature, longer living and more highly replicating cells. Neoplastic transformation could then be triggered and, with further division, the emergence of a carcinoma. This hypothesis explains the association of liver cell carcinoma with long-term HBsAg carriers and, since these are principally men, the observation that most liver cell cancer patients are male. It also provides an explanation for the relationship with cirrhosis, because actively dividing cells will increase the chances of viral DNA integration. The finding of alpha-fetoprotein among the liver tumour cells indicates that immature rapidly dividing cells are involved.

2 Cirrhosis: an association between non-Hepatitis B virus cirrhosis and liver cell carcinoma is recognized. Over two-thirds of the patients in the UK will have alcohol-related cirrhosis and most are male. The cirrhosis is well established with regenerative nodules and the tumour is often multicentric. Dysplastic cells, among both non-neoplastic liver cells and in early cirrhosis, support the concept that the cancer arises from an aberration of regeneration.

3 Other factors: aflatoxin is the toxin from *Aspergillus flavus* which contaminates ground nuts, a stable part of the diet of a large number of Africans. It is clearly related to liver cell cancer both among domestic turkeys and in experimental studies. *Haemochromatosis*, a condition associated with increased iron absorption, and the high iron content of the diets of some Africans are also co-factors in some patients.

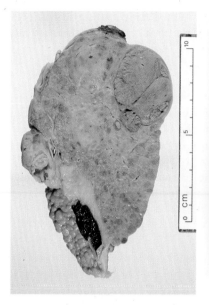
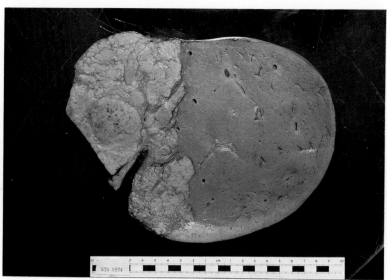

Fig. 6.23 Liver cell carcinoma; (*above right*) in a liver without cirrhosis and— (*above left*) in a liver with cirrhosis.

APPEARANCES

The tumour is seen both as a single mass, most often in the non-cirrhotic liver, and as a multinodular and multifocal tumour when related with cirrhosis (Fig. 6.23). Multicentric tumours in non-cirrhotic livers in Africa demonstrate that this division is not absolute. The distinction between a multifocal primary tumour and a primary growth with intrahepatic spread may not always be possible but when one nodule is notably larger than its fellows and these lie as satellites, intrahepatic spread is more likely. Differentiation from metastatic carcinoma in these circumstances can be aided by the presence of bile, a feature of a minority of liver cell carcinomas, and by the demonstration of alpha-fetoprotein and alpha-1-antitrypsin within liver tumour cells. Raised serum alpha-fetoprotein levels also occur in just over one-quarter of patients with liver cell carcinoma.

The liver is enlarged and the right lobe affected more than the left. Bile production or obstruction to bile flow within or outside the liver can lead to bile staining of the tumour and of the liver. If cirrhosis is present, this is invariably of the macronodular type.

Spread. Intravascular spread is very common with a 95% incidence in some angiographic studies, and accounts for the extrahepatic spread to the lungs in 60–80% of patients at death. Lymphatic spread with portal lymph node involvement is seen in about one-third of patients but seedling spread into the peritoneum is rare.

Complications

Death may follow from hepatic failure, infection or gastrointestinal haemorrhage. Portal hypertension from venous occlusion by the tumour and the subsequent appearance of varices and bleeding diatheses from liver failure are all factors contributing to haemorrhage. Intra-abdominal rupture of the tumour is an unusual event.

Cholangiocarcinoma

This carcinoma forms one in five primary liver tumours and, apart from in South East Asia, is much less common than liver cell carcinoma. The tumour arises from the biliary epithelium and affects both sexes equally with a maximum incidence at 60—70 years. Liver fluke (*Clonorchis sinensis*) infection is a pathogenetic agent in Asia but in the majority of patients no causative factors have emerged. Neither gall-stones nor cirrhosis are related.

APPEARANCES

The tumour is a slowly growing adenocarcinoma. It is often associated with substantial fibrosis which can, in X-ray studies and biopsy specimens, cause confusion with sclerosing cholangitis. The tumour may be confined within the liver, to the hilum of the liver or to the common bile duct or its intrapancreatic portion. In the latter site it may be difficult to distinguish from a carcinoma of the ampulla of Vater. Metastases within the lungs, bones and lymph nodes are seen in approximately half the patients autopsied.

Metabolic disorders

Congenital disorders associated with abnormalities of the normal metabolic pathways are rare and may be confined to the liver or

Table 6.11 Examples of metabolic disorders

Disorder	Inheritance	Marker in liver cell	Liver involvement	Non-hepatic features
Alpha-1-antitrypsin deficiency (AlAT)	Autosomal co-dominant	AlAT globules	40—50% of childhood cirrhosis and hepatitis Cirrhosis in adults Liver cell carcinoma	Emphysema Pancreatitis
Cystic fibrosis/ Mucoviscidosis	Recessive	Mucin plugs in intrahepatic bile ducts	Biliary fibrosis and cirrhosis Increased mucus in bile secretions	Bronchitis Increased sweat chloride Malabsorption
Wilson's disease	Recessive	Copper Mallory bodies	Chronic active hepatitis Fatty Cirrhosis	Corneal Kayser—Fleischer rings CNS features
Haemochromatosis	Recessive	Iron	Cirrhosis Liver cell carcinoma	Iron deposition in heart and pancreas
Glycogen storage disease (10 types)	Recessive	Glycogen	Cirrhosis	Differing organs depending upon the pattern of enzyme deficiency

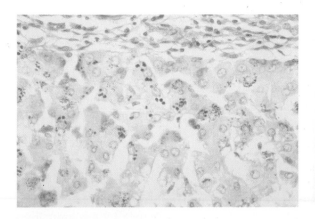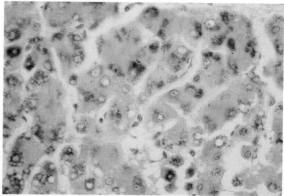

Fig. 6.24 Alpha-1-antitrypsin in a liver demonstrated (*above left*) non-specifically as diastase resistant periodic acid positive granules and (*above right*) specifically with labelled antibody.

associated with similar biochemical defects in other organs (Table 6.11). They can be revealed by liver biopsy but structural changes are not always present. In some there is a non-specific accumulation of fat and, rarely in others, diagnostic substances such as alpha-1-antitrypsin (*alpha-1-antitrypsin deficiency*) (Fig. 6.24) and copper (*Wilson's disease*). The basic cause for the individual defect in most patients remains unknown although many are autosomal recessive disorders.

APPEARANCES

The liver may remain macroscopically normal or develop hepatitis, fibrosis and even cirrhosis.

Further reading

Hall, P. (1985). *Alcoholic Liver Disease:Pathobiology, Epidemiology, and Clinical Aspects*. Edward Arnold: London.

Lieber, C.S. (1977). Pathogenesis of alcoholic liver disease: an overview. In: *Alcohol and the Liver*. Ed. by Fisher, M.M., Rankin, J.G. pp. 197–259. New York: Plenum Press.

London, W.T. (1981). Primary hepatocellular carcinoma — etiology, pathogenesis and prevention. *Hum. Pathol.* **12**, 1985–97.

MacSween, R.N.M., Anthony, P.P. and Scheuer, P.J. (1987) (Editors). *Pathology of the Liver* (2nd Edition). Churchill Livingstone: Edinburgh.

Wright, R., Millward-Sadler, G.H., Alberti, K.G.M.M. and Karran, S. (1985) (Editors). *Liver and Biliary disease. Pathophysiology, Diagnosis and Management* (2nd Edition). W.B. Saunders Co. Ltd.: London, Philadelphia, Toronto.

7 Pancreas

Pancreatic disorders are manifest predominantly by dysfunction of the exocrine or endocrine component and rarely by a combination of both. Nevertheless these two functions are closely interrelated and careful testing of each in any pancreatic disorder can reveal unsuspected abnormalities. In diabetes mellitus, the most important endocrine abnormality, subtle degrees of malabsorption are sometimes found indicating exocrine involvement; conversely, in pancreatitis there is evidence of altered glucose metabolism. Systemic complications form an important part of any pancreatic disorder and also reflect the endocrine and exocrine functions as well as the importance of normal pancreatic function.

The pancreas, lying between the stomach and the vertebral column, is not directly accessible for clinical examination and biopsies may produce fistulae or infection. Fine needle aspiration overcomes some of these difficulties and modern radiological techniques provide methods for localizing disorders. Confirmation of these may come from the demonstration of biochemical changes although many are non-specific. All these factors contribute to delay in recognizing some pancreatic disorders and are a major factor behind the high mortality of pancreatic cancer.

Pancreatitis

Inflammatory disease of the pancreas has many causes but is most often due to either biliary calculi or an excess of alcohol. The disease is manifest clinically by the extremes of acute and chronic disease with a common end result of destruction, principally of the exocrine tissues. The two clinical extremes may not represent one but two disorders, a viewpoint supported by the differences in age distribution, cause and natural history (Table 7.1). Even so, the division is not absolute and the patient with chronic disease can experience acute disease, and vice versa. Recognition can be difficult and the diagnosis is often missed since there is no single specific investigation or even group of investigations.

Causative factors (Fig. 7.1)

1 *Autodigestion.* Although the pathogenesis is uncertain the final event is the release of pancreatic enzymes with local and even systemic autodigestion. This process is normally protected against

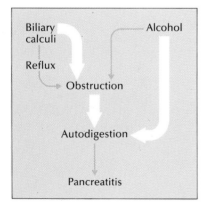

Fig. 7.1 Pathways for injury in pancreatitis.

by synthesis of these enzymes as inactive forms separated from the cytoplasm by membranes and seen as *zymogen granules*. In addition protease inhibitors occur in the acinar cells, the pancreatic secretions and the serum, which antagonize the active enzymes. Beta-2-macroglobulin and alpha-1-antitrypsin are two such agents, and deficiencies of either can, in rare instances, result in pancreatitis. The continuous flow within the pancreatic duct associated with mucus secretion also reduces the opportunity for autodigestion.

2 *Obstruction.* Experimentally, obstruction from ligation of the main pancreatic duct can produce pancreatitis and this mechanism is thought to contribute to the pancreatitis associated with gall-stones. Biliary calculi (Fig. 7.2) may produce pancreatitis either by direct blockage of the ducts with secondary fibrosis and stenosis or by inducing spasm. This is especially so if the obstruction is within the common bile duct or beyond this, rather than in the cystic or hepatic ducts. In addition the increased intraduct pressure from obstruction may contribute to pancreatitis, as demonstrated in dogs. If obstruction is important, stones should be found in the biliary tree of most patients. Surgical and autopsy studies have only shown small increases in incidence but a careful analysis of stools reveals stones eight times more frequently in pancreatitis patients than in controls. Further compelling evidence of an association with obstruction is that removal of the calculi or relieving any obstruction cures many patients.

Table 7.1 Classification of pancreatitis

Type	Clinical course	Age group	Major cause	Natural history
Acute Acute relapsing	Severe fulminant	60−70	Gall-stones 60%	Rapid death or complete return of normal function
Chronic Chronic relapsing	Mild to severe	30−40	Alcohol 40%	Permanent, often progressive, changes in function

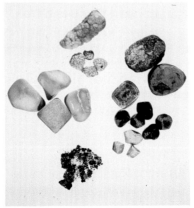 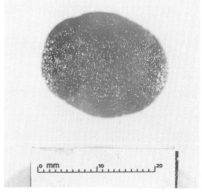

Fig. 7.2 Gall-stones, an important cause of pancreatitis. (*Left*) Mixed types and pigment types (bottom). There is a wide spectrum of appearances to the mixed types. These are formed from calcium salts which are deposited in layers as seen in the sectioned calculus centre. (*Right*) Cholesterol type. These are opaque, generally large and single.

3 *Anatomical features.* The anatomy of the opening of the pancreatic duct may affect the appearance of the disorder. A wide range of variations occurs although the most common are entry of the pancreatic duct to the duodenum either via a pathway shared with the common bile duct or a separate but parallel entry with the common bile duct. The particular anatomical pattern will affect the localization of any obstruction and affect the reflux of pancreatic secretions and bile into the pancreatic duct.

4 *Reflux.* Calculi, spasm or some of the anatomical variants of the opening of the pancreatic duct may all predispose to reflux of either bile or pancreatic juice or both. Refluxed juices first damage the lining of the ducts and later the supplying acini. The bile has a detergent effect and releases, and thus activates, the pancreatic enzymes.

5 *Alcohol.* Alcohol given to animals either as single large doses or as repeated doses over long periods produces effects on the pancreas that are not directly analogous to those in man. Random alcohol loading reduces pancreatic secretions while chronic administration increases the protein content. The protein content does, however, diminish with a persistent alcohol intake over several years while the water and bicarbonate concentrations increase. None of the these changes are directly produced within the pancreas but are probably mediated via the cholinergic nervous system and gastrin secretion. In man, the earliest change related with alcohol is that of hyaline protein-rich casts within the ducts. This result could obviously arise from changes in the secretions analogous to those observed experimentally. The casts may produce obstruction and reflux as well as provide a focus for calcification and stone formation via the formation of esters.

The amount of alcohol needed to produce pancreatitis is quoted as 150−170 g of pure alcohol per day, which is equivalent to 4−7 pints of beer or 14 measures of spirit. Nevertheless there is individual variation, just as there is in the development of alcohol-associated cirrhosis. The younger age group with pancreatitis compared to that for alcoholic cirrhosis indicates a shorter period of alcohol abuse and estimates vary between 16 to 18 years in contrast to the average 30-year period that precedes liver damage. Epidemiological support for a role for alcohol revolves around the high incidence of pancreatitis in areas where alcohol abuse is highest. The disease occurs more in cities and, within the UK, more in Glasgow and Edinburgh than London. There is a high prevalence in the Skid Row area in New York and amongst the wine drinking communities, especially the French. Pancreatitis is an occupational hazard for publicans and those in the brewing industry.

6 *Miscellaneous.* A range of other factors are recognized with some in contrast to those discussed, primarily affecting the acinar cells and others with no clear site of injury (Table 7.2).

Development

Biliary calculi, reflux of secretions and alcohol can initiate autodigestion and, in some patients, all three factors may be to blame.

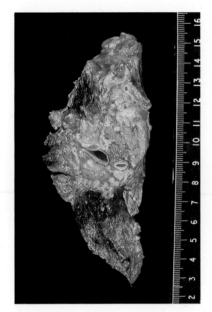

Fig. 7.3 TS of a pancreas with acute pancreatitis. The black areas include altered blood from haemorrhage, and the yellow and white regions, necrosis. The main duct (centre) is patent.

All the many pancreatic enzymes can be involved and, while *in vitro* a distinct effect for each is demonstrable (Table 7.3), the tissue changes are the end product of their combined action. Autodigestion necessitates a breakdown in the balance between activators and inhibitors and the release of trypsin from trypsinogen. Trypsin activates most of the other enzymes both within the acinar cells as well as in the tissues and serum. The clotting and fibrinolytic systems are similarly affected and local and systemic changes follow.

APPEARANCES

These depend very much upon the stage at which the organ is examined. Oedema is most obvious in the early stages of the acute disorder and haemorrhage and necrosis later (Fig. 7.3). Descriptive terms such as acute interstitial and acute haemorrhagic pancreatitis have been used for these but they contribute little if anything to an understanding of the disorder. All the changes, as well as the concomitant cellular infiltrate, cause enlargement of the gland which may either be localized or widespread. The necrosis produces a characteristic yellow colour and calcification not infrequently follows. Calculi within the biliary tract or the ducts of the head of the pancreas should be looked for.

Table 7.2 Causes of pancreatitis with postulated sites of action

Viruses (2.4% of mumps; ? Coxsackie)	
Drugs (steroids; thiazides; azathioprine;? contraceptive pill)	
Ischaemia (polyarteritis)	Acinar injury
Nutritional deficiency	
Trauma (incl. post-operative, endoscopy and post-gastrectomy)	
Gall-stones	
Cystic fibrosis	Duct obstruction
Alcohol	
Hereditary factors (congenital–familial)	
Hypercalcaemia	Unknown
Hyperlipidaemia	

Table 7.3 Pancreatic enzymes and their principal actions

Trypsin	Shock, proteolysis, coagulopathies; kinin release
Chymotrypsin	Proteolysis
Elastase	Proteolysis, elastolysis; haemorrhage
Lipase	Fat necrosis, hypocalcaemia
Phospholipase A	Phospholipid hydrolysis; lysolecithin formation; shock lung
Kallikrein	Kinin release
Kinin; histamine	Oedema; pain; vasodilation shock; increase of vascular permeability
Myocardial depressant factor	Reduced cardiac output

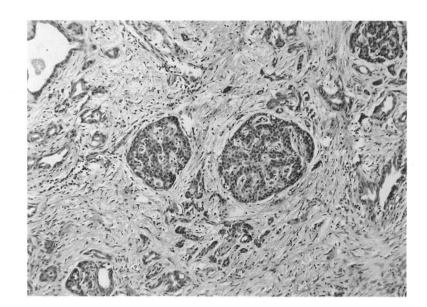

Fig. 7.4 End effects of chronic pancreatitis. Only the islets are recognizable. The acinar tissue and ducts are almost entirely replaced by fibrous tissue.

If chronic pancreatitis is present the gland is small, hard and extremely tough (Fig. 7.4). The ducts may be dilated and cysts found. Within the ducts there may be calculi. Superimposed acute changes may also be present.

Complications

Local complications include pseudocyst formation. A pseudocyst, in contrast to a true cyst, is one in which there is no epithelium. These cysts develop within the pancreas, retroperitoneally and anteriorly between the pancreas and stomach, duodenum and colon. Infection and abscess formation can supervene. Fat necrosis locally in the mesentery, omentum and peritoneum is invariable in acute disease (Fig. 7.5). This may be associated with calcification and a brownish, protein-rich, peritoneal fluid, an ideal medium for the growth of organisms. Endocrine involvement may contribute to hyperglycaemia but this is partly due to release of stress hormones and partly to islet dysfunction.

Systemically kidney, liver, lung and heart failure with effusions and thrombosis can all appear. The underlying mechanisms are complex with shock, disseminated intravascular coagulation and dispersed pancreatic enzymes all playing a role. Additionally, in the lungs surfactant may be altered, hyaline membranes form and adult respiratory distress syndrome result. The impaired respiratory movements from the abdominal distension and the pain of the disease will also contribute to infection and progressive respiratory distress. Malabsorption is inevitable in chronic disease but persisting diabetes mellitus is uncommon. Hypocalcaemia can develop in acute pancreatitis from the loss of calcium within the foci of fat necrosis as well as from changes between extracellular and intracellular calcium. Hypoproteinaemia results principally from protein

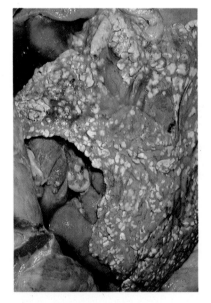

Fig. 7.5 Fat necrosis in the greater omentum complicating acute pancreatitis. There are similar changes in the fat around the caecum and colon (right).

loss into the peritoneum but will also be affected by liver and kidney failure and contributes substantially to infection.

Cancer is rare except in familial chronic pancreatitis. This disorder is associated with a 20% incidence of malignancy and it may be suspected from the young age of the patient.

Diabetes mellitus

Diabetes mellitus was recognized long before the modern era of medicine and was recorded by Hippocrates and described amongst Hindu civilizations. The isolation of insulin dramatically altered the outlook for many of the sufferers but has, in turn, opened the way for the widespread complications of the disorder to appear. These, rather than the immediate metabolic consequences, are the cause of the present morbidity and mortality of the disease. Attempts to reduce both have stimulated a search for better control by such means as transplantation, immunosuppression and improved insulin administration including continuous insulin infusion, all aimed at reproducing the normal biochemical profile of glucose. As a consequence, knowledge of the pathogenesis of the disorder and of its complications has increased. Even so, an acceptable definition of diabetes is still elusive since differences between normal and abnormal blood glucose levels are arbitrary. In the future, diagnosis and definitions may depend more upon immunological findings and DNA abnormalities which provide markers for the disorder.

Classification

These have been subject to numerous changes mainly because of valid criticisms of the inexact criteria applied. Uniform to all the terminology suggested has been the division into primary, when there is no other disease present, and secondary diabetes, when other disorders are the cause (Table 7.4). The primary group is currently subdivided into two main types, Types I and II. Type I diabetics can be further subdivided according to the principle postulated cause. In Type I(a), the classical juvenile form, viruses may be primarily involved while in Type I(b), autoimmune mechanisms predominate.

Pancreatic islets. These can be studied immunocytochemically by light and electron microscopy (Fig. 7.6). Labelled antibodies to the hormones of all four main cell types show that each cell synthesizes only a single hormone (Fig. 7.7). The cells are best referred to by the hormones they produce but the older terminology giving an alphabetical prefix still persists. The cells are arranged in a fixed manner one to another within the islets as lobules separated by vascular spaces in a fashion analogous to the renal glomerulus (Fig. 7.8). This arrangement facilitates paracrine action particularly of somatostatin cells and probably also the balance between release of insulin and its antagonist, glucagon. Insulin cells predominate in the centres of the islets and form 60–80% of each islet's cell

Table 7.4 Classifications of diabetes mellitus

Primary
Type I
  Growth onset
  Juvenile
  Insulin dependent
  Islet cell antibody associated

Type II
  Maturity onset
  Adult
  Non-insulin dependent

Secondary
  Surgical removal (>95%)
  Pancreatitis
  Haemochromatosis
  Mucoviscidosis
  Tumour
  Endocrine disease (Cushing's;
    acromegaly;
    phaeochromocytoma)

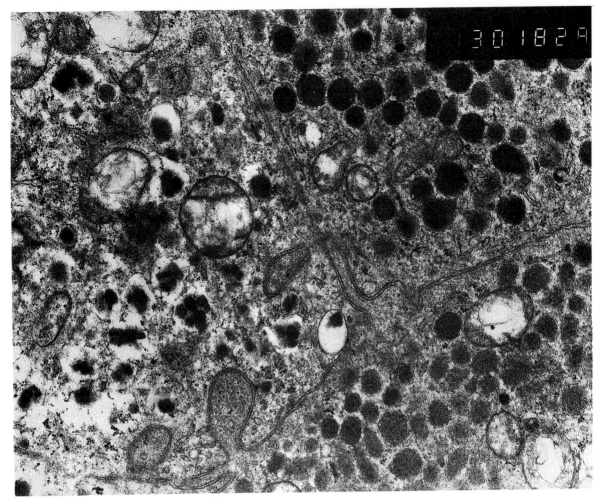

Fig. 7.6 Ultrastructural appearances of islet cell granules. The crystalloid forms are insulin-producing, the dense oval glucagon-producing and the less dense associated with somatostatin.

population. Within the ventral or uncinate lobe of the head of the pancreas, pancreatic polypeptide cells are found in greater numbers than elsewhere; the proportion of other cell types is similar in all regions.

Changes in the numbers of cells occur in diabetes and differ according to the type. A gross reduction in the insulin cells is found in Type I diabetes although the ratios between other cell types are maintained. Insulin replacement is therefore invariably necessary. In Type II diabetes insulin cells are decreased and the glucagon cell mass increased so that treatment may not require insulin. Hormone producing cells develop from the ducts and are occasionally found adjacent to some ducts, a process termed *neoformation*. This phenomenon may compensate for loss of insulin cells and the rarity of mitoses amongst islet cells. Mitoses are seen but the few cells proliferating at any particular time do so rapidly and with age this becomes more infrequent. This poor regenerative response may influence the development of diabetes, especially Type II.

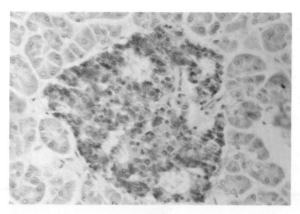 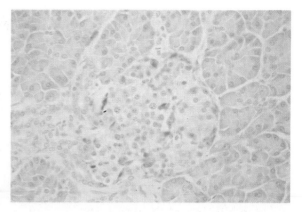

Fig. 7.7 Normal pancreatic islet labelled with antibody to (*above left*) insulin and (*above right*) glucagon. The glucagon-containing cells are arranged peripherally and the insulin cells centrally.

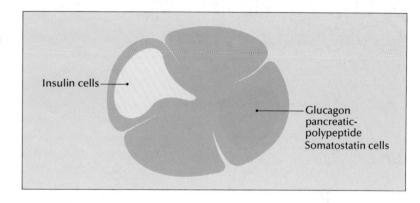

Insulin cells

Glucagon pancreatic-polypeptide Somatostatin cells

Fig. 7.8 Hormone cell distribution in islets.

Causative factors

Type II Diabetes. Type II disease is the most common form of diabetes but is nonetheless largely unexplained. It is a disorder of developed countries and runs in families, although with no HLA pattern. There are no immunological or viral associations. These diabetics are commonly obese and elderly and it has been postulated that the obesity produces insulin resistance and secondly insulin cell exhaustion (Fig. 7.9). This end point may also be reached from insulin cell dysfunction from either age or hereditary factors. Alternatively, it is suggested that either insulin resistance arises from the central nervous system or other extrapancreatic site, since the *in situ* content of insulin in the pancreas is normal, or that the amyloid (Fig. 7.10), often found between the insulin secreting cells and adjacent capillaries, impairs insulin release by disrupting the islet architecture.

Type I Diabetes. Hereditary, immune reactions and virus infection are all believed to play a role in the development of Type I diabetes (Fig. 7.11).
1 *Hereditary factors.* HLA studies clearly show a risk for those with HLA B8 DRW3 or HLA B15 DRW4 and a higher risk for those with both of these haplotypes, such individuals lacking the gene

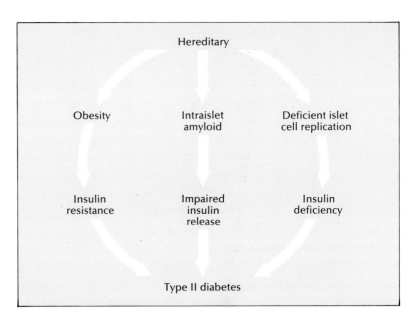

Fig. 7.9 Factors leading to Type II diabetes.

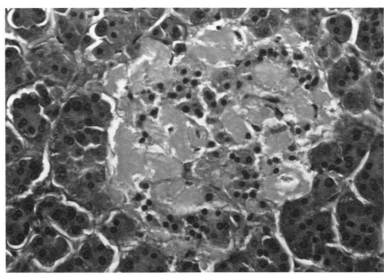

Fig. 7.10 Islet with substantial amyloid deposition, seen as the amorphous eosinophilic material. The patient had Type II diabetes mellitus.

protecting against the disorder. The same HLA patterns are common to autoimmune disorders and provide the link between the hereditary and immune factors involved in Type I diabetes.

2 *Immune factors.* Appearance of circulating antibodies, changes in cell mediated responses and some histopathological findings all clearly implicate humoral and cellular immune reactions in Type I diabetes.

A suggested sequence is that autoantigens appear and, in the presence of an abnormal T-suppressor-cell pathway, these interact with B-cells and complement to destroy the insulin cells. The autoantigens may appear because of either a hereditary predisposition (HLA-associations) or environmental factors (viruses) or both. The

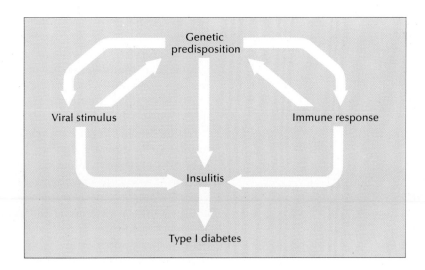

Fig. 7.11 Factors leading to Type I diabetes.

alternative possibility is that the abnormal immune reactions are incidental or secondary to the disorder.

Islet cell antibody is the most important humoral antibody and is found in virtually all patients at diagnosis and at varying periods before and after the onset of the disorder. It is also found in 0.5% of the general population. The antibody, IgG, is against all islet cells and not specifically the insulin cell. There are two types, one against the cell cytoplasm and the other, which is complement fixing, against the cell membrane.

Insulin antibodies develop but are rarely of any clinical significance and are usually secondary to insulin therapy. They should cease to appear as human insulin preparations are more widely adopted. Some, however, do follow certain viral infections and are true auto-antibodies.

Anti-insulin receptor antibodies are even more rare and are largely confined to patients with acanthosis nigricans, a pigmentary skin disorder, and are not associated with Type I diabetes.

Auto-antibodies which reflect the auto-immune status of the disorder appear. They are found mainly in female patients and directed particularly against the adrenals and thyroid with or without clinical manifestations.

Cell mediated responses to both the pancreas and the islets occur but these are of uncertain significance.

Suppressor T-cell levels are persistently higher than in normal subjects, and may be the result of therapy, infections and other complications. They are also, however, seen in identical twins before the development of the disorder.

Lymphoid infiltrates are found during the early stages of the disorder surrounding some islets. These include eosinophil polymorphs but are not associated with plasma cells or follicle formation, in contrast to those in other auto-immune disorders. Similar changes also develop in the pancreases of neonates of diabetic mothers.

Some *immunosuppressive drugs*, particularly Cyclosporine A, produce a transient remission of diabetes both experimentally and clinically.

3 *Viral factors.* The viruses implicated with diabetes are the cytomegalo, mumps, rubella and Coxsackie B viruses. Recently a multinational study has provided no evidence for a role of any of these other than Coxsackie B_4. The study does not resolve the dilemma of whether the diabetic is genetically susceptible to an infection causing the disease or whether the incidental virus infection unmasks the inherent disease. In either event insulin cell damage may also arise from repeated infections from a range of viruses. This would be consistent with the appearance of islet cell antibody years before the onset of diabetes, the viral insult releasing auto-antigens from the islet cells and exciting an auto-immune response. Seasonal incidence, Spring and Autumn, and the young age of onset of the disorder which corresponds with starting school and a wider exposure to viral infections add support to these concepts. Experimentally the M variant of the encephalomyocarditis virus which is similar to the Coxsackie virus produces diabetes.

APPEARANCES

Structurally, without immunocytochemistry, there may be little abnormal in the pancreas whatever the type of diabetes. Immuno-cytochemistry demonstrates the hormones present but lack of stain-ing is not always indicative of absent synthesis. The hormones may be lost prior to examination or none may be stored due to substantial physiological demands. Excessive fat deposition is often remarked upon, especially in the pancreases of Type II diabetics. This also occurs in non-diabetics but is not confined to obese subjects. Similar remarks apply to atherosclerotic changes but when these are in a young person they can be regarded as possibly indicative of dia-betes. If the diabetes is secondary the features of pancreatitis, tumour or haemochromatosis will be found.

Systemic effects and complications

Either type of diabetes mellitus can be complicated by a wide range of changes affecting many different tissues. These changes are, however, more common with Type I diabetes where, because young patients are involved, the consequences are often more debilitating. Apart from the association with diabetes no other genetic factors are involved. The relationship between complications and severity, as measured by insulin dosage, and the effectiveness of control of the disorder, as judged from urine and blood levels of glucose and ketones, is not always clear-cut. Patients with brittle diabetes, a form extremely difficult to control, often produce few complications while others with apparently well-controlled diabetes may develop a wide spectrum of complications. Conscientious urine testing and appropriate insulin dosage together with strict adherence to diet have not been uniformly associated with a decreased incidence of complications. This observation may reflect our lack of understanding of the normal physiological and biochemical carbohydrate metabolism or equally the ineffectiveness of modern therapy in replacing these responses. The only factor clearly related to the appearance of complications is the age at diagnosis of the disease. More complications can be anticipated in a young patient and then often at a fairly short interval after the onset. Pregnancy may lead to a worsening of established complications as well as the appearance of others.

Infection, renal disorders and a micro- and macro-angiopathy are the most important complications but tumours and non-specific changes can also afflict the patient and cause death.

1 *Infection*. This remains an important cause of diabetic coma despite antibiotics. All micro-organisms are potentially involved but some of the most common are staphylococcal and *Candida* infections. Tuberculosis, a frequent hazard in the past, still appears. Why diabetics should be the subjects of increased infection is not clear but a number of factors probably contribute. Among these are:

(a) the patient's nutritional status with a negative nitrogen balance and impaired protein synthesis;
(b) relative dehydration, so removing any dilution effect on organisms as well as impeding antibody responses;
(c) reduced macrophage activity and impaired immunoglobulin production and T-cell responses;
(d) vascular insufficiency from the micro- and macroangiopathy.

Excess glycogen within the tissues is commonly believed to be important since this may act as a medium for micro-organisms and facilitate their growth. This contribution is probably over-stressed since glycogen is not important for either staphylococcal or tuberculous infections; it may play a role in the incidence of *Candida* infections.

2 *Renal disorders*. Urinary tract infections, hypertensions and a specific glomerular disorder (diabetic glomerulosclerosis), as well as glomerulonephritis in any of its forms, develop and any of these may occur alone or in combination. Potentially they can all lead to renal failure but this most often follows from diabetic glomerulosclerosis.

Urinary tract infection. In female diabetics this is said to be twice as common as in non-diabetic women. When the kidneys are involved there is a high incidence of bilateral papillary necrosis. An autonomic neuropathy affecting the bladder and its emptying is a significant underlying factor in some patients.

Hypertension. The effects are comparable with those in the non-diabetic. Similar causes also apply but additionally there is the impact of micro- and macro-angiopathy. Whether there is increased incidence is contested amongst different authorities, in part depending upon the definitions used, the populations studied and the presence of other renal disorders.

Diabetic glomerulosclerosis or the Kimmelsteil—Wilson kidney. This is the renal disorder that is unique to diabetes mellitus, occurring in both types although more common in the Type I disorder.

The cause(s) remains unclear although the disorder is widely regarded as a manifestation of micro-angiopathy. A sequence of functional changes can be correlated with the structural and clinical sequelae. Local plasma flow increases corresponding with dilatation of arterioles and altered basement membrane permeability. This is reflected by enlarged kidneys, a change involving all parts of the nephron but with no increase in the basement membrane thickness. The urine includes albumen and the condition is incompletely reversible. Only one-third of diabetics in this stage progress to the second phase which is clinically silent. During this, basement membrane thickening and vascular hyalinization develop and progress and there is also some increase in the mesangial matrix. The final phase occurs in about 30% of diabetics. Increasing numbers of nephrons stop functioning, culminating in kidney failure and the appearance of the fully developed lesions of glomerulosclerosis.

Diabetic glomerulosclerosis is a microscopic diagnosis which depends upon identifying some or all of the principal lesions (Figs 7.12–7.14). These lesions have been recognized within eighteen months after the appearance of diabetes and are found with increasing incidence during the subsequent 20–30 years. Thirty per cent of these patients will develop progressive renal failure and eventually need intermittent dialysis or transplantation. Males are more affected than females and retinopathy and neuropathy are frequent accompaniments.

Grossly, at any phase, the involved kidneys are indistinguishable from those of glomerulonephritis. The distinguishing features are:

(a) There is invariably unequal involvement of the kidneys, even though both are affected.

(b) Glomerular changes are not found either in all glomeruli or to the same extent in those involved and all the glomerular lesions are not always present within one kidney.

(c) There are no dense or lucent ultrastructural deposits.

(d) There are no consistent immunofluorescent findings. Mesangial deposits of fibrinogen, complement and immunoglobulins occur but may represent phagocytosis by the mesangial

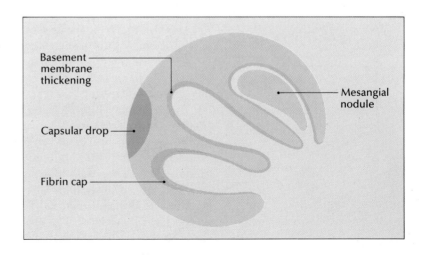

Fig. 7.12 Glomerular lesions of diabetic glomerulosclerosis.

cells. Circulating antibodies and immune complexes are both absent.

3   *Microangiopathy*. Hyaline thickening of the walls of small vessels and capillaries is the basis of this complication which is found in all diabetics. It is similar to that occurring with age in non-diabetics but differs in that young age groups are also affected. This complication is most obvious in the retinal vessels resulting in blindness (Fig. 7.15), the small heart vessels contributing to a cardiomyopathy, the vessels associated with nerves of all types contributing to neuropathy and within the kidneys as part of the diabetic nephropathy. Hyperglycaemia, hypertension, basement membrane thickening, changes in endothelial function and reduced blood flow are all believed to play a part. Increased platelet stickiness may also be involved as a final event and cigarette smoking and ageing will aggravate the disorder.

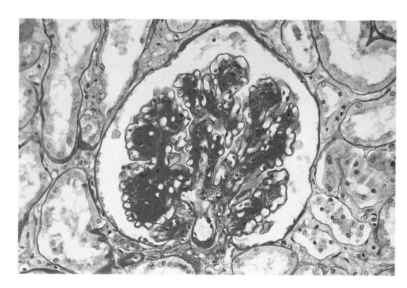

Fig. 7.13 Glomerulus with the nodular form of diabetic glomerulosclerosis. The nodules arise from an increase in mesangial matrix. There is a mild aneurysmal dilatation of the glomerular capillaries.

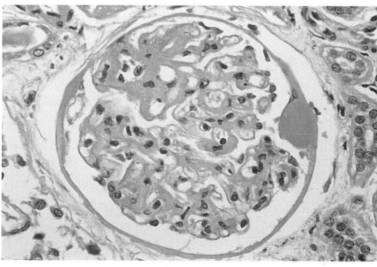

Fig. 7.14 Glomerulus with the diffuse membranous pattern of diabetic glomerulosclerosis due to thickening of the basement membranes. A large capsular drop lies on the membrane of Bowman's space.

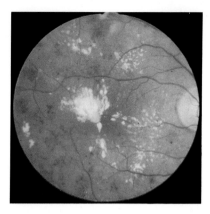

Fig. 7.15 Ophthalmoscopy appearances typical of diabetes mellitus with the disc right. The yellow plaques are fatty organized exudates which by replacing the macula have produced blindness. The red foci are haemorrhages which, like the plaques, are the result of the increased vascular permeability. The vessels appear normal and there are no microaneurysms.

The natural progression of micro-angiopathy is easily followed in the retinal vessels. A patchy increase in the blood flow develops first and this is associated with dilatation of venules. Dilatation is accompanied by later constriction of the arterioles and capillary closure. Ultimately there is sclerosis of vessels of all types.

4   *Macroangiopathy.* This is the development of atherosclerotic lesions. In diabetics these appear in younger age groups and women more than in controls. Type II diabetics can also be more severely affected than other patients but the features, sites and other aetiological factors are similar to those for the non-diabetic (Fig. 7.16). The most important results are coronary artery disease often associated with painless infarction, cerebral infarction and haemorrhage and peripheral vascular disease with gangrene. In addition there will be ischaemia to many other tissues which will promote infections and contribute to neural degeneration and various neuropathies.

Tumours

Adenocarcinoma is the most common tumour in the pancreas and the principal peri-ampullary carcinoma (Table 7.5; Fig. 7.17). Benign exocrine tumours, cystadenomas, are rare and invariably incidental findings. Endocrine tumours are uncommon and are examples of tumours whose malignant potential can only be gauged by their clinical behaviour. They are hormone producing, the hormone corresponding to the cell of origin.

Exocrine

The adenocarcinomas arise from the pancreatic ducts but, since the acinar cells develop from the duct epithelium, de-differentiation

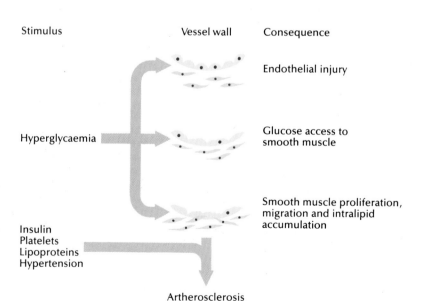

Fig. 7.16 Postulated effect of diabetes on atherosclerosis.

to an acinar type may be involved. Over 65% of carcinomas occur in the head of the pancreas, reflecting the higher proportion of duct tissue relative to the rest of the gland. Males are predominantly affected and there is an increasing incidence. This has been related with cigarette smoking but nitrosamines and coffee drinking may also be involved. Diabetics and those with familial pancreatitis, ataxia telangiectasia and haemochromatosis all have an increased risk as do those with chronic pancreatitis. There are no specific markers for the tumour although a number of non-specific tumour antigens including carcino-embryonic antigen and alpha-fetoprotein appear. Metastases have invariably developed by the time of diagnosis and the prognosis is correspondingly poor. Less than 1% of patients survive for more than 5 years.

APPEARANCES

The tumour is recognized as a hard sclerotic mass and there is a wide range of microscopic appearances (Fig. 7.18). A fibrotic stroma is common and this may surround intact islets in a fashion analogous to that seen in chronic pancreatitis.

Complications

Spread is predominantly local and often perineural. Pancreatitis and a migrating thrombophlebitis both occur and, within a small number of patients, panniculitis, polyarthritis and eosinophilia.

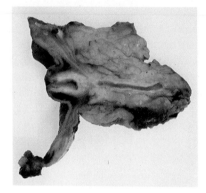

Fig. 7.17 Early ampullary carcinoma surrounding the duct opening into the duodenum. There is no infiltration into the pancreas at this stage.

Endocrine

These tumours are extremely rare. They may be found incidentally during autopsy or laparotomy or are diagnosed from their hormonal effects. These are not always evident since each hormone has an antagonist and any systemic effect reflects an imbalance between the two. Functional effects may also be absent with tumours in their early phases because too little hormone is produced or, at any stage, because that produced is not biochemically identical to its normal counterpart. More than one hormone is usually formed by an individual tumour although clinically the effects of only one hormone predominate. However, each cell within the tumour only synthesizes a single hormone.

The hormones are recognized by combination of blood and tissue analyses including immunohistochemistry incorporating hormone antibodies. Similar techniques can be used ultrastructurally to localize the hormone with its granule. Ultrastructural appearances of granules cannot be confidently related with a specific hormone since these alter if there is active secretion and with the demands made for that hormone. Tumours may include no granules if maximum secretion is occurring and their granules are also unlikely to mimic exactly those in normal cells.

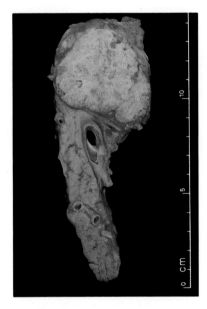

Fig. 7.18 Large adenocarcinoma replacing most of the head of the pancreas.

Classification

Listing the hormones within the tumour provides the best system of nomenclature. Formerly the tumours were associated with clinical syndromes (one of the best known being the Zollinger–Ellison syndrome), or called *islet cell tumours*. The latter term is inappropriate since tumours can arise independently of the endocrine cells in the islets and further, some of the hormones produced are not synthesized within normal islets.

APPEARANCES

Endocrine tumours are found throughout the length of the pancreas and do not have a higher incidence in any one part. Single and multiple tumours occur and if the tumour is over 0.5 g hormonal effects can be anticipated. There is no way of distinguishing benign from malignant tumours other than by recurrence after excision or the development of metastases. Metastases occur particularly in the portal lymph nodes and liver. Secondary tumour in endocrine glands must be distinguished from primary adenomas. Multiple dispersed adenomas are often familial and form the rare pluriglandular or multiglandular syndromes which can involve the pancreas.

Further reading

DCCT Research Group (1988). Are continuing studies of metabolic control and microvascular complications in insulin-dependent diabetes mellitus justified? *New Eng. J. Med.* **318**, 246–9.

Frey, C.F. (1986). Classification of pancreatitis: state-of-the-art 1986. *Pancreas* **1**, 62–8.

Krolewski, A.S., Wappam, J.H., Rand, L.I. and Kahn, C.R. (1987). Epidemiologic approach to the etiology of Type I diabetes mellitus and its complications. *New Eng. J. Med.* **317**, 1390–8.

Morley, A.R. (1988). Renal vascular disease in diabetes mellitus. *Histopathology* **12**, 343–58.

Volk, B.W. and Wellmann, K.F. (1977) (Editors). *The Diabetic Pancreas.* Plenum Press: New York and London.

8 Urinary tract

The urinary tract is the pathway for urine to pass from the renal papillae to the environment. It is lined throughout by transitional epithelium and has an abundant vasculature. This, unlike that to the kidney, is not confined to restricted areas and hence if disease affects a part this is easily compensated for and vascular disorders of the urinary tract are thus rare. Infection within parts of the urinary tract, in contrast, is common and may occasionally produce secondary disorders in the kidney. Any abnormality of the tract may provoke infection but obstruction, tumours, calculi and diverticulae are well-recognized causes.

Infection, reflux and pyelonephritis

Urinary tract infection is used synonymously with pyelonephritis, believed to be the end result and invariable consequence of urinary tract infection. Formerly pyelonephritis was given a very guarded prognosis and, even as recently as 1979, listed as the second cause for end-stage renal disease and as the reason for 20% of patients requiring either dialysis or renal transplantation. Long-term studies, particularly among girls and women, show that this sequence is not inevitable and even extremely rare or non-existent. It has also emerged that reflux of urine from the bladder into the upper urinary tract occurs and produces morphological changes similar to those attributed to urinary tract infection and labelled pyelonephritis. Pyelonephritis, especially in its chronic form, is now questioned and no longer confidently ascribed to infection. It is possible that all such diagnoses may in future be categorized as reflux nephropathy.

Urinary tract infection

This can involve the renal calyces and pelves, the ureters, the bladder and, in the male, the prostate (Table 8.1). Among these it is in the bladder that infection predominates, producing *cystitis*. The patient can be free of symptoms despite severe bacturia but alternatively there will be frequency and pain on micturition and even frank pus and blood. Loin pain and non-specific systemic effects occur but do not imply that the infection has spread to the ureters and kidney. Clinically it is impossible to localize renal tract infection and a diagnosis of cystitis rests upon the premise that infection most probably affects the bladder. Tests localizing the site are not

Table 8.1 Disorders leading to urine infection

Obstruction	See Table 8.4
Functional disorders	Reflux. Neurogenic bladder
Metabolic disorders	Hypercalcaemia. Hypokalaemia
	Hypergammaglobulinaemia
Trauma	Catheterization

universally accepted and the only indisputable test is the demonstration of bacteria in urine taken from known areas of the urinary tract, an impracticable procedure clinically.

Bacteria within the urine (*bacturia*) are the ultimate evidence for infection. However, the presence of organisms is often due to contamination arising during the collection of the specimen. Kass established that over 100 000 organisms/ml of urine is clear evidence of urinary infection and levels below this of contamination. This figure forms the basis of all reputable studies of urinary tract infection. The organisms and the factors favouring these and their establishment within the urinary tract are largely matters for microbiologists but include the following.

The organisms

Table 8.2 Common organisms underlying urine infection

	%
E. coli	70–80
Proteus	9
Staphylococcus albus	6
Klebsiella	3
M. tuberculosis	
Others	

1 *Escherichia coli* and even certain subtypes are those invariably responsible. Others are also predominantly Gram-negative (Table 8.2).

2 A single organism is the rule. More than one organism presents the possibility of obstruction, and underlying anatomical abnormality or foreign body.

3 The organisms often come from the faeces, the urinary serotypes mirroring these. Why *E. coli* which forms only a small proportion of the total faecal population and not other members predominates is unclear.

4 Instrumentation, including catheterization and cytoscopy, carries a risk of urinary infection and must never be performed without firm indications and rigorous asepsis.

5 Infection in any part of the urinary tract is usually ascending. Bacteria spread against the urinary flow and, in the ureters, against peristalsis. Bacterial adherence factors, the proximity of anus and, in the female, the introitus, the front-to-back closure of the urethra, the anatomically short female urethra as well as any reflux, obstruction or instrumentation encourage this spread.

6 Repeated infections may be difficult to distinguish from persistent infections (Table 8.3). The former usually involve faecal flora and the latter other organisms and often multiple organisms.

Table 8.3 Causes of persistent urine infection

Calculi
Chronic prostatitis
Bladder diverticula
Ureteric stumps following nephrectomy
Necrotic renal papillae
Pericalyceal diverticula

Urine

1 The continuous flow of urine is the single important factor impairing infection.

2 Urine is a sterile medium but one that is ideal for bacterial growth.

3 The osmolarity and low pH and the secretion of IgA within the transitional epithelium counteract bacterial colonization. Body temperature, the absence of inflammatory and mononuclear cells and of immunoglobulins and complement as well as the presence of proteins and sugars enhance bacterial growth.

4 Complete emptying of the bladder is impossible and residual urine will always be trapped within the bladder folds.

5 Prostatic fluid includes antibacteriacidal substances which empty into the bladder after micturition. It is unknown whether the peri-urethral glands in the female form a similar function.

Patients

1 Women and girls are predominantly infected and especially during pregnancy. Sexual intercourse is associated and more than one infectious episode may warrant investigation.

2 Infection in pregnancy can result in acute pyelonephritis but this does not become chronic or cause persistent renal dysfunction.

3 Infection in girls and women, even if repeated, does not alone result in either pyelonephritis or end-stage renal failure.

4 Infection in boys is uncommon and requires careful examination for a cause. In men, infection generally follows prostatic obstruction but neither renal involvement nor end stage renal failure are inevitable.

APPEARANCES

The effects of infection are most often seen by the urologist. At autopsy there are inevitably similar features following catheterization before death. The urine may be clear or turbid. The bladder epithelium is reddened, haemorrhagic and oedematous (Fig. 8.1). The histopathologist subdivides the inflammatory patterns but most have no importance clinically.

Reflux

Urine flows from the nephrons into the calyceal—pelvic system, down the ureters and into the bladder. With normal hydration, a constant rate of 2 ml/min is maintained. When micturition occurs sphincters around the lower ends of the ureters close and prevent urine from the contracting bladder flowing in a retrograde manner up the ureters. If the sphincters are incompetent *vesico-ureteric reflux* occurs either solely into the lower parts of the ureters, or into the calyceal—pelvic systems. Further reflux (*intrarenal reflux*) into the collecting ducts depends upon their position and the pressure achieved by the vesico-ureteric reflux within the calyceal—pelvic system. Papillae particularly at the poles of the kidney, *compound papillae*, have concave tips with the collecting ducts confined to these regions. Increased intrapelvic pressure distends these tips, so

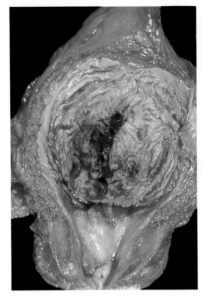
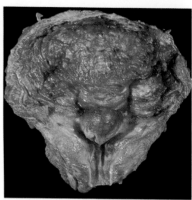

Fig. 8.1 Effect of urinary infection; (*left*) in a woman who had a catheter *in situ* some weeks prior to death: (*right*) in a man with benign enlargement of the prostate. The mucosa bladder is inflamed; note also its normal trabeculation.

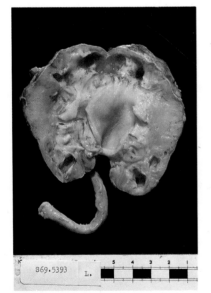

S69.5393   L.   5 4 3 2 1

Fig. 8.2 Contracted kidney, probably from long-standing reflux. At either pole the calyces are distended and the overlying parenchyma thinned. In contrast the calyces and tissue in the centre are uninvolved.

opening the collecting duct apertures and facilitating reflux of urine. *Simple papillae*, invariably in other areas, have convex tips with their collecting ducts opening over all parts of the papillae and are therefore less prone to reflux. These reflux patterns can be demonstrated by micturating cystograms and are affected by urine flow and hydration. They occur unilaterally or bilaterally and may be intermittent or persistent.

Causes

Vesico-ureteric reflux is demonstrable in over 50% of newborn infants as well as in patients with any muscular weakness of the ureteric sphincter. Cystitis, bladder wall hypertrophy, congenital defects of the bladder and neuropathies are all causes for such a weakness. Intrarenal reflux follows either from severe vesico-ureteric reflux or from obstruction within the urinary tract. Obstruction follows from lesions outside the urinary tract, within the wall and the lumen and in each part different causes predominate (Table 8.4). Prostatic enlargement is the main reason for urethral obstruction, bladder tumours for bladder obstruction and calculi for ureteric and pelvic obstruction.

APPEARANCES

Vesico-ureteric reflux propels urine into the ureter and, if this is sufficiently severe, dilatation of the polar calyces follows, the upper more than the lower. A secondary effect is intrarenal reflux with scarring in the involved parenchyma and compensatory hypertrophy of the uninvolved adjacent tissue (Fig. 8.2). Since the affected nephrons feed into the renal papillae lying over the dilated calyces scars are confined to these areas. This pattern of scarring, with and without

Table 8.4 Some causes of urinary tract infection

Luminal	Tumours
	Calculi
	Infection
Mural	Congenital valves
	Megaureters
	Pelvic−ureteric junction stenosis
	Strictures
Extramural	Prostatic hypertrophy
	Pelvic neoplasms (rectal, cervical, etc.)
	Idiopathic retroperitoneal fibrosis

infected urine, has been produced experimentally in pigs and followed in children and adults but rarely with any detrimental effect upon renal function. A small percentage of patients may develop hypertension and others proteinuria.

Pyelonephritis

Clinicians have, as with reflux, relied upon radiology for the diagnosis. Radiologists and histopathologists recognize scarred kidneys with deformed calyces and pelvis and one kidney more involved than the other (Fig. 8.3). It is on these appearances that the diagnosis of pyelonephritis rests. The difficulties in interpretation are reflected by the wide indices amongst autopsy series, 33% to less than 1%. Non-obstructive and obstructive forms occur but in either urinary tract infection is considered the cause. The microscopic findings are similar in either form and reflect chronic inflammation with destruction of nephrons and compensatory changes among those surviving (Fig. 8.4). They can simulate a wide variety of other conditions often referred to as interstitial nephritis.

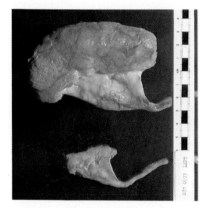

Fig. 8.3 Kidneys of a patient with end-stage renal failure and a history of urinary tract infection. There is unequal shrinkage of the kidneys but both have scarred surfaces, appearances compatible with a diagnosis of chronic pyelonephritis.

Fig. 8.4 Distended renal tubules with acute inflammatory cells in their lumina and in the interstitial tissue. Other tubules are atrophic and the interstitial tissue is increased. Features consistent with acute and chronic inflammation seen with pyelonephritis.

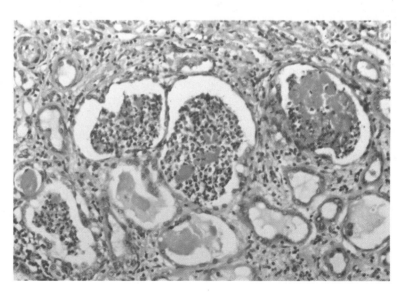

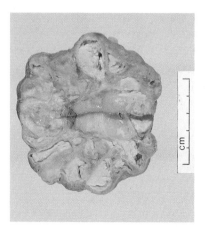

Fig. 8.5 Renal tuberculosis. Caseous material fills the pelvis and calyces as well as replaces much of the renal parenchyma.

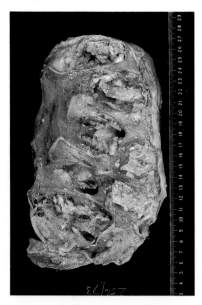

Fig. 8.6 Acute pyelonephritis. The kidney is grossly enlarged and the pelvi–calyceal system filled with green pus. This patient had received no antibiotic therapy since the condition was unrecognized.

Source of infection

Infection may reach the kidney via the blood stream or lymphatics or within the urine.

1 The substantial vasculature of the kidneys encourages haematogenous infection. This occurs if the patient has a septicaemia but only if there is also outflow obstruction. Multiple renal abscesses in staphylococcal septicaemias, *Candida* abscesses in systemic candidiasis and renal tuberculosis (Fig. 8.5) are all the result of vascular dissemination in the presence of a reduction in urine flow. The number of such infections is nevertheless exceedingly small when compared with the number of patients with septicaemias.

2 Lymphatic spread of infection is in theory possible but has not in practice been convincingly shown.

3 Urinary infection is common, especially in girls and women, and thus could cause pyelonephritis. Acute pyelonephritis complicates the bacturia of pregnancy in 20–40% of women but does not progress to a chronic end-stage disorder. The physiological dilatation of the upper urinary tract as well as increased multiplication of rates of *E. coli* in pregnant patients lie behind this infection. Uncomplicated bacturia also does not produce chronic pyelonephritis but urinary infection secondary to obstruction might play a part in renal parenchymal damage. An effect of obstruction is reflux which localizes the parenchymal damage, and any infection then perpetuates and accelerates the damage. Patients with renal tract obstruction have infected urine and can progress to irreversible renal failure. Those without obstruction but with reflux and infected urine may similarly develop scarred kidneys.

APPEARANCES

Acute pyelonephritis because of effective therapy is rarely encountered by histopathologists. The kidney is enlarged with small abscesses scattered over the surface. The cortex and medulla include multiple red and white streaks where parts of the nephrons are filled with pus and surrounded by acute inflammation (Fig. 8.6). The mucosa of the calyces and pelves are inflamed and include adherent pus. Pus may distend the entire calyceal–pelvic system and spread down the ureter. The right side is more involved than the left in the pregnant woman because the gravid uterus rotates towards this side and partly compresses the right ureter.

Chronic pyelonephritis produces a scarred, contracted kidney reminiscent of that with reflux but more severely affected (Fig. 8.7). The calyces are dilated and club-shaped with their proximal parts flattening the renal papillae and overlying parenchyma. The surrounding parenchyma shows compensatory hypertrophy and the overall effect is a shallow surface depression to which the capsule is firmly adherent. These changes are most marked at the renal poles and are more severe in one kidney than the other. Other observations are thickening of the walls of the pelvis and calyces, apparent increase in the pericalyceal fat and thickening of the walls of the

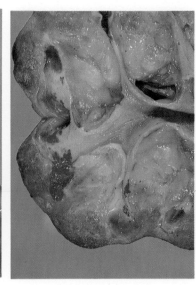

Fig. 8.7 Chronic pyelonephritis; (*left*) the unevenly and in places deeply scarred surface; (*right*) the club-shaped deformity of the calyces with thinning of the overlying parenchyma and increase of that between the calyces.

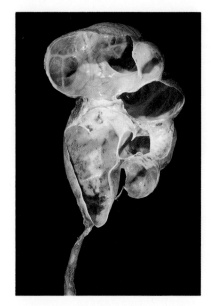

Fig. 8.8 Hydronephrosis arising from stenosis at the pelvi–ureteric junction. The parenchymal loss and destruction has arisen from the pressure of the obstructed urine and infection.

intrarenal vessels. Necrosis of the renal papillae may be found particularly if the patient also has diabetes mellitus.

When the disorder is associated with renal tract obstruction the site of this and its duration determine the degree of calyceal, pelvic and ureteric dilatation (Fig. 8.8). The kidneys include substantial parenchymal loss irregularly dispersed over the entire kidney contributed to by pressure and infection. A distinctive variant of obstructive pyelonephritis is *xanthogranulomatous pyelonephritis*. Lobulate yellow masses replace parts of the kidney and calculi and calcification occupy, respectively, the calyceal–pelvic system and parenchyma. At light microscopy there are numerous granulomas including many fat-filled foamy macrophages.

Calculi

These are found in all parts of the urinary tract. They can be asymptomatic or associated with obstruction and infection. Infection, dehydration, hypercalcuria and desquamated material and blood clot are implicated in their formation (Table 8.5). The centre of the

Table 8.5 Common types of urinary calculi

Type	Appearance	Precursors
Calcium phosphate	Grey-white. Smooth. Crumbling	Urea splitting organisms (Proteus) and prolonged immobilization
Calcium oxalate	Brown-black Spiny. Hard	Primary hyperoxalosis in very few patients
Uric acid	Yellow-brown Smooth. Hard	25% related to gout

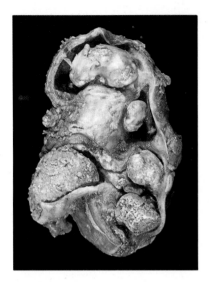

Fig. 8.9 Numerous calculi within the calyces and pelvis. The renal tissue loss has arisen from the combination of obstruction to the urine flow and infection.

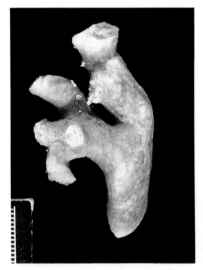

Fig. 8.10 Staghorn calculus from a child's kidney. The pattern of the calyces and pelvis is easily recognized.

calculus is formed by one of several crystalloids and provides a nidus for infection which leads to further enlargement. The most common form of calculus is the mixed calcium phosphate type provoked particularly by alkaline urine while others include oxalate, uric acid, cystine and xanthine, all promoted by acid urine. The calculi can be gritty or fill the surrounding viscus (Fig. 8.9). *Staghorn calculi* (Fig. 8.10) which mirror the calyceal−pelvic system are examples in the latter category but similar large calculi also occur in the bladder. Possible complications are hydronephrosis and ascending infection.

Tumours

Transitional cell carcinomas

Transitional epithelium lines the entire urinary tract from the calyces to the terminal end of the urethra. Tumours can arise from all parts but do so most commonly in the bladder (Fig. 8.11). Transitional cell carcinoma of the bladder forms 2−7% of all adult cancers and almost 90% of bladder tumours. The urethra is rarely affected. Originally benign papillomas and carcinomas were distinguished but it is now accepted that this is not possible and all transitional tumours are regarded as carcinomas. Men are more affected than women and most develop between 40 and 80 years. Clinically they cause painless haematuria and the possibility of this carcinoma

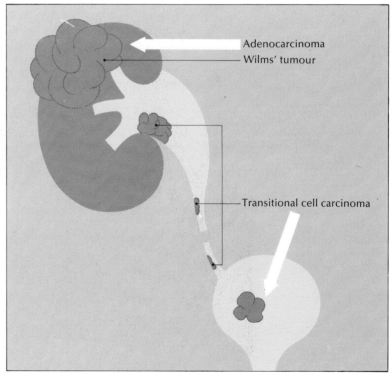

Fig. 8.11 Kidney and urinary tract tumours.

must be considered in any patient with haematuria. Dysuria from infection and obstructive symptoms are usually late presentations.

Causes

Although causes for most are unknown it has long been recognized that those in the analine dye industry are at risk. Other risk industries are those involving rubber, cable, plastics and gas manufacture where the carcinogens are β-naphthylamine, benzidine, magenta and 2-acetylaminofluorene but a latent interval, as long as 40 years, may intervene. Other precursors are abnormal tryptophane metabolites, phenacetin abuse (especially allied with pelvic tumours in women), Thorotrast in retrograde pyelography, smoking and persistent urinary tract infections. A geographical link is with *Balkan nephropathy*, interstitial nephritis confined to areas of Bulgaria, Rumania and Yugoslavia. The high incidence in the bladder as opposed to the pelvis and ureters (25:5:1) probably reflects the larger surface area and the longer exposure to carcinogens related with urine storage.

APPEARANCES

An *in situ* phase can occur when the epithelium is thickened and reddened often with a velvety pattern down the cystoscope. Frank tumour can range from papillary, with delicate pink fronds similar to a sea anemone, to ulcerated and partly necrotic infiltrating growths (Fig. 8.12). One tumour pattern may persist but in about 20% a change to a more complex form is seen and up to 70% become invasive within five years. About 30% of patients have multiple

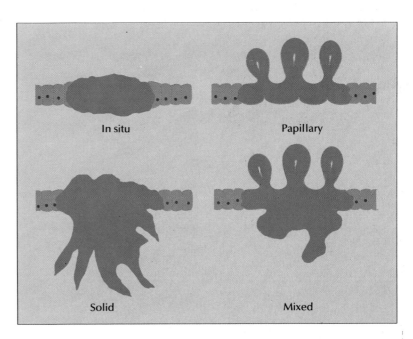

Fig. 8.12 Patterns of transitional cell carcinoma.

In situ

Papillary

Solid

Mixed

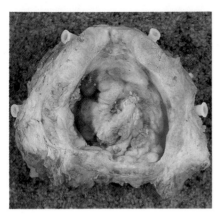

Fig. 8.13 Transitional cell carcinoma of the bladder involving the entire mucosa.

tumours which may be due to seedling spread or multiple primary growths.

In the bladder, tumours mostly develop in the trigone and may obstruct the ureteric openings (Fig. 8.13). Diffuse involvement occurs in the renal pelvis and sometimes causes obstruction (Fig. 8.14). Transition to squamous cell carcinoma occurs and the tumour is then less responsive to chemotherapy and radiation. Other factors worsening the prognosis are poor cytological differentiation, local invasion, tumour beyond the urinary tract and, in the bladder, tumour in the dome or on the anterior wall.

Spread

Direct, lymphatic and vascular spread occur. Invasion within the bladder wall and ureter increase the possibility of lymphatic spread because of their many lymphatics. Local spread in the bladder can result in ureteric obstruction and ascending infection. More widespread local invasion culminates in a frozen pelvis with tumour eroding into the adjacent organs, pelvic bones and the sacral and lumbar nerve plexuses.

Metastatic tumours

Carcinomas and lymphomas are important sources of metastases. These may involve and obstruct the urinary tract via the intramural lymphatics or peri-ureteric tissues or produce obstruction from enlarged involved lymph nodes, particularly the para-aortic.

Squamous cell carcinomas

These are uncommon and must be distinguished from squamous

Fig. 8.14 Transitional cell carcinoma associated with obstruction to the urinary tract; (*left*) in the renal pelvis; (*right*) in the ureter.

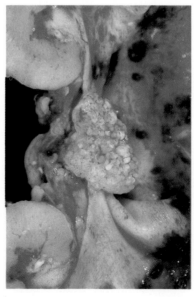
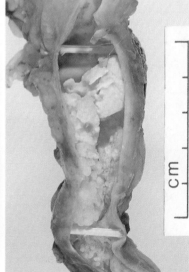

change within a transitional cell carcinoma. Prolonged infection, calculi and, in Egypt, chronic schistosomiasis, are the invariable precursors with preceding squamous metaplasia.

Miscellaneous

Paragangliomas, embryonal rhabdomyomas and adenocarcinomas all occasionally occur within the bladder.

Further reading

Chisholm, G.D. and Williams, D.I. (1982) (Editors). *Scientific Foundations of Urology* (2nd Edition). William Heinemann Medical Books Ltd: London.

Francois, B. and Perrin, P.P. (1983) (Editors). *Urinary Infection*. Butterworths: London and Boston.

Heptinstall, R.H. (1983) *Pathology of the Kidney* (3rd Edition). Little, Brown and Co:Boston.

Risdon, R.A. and Turner, D.R. (1980). *Atlas of Renal Pathology*. MTP Press Ltd: Lancaster.

9 Kidney

Systemic effects of renal failure

Glomerulonephritis
- The normal glomerulus
- Light microscopy terminology
- Ultrastructural terminology
- Immunofluorescence studies
- Ancillary immunological studies
- Mechanisms of injury

Glomerular changes and systemic disease

Vascular disorders
- Anatomy
- Vascular impairment
- Disorders
- Hypertension
- Renal artery stenosis
- Ischaemic lesions

Cystic disease

Interstitial nephritis

Analgesic nephropathy and papillary necrosis

Transplant kidney

Tumours
- Adenocarcinoma
- Wilm's tumour (nephroblastoma)
- Other tumours

Renal transplantation shows that normal renal function can be maintained by a single kidney and demonstrates the normal reserve function available. The kidneys remove waste and harmful materials and maintain the normal fluid balance; they also control the blood pressure and secrete hormones such as erythropoietin. These functions depend upon a normal structure, adequate blood perfusion and a patent urinary tract without which renal failure results. Glomerulonephritis is the most important disorder causing renal failure at any age with ascending infection, reflux nephropathy and adult polycystic disease as the other main causes. The blood supply can be embarrassed with similar effects by arteriosclerosis but more important are the consequences of hypertension, blood loss and shock. Kidney tumours, although common, rarely produce renal failure.

Renal failure may arise from systemic disorders. Chief among these is Type I diabetes mellitus and less commonly amyloidosis and connective tissue disorders. Less well understood is renal failure developing from cardiac, pulmonary and hepatic diseases which may be contributed to by drugs used to treat these conditions (Fig. 9.1).

Clinically renal failure is reflected by a number of syndromes (Table 9.1), none of which are diagnostic for any one cause of renal failure. Great reliance diagnostically is consequently placed upon the renal biopsy. Unfortunately, there are few opportunities to reverse renal failure and restore normal function. It is also regrettable that adequate preventative measures can be taken for only a few disorders. These hinge either on genetic counselling, as for congenital adult polycystic disease, or on the avoidance of occupations allied to some tumours.

Table 9.1 Common clinical presentations of glomerulonephritis

Acute nephritic syndrome
Nephrotic syndrome
Haematuria
Proteinuria
Haematuria and proteinuria
Chronic renal insufficiency
Acute oliguric renal failure

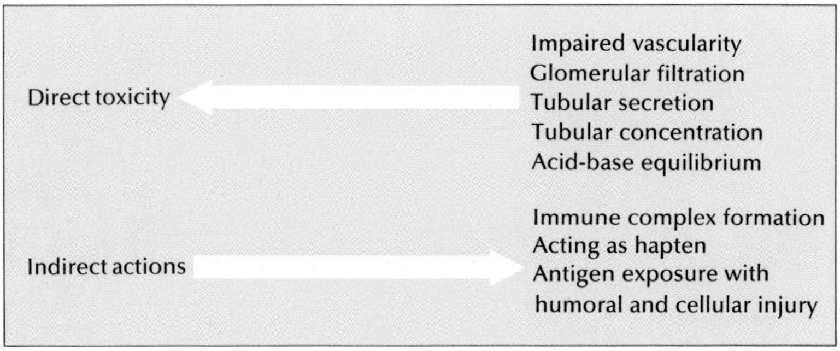
Direct toxicity
Impaired vascularity
Glomerular filtration
Tubular secretion
Tubular concentration
Acid-base equilibrium
Indirect actions
Immune complex formation
Acting as hapten
Antigen exposure with
humoral and cellular injury

Fig. 9.1 Drugs and the kidney.

Systemic effects of renal failure

A wide spectrum of systemic changes accompany renal failure. These were attributed to the raised urea and referred to as *uraemia*. This term persists although it is realized that urea is not the cause and that similar levels of urea are tolerated by normal individuals. The basis for the changes remains uncertain but it is clear that many factors are involved including acidosis and the electrolyte abnormalities basic to renal failure. In addition hypertension, clotting abnormalities, secondary immunosuppression from renal failure and malnutrition are implicated as well as changes in hydration and hormone secretion and the effects of therapy. Long-term dialysis and transplantation have both resulted in modifications to some structural changes and in the introduction of others.

APPEARANCES

All organs can be affected but rarely is this so in each patient. Fibrinous pericarditis, atherosclerosis and cardiac hypertrophy are all common. Pulmonary oedema is invariably present and has a high fibrin content and readily undergoes organization. These features were interpreted as unique and termed *'uraemic lung'* but it is now appreciated that any form of chronic pulmonary oedema produces comparable changes. Haemorrhage, with and without focal or diffuse ulceration, occurs within the gastrointestinal tract and inspissated secretions block exocrine organs, particularly the salivary gland and the pancreas. Hepatitis, potentially from a multitude of causes including the hepatitis viruses, is seen but is more common after dialysis or transplantation. Both treatments render the patient susceptible to infections although these also develop in any patient with renal failure. The lungs are the main site with death from bacteria and fungal pneumonia. Similar infections as well as viral are seen in the brain where a metabolic encephalopathy is also evident. The haemorrhagic propensity of renal failure is heightened by dialysis and transplantation and diffuse or localized haemorrhage within one or many organs is generally found at autopsy. Bone disease presents one of the more perplexing problems since it can be the end result of the combination of osteomalacia, osteoporosis and hyperparathyroidism, all of which are aggravated by dialysis and renal transplantation. Bone changes are collectively referred to as *renal osteodystrophy*.

Glomerulonephritis

This is a group of disorders in which injury centres upon the glomerulus. There is generally uniform involvement of all glomeruli in both kidneys, although rarely the disease is focal. In both cases immune mechanisms involving either complexes or direct antibody damage are believed to underlie the changes. The antigen, however, has only rarely been identified. Experimental studies provide the evidence for these beliefs, although their translation to clinical nephrology may have been too literal and too readily accepted. The concept of immune damage makes it essential to incorporate antibody studies in the diagnosis of glomerulonephritis and often electron microscopy. As a result a variety of potential classifications of glomerulonephritis have emerged (Table 9.1), none consistently relating with others or with clinical findings. The inclusion of glomerular lesions of certain systemic disorders within these classifications provides further difficulties as do differences in survival seen among individuals sharing comparable changes.

Presentation

World-wide, glomerulonephritis is the principal reason for maintenance dialysis or renal transplantation. At this juncture end-stage or irreversible renal failure has been reached but prior to this varying degrees of renal impairment will have been experienced, some of which may be asymptomatic. Proteinuria and haematuria, either isolated or combined, are the most common indices of renal failure. The failure may be brief or extend over years but the pattern can be pigeon-holed into one of several categories, the best known being the nephrotic syndrome (Table 9.1). This categorization is not always precise, since clinically variants occur and with time the categorization invariably alters. A further difficulty is that no category consistently relates with a specific structural change. It cannot therefore be assumed from the presentation that a specific spectrum of glomerular changes will be present nor, and as importantly, vice versa.

Diagnosis

To record the glomerular features a biopsy is essential. If glomerular assessment is left until nephrectomy or autopsy the disorder may be too advanced for a precise structural description and it is only following the introduction of biopsies that the various types of glomerulonephritis have emerged. The natural history of these, even so, is often still unclear and is now confused and altered by therapy. Geographical differences as well as age and hereditary are further factors influencing the prognosis.

The normal glomerulus

Each is globular with a capillary deeply concertinaed into lobes lying within the urinary space (Fig. 9.2). This space is bounded by an epithelial-lined capsule (*Bowman's capsule*) and separated from the capillary by a visceral epithelium. The capillary lumen is covered by a fenestrated endothelium and the body of the cell housing the nucleus lies opposite to the capillary bordering the urinary space. This free border and its outer epithelial cells and inner endothelial cell processes receives additional support from a basement membrane with three distinct zones, inner, central and outer. The body of the endothelial cell is directly associated on its non-luminal sur-

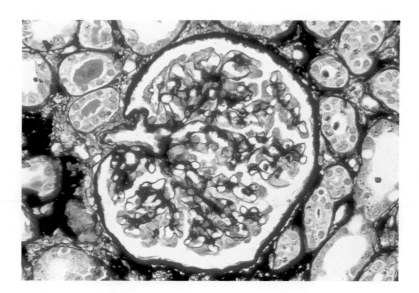

Fig. 9.2 Normal glomerulus. The basement membrane is stained black. The lobular pattern, capillaries, epithelial and endothelial cells can be identified. Most of the surrounding tubules are proximal convoluted tubules.

face with the supporting core of each lobule, the *mesangium*, formed from a matrix and phagocytic cells. The matrix is in direct continuity with the inner part of the basement membrane. An afferent arteriole brings blood to the glomerulus and blood leaves via an efferent vessel, both lying at the hilum. Filtrate within the urinary space drains directly into the proximal tubule at the pole opposite the hilum.

Light microscopy terminology

Usually glomerulonephritis affects all glomeruli equally and may be referred to as *diffuse* (Table 9.2) but since most examples are diffuse this prefix is rarely used. Uncommonly the distribution is not uniform and it is then termed *focal*.

When renal tissue is examined by light microscopy the glomerulus is seen in one plane and its globular form easily overlooked. There are forms of diffuse glomerulonephritis in which not all of the lobules are equally involved and on a random section some glomeruli appear normal. Serial sectioning would reveal some abnormal lobules in these glomeruli and so confirm a diffuse disorder. Such a disease is aptly termed *segmental* and its distinction from the much more rare focal disease must be appreciated. Other terms are not universally accepted and their usage contributes to some of the misunderstanding and mystique surrounding the nomenclature of glomerulonephritis.

Proliferative is used for an increase in cell numbers within either the whole or part of the glomerulus (Fig. 9.3). It refers to all cell types but strictly does not apply to an increase in cell size, the only change in some types of glomerulonephritis. Illogically it is used when thickening of the basement membrane is predominant. The term has become less appropriate following the demonstration that much of the cellular 'proliferation' within the urinary space is due to macrophage infiltration and not parietal epithelial proliferation.

Table 9.2 Patterns of diffuse glomerulonephritis and common clinical course

Immune complex types	
1 Proliferative Endocapillary proliferative Post-streptococcal IgA nephropathy	Variable with the best outlook when proliferation is confined to the mesangium. There is normal long-term renal function for many patients
2 Membranoproliferative Mesangiocapillary	Gradual deterioration in renal function
3 Membranous	9% of adult glomerular disease. Slow progression to irreversible renal failure
Antiglomerular basement membrane type	
Rapidly progressive Crescentic Extracapillary	Majority lead rapidly to irreversible renal failure
Unrecognized cause	
1 Minimal change Lipoid nephrosis	Most common pattern between 1 and 5 years with invariable complete resolution
2 Chronic sclerosing End-stage Unclassified	Progressive renal failure

Lobular is used when proliferation was confined to the mesangial regions. This is found following exposure to any stimulus and consequently part of any form of glomerulonephritis. Lobular has also been applied to glomerulonephritis combining this feature and basement membrane thickening as well as the more common name *mesangiocapillary glomerulonephritis* or, less popularly, *membrano-proliferative glomerulonephritis* (Table 9.2, Fig. 9.4).

Extracapillary refers to proliferation of parietal epithelial cells and macrophage infiltration within Bowman's space, thereby producing a *crescent* (Fig. 9.5). *Crescentic* or *extracapillary glomerulo-nephritis* are thus synonymous terms and include *rapidly progressive glomerulonephritis* (Table 9.2).

Endocapillary may be applied to proliferation of predominantly the endothelial cells. The weakness of the term is that this is probably an uncommon phenomenon, the more frequent change being enlargement of these cells. It is also used, inappropriately, when mesangial cell processes extend into the capillary walls beneath the endothelial cells.

Exudative refers to the infiltration of neutrophil polymorphs and the appearance of fibrin, phenomena accompanying some acute glomerulonephritides, especially after streptococcal infection (Table 9.2, Fig. 9.6).

Sclerosis is the final appearance of glomeruli in glomerulonephritis in which resolution has failed although in a few sclerosis is the dominant feature from the inception of the disease. All cellularity is lost and the glomeruli appear as hyaline balls. The change is eventually seen in most kidneys in end-stage renal failure and, without previous biopsies, no idea of preceding histology is possible.

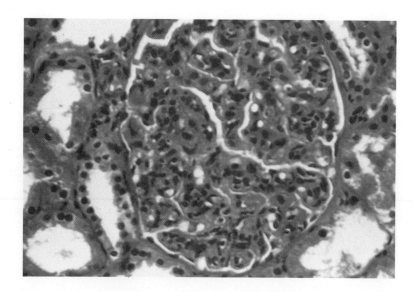

Fig. 9.3 Glomerulus from a kidney with acute proliferative glomerulonephritis. There is an increase in the cellularity of the glomerular tuft causing this to enlarge and fill Bowman's space and also compress the capillaries. Similar changes involved all the glomeruli within the biopsy.

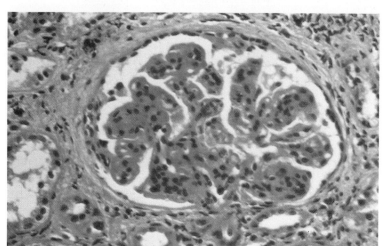

Fig. 9.4 Mesangiocapillary glomerulonephritis. The lobules of the glomerulus are clearly apparent and within the centres of these there is an increase in stroma and cells.

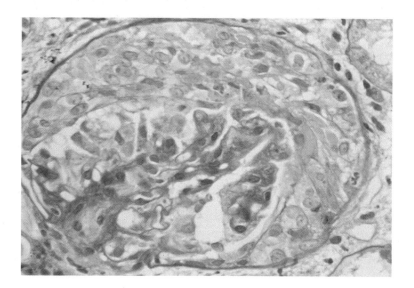

Fig. 9.5 Crescent formation in glomerulonephritis. Similar changes were seen in the other glomeruli in the biopsy.

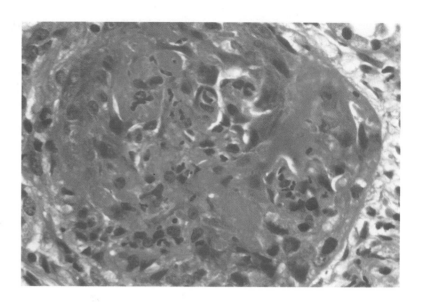

Fig. 9.6 Glomerulus with proliferative changes, infiltration of neutrophil polymorphs and fibrin deposition. All of these features were seen in the other glomeruli in the biopsy.

The terms *chronic sclerosing glomerulonephritis, unclassified glomerulonephritis* or *end-stage renal disease* are often used in these circumstances (Table 9.2).

These terms are used to describe and classify diffuse glomerulonephritis and some are also appropriate to some forms of diffuse segmental glomerulonephritis. Two clear-cut histological forms of glomerulonephritis are not embraced by any of this terminology: *Membranous glomerulonephritis*, in which membrane thickening is the sole feature (Table 9.3, Fig. 9.7); *Minimal change disease*, a form with no structural changes in the glomeruli at light microscopy (Table 9.2). In theory this should be easily identified but in practice it may be difficult to rule out an early proliferative disorder.

Prognostic features

The likely course is almost impossible to predict structurally or

Table 9.3 Antigens identified in immune complex glomerulonephritis

Exogenous antigen	
Bacterial	α and β streptococci; staphylococci; enterococci; *T. pallidium*; *M. leprae*
Viral	Hepatitis B; cytomegalo; Epstein–Barr; measles
Parasitic	*P. malariae* and *falciparum*; *S. mansoni*; *T. gondii*
Drugs	Gold, penicillamine, mercury, heroin, vaccine serum
Endogenous antigen	
Nuclear	Lupus erythematosus
Tumour	Carcinomas and lymphomas
Immunoglobulin	Cryoglobulinaemia
Renal	Kidney tubules
Thyroid	Thyroiditis

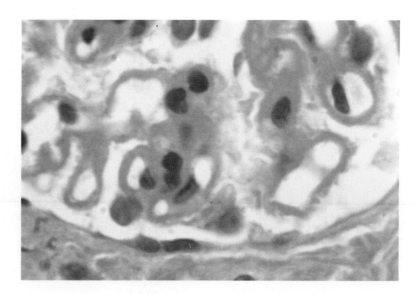

Fig. 9.7 Part of a glomerulus with marked and fairly uniform thickening to the basement membrane. A similar change affected all the glomeruli examined.

clinically. Morphological changes, especially associated with a potentially bad prognosis, are:

1 crescents in more than 70% of glomeruli;

2 marked atrophy of tubules, irrelevant of the glomerular features.

Findings that may imply a good prognosis include:

1 minimal change disease, especially in children;

2 diffuse proliferative glomerulonephritis with few or no crescents and no basement membrane thickening.

Prognosis with segmental glomerulonephritis was considered good but with longer-term follow-up this is less certain for all patients.

Ultrastructural terminology

Deposits

Tissue for electron microscopy is stained with lead citrate and osmium tetroxide. Some structures stain black or shades of grey while others are unstained. The stained areas are referred to as *dense areas* and the unstained as *lucent areas*. Some forms of glomerulonephritis are associated with deposits in the basement membrane and these, although invariably dense, can be lucent (Fig. 9.8). The deposits are generally focal but with progression they enlarge and become less dense. A variant is *dense linear deposits* which are also found in the basement membranes of the tubules and are confined to a few patients with membranoproliferative glomerulonephritis. Deposits may be found in the central part of the basement membrane or beneath the endothelial and epithelial cells forming *intramembranous, subendothelial* and *subepithelial deposits* or *humps* (Figs 9.8, 9.9). Any form of glomerulonephritis has deposits only within one of these sites and invariably the basement membrane is also thickened. In some the humps project from the surface of the

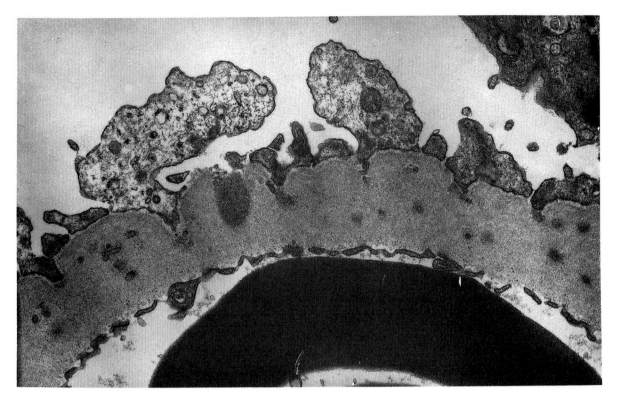

Fig. 9.8 Dense deposits within a thickened basement membrane demonstrated by electron microscopy.

basement membrane. The early phases of membranous glomerulonephritis are characterized by regular subepithelial deposits separated by projecting areas of the basement membrane, both thickening this and seen as spikes from these areas at light microscopy (Fig. 9.10).

Dense deposits also occur in the mesangial regions particularly with disorders accompanying certain systemic diseases (Fig. 9.11). In these there are often also deposits in the basement membrane, although in *IgA nephropathy (Berger's disease)*, the deposits may be confined to the mesangial regions.

Podocyte fusion

The body of the visceral epithelial cells is separated from the basement membrane by a number of projections, *foot processes* or *podocytes*. Transmission electron microscopy shows that these extend from the cell and are covered by the plasma membrane with a space intervening between each podocyte and the next. Scanning electron microscopy reveals a more complex state with the podocytes of surrounding epithelial cells interdigitating with one another. Any glomerular injury can lead to swelling of the podocytes which, with the transmission electron microscope, gives the impression that adjacent podocytes have fused, but in reality the interdigitating pattern has been displaced by the expanded foot processes (Fig. 9.9). The basement membrane consequently becomes covered by

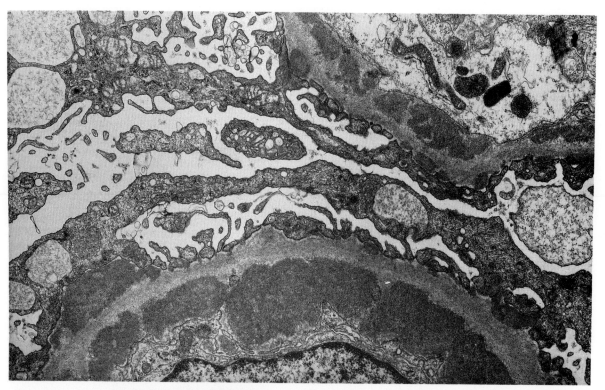

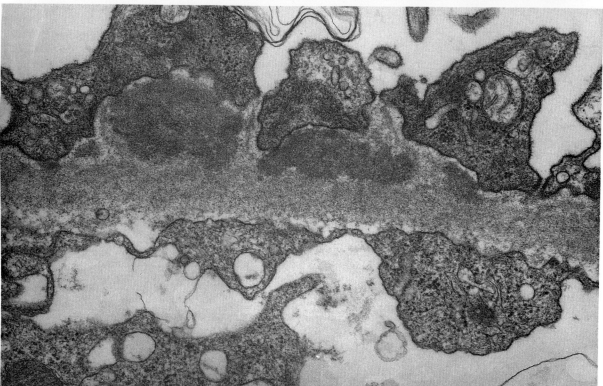

Fig. 9.9 (*Above*) Subendothelial dense deposits with a few subepithelial dense deposits. There is fusion of many of the foot processes of the epithelial cells; (*below*) subepithelial dense deposits producing humps.

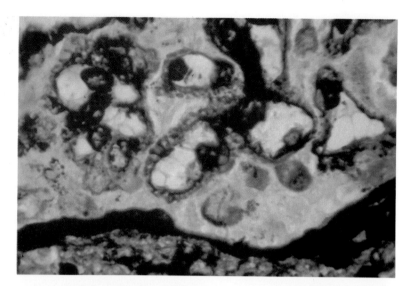

Fig. 9.10 Part of a glomerulus from a kidney with membranous glomerulonephritis. The spikes from the basement membranes (stained black) are easily seen.

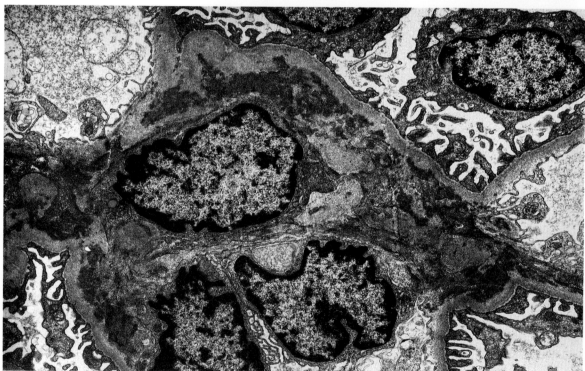

Fig. 9.11 Dense deposits in the mesangial region of a kidney from a patient with systemic lupus erythematosus.

the epithelial cell cytoplasm, separated only by the plasma membrane. This appearance is common to all glomerulonephritis and is the only structural change in minimal change glomerulonephritis.

Immunofluorescence studies

An essential part in the diagnosis of glomerular disease is the recognition of antigens trapped within the glomerulus. These may

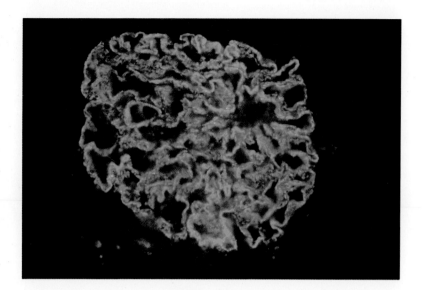

Fig. 9.12 Green fluorescence in a glomerulus from antibody to IgG. The fluorescence outlines the glomerular capillaries and has a granular pattern compatible with immune complex deposition.

be deposited either free or as preformed immune complexes with their antibody or they may be trapped within the basement membrane with the subsequent formation of immune complexes.

The antigen is demonstrated by specific antibodies or more often by antibodies to the human immunoglobin forming the immune complex. If any of the complement components or fibrinogen are also involved these can be shown by anticomplement or antifibrinogen antibodies. Fluorescence dye giving a bright green fluorescence under ultraviolet light is usually used to label the antibodies but necessitates frozen or cryostat sections of tissue. An alternative approach, using paraffin wax sections of tissue, is to label antibodies with peroxidase or other enzymes which can then be seen with a light microscope.

Immune complex disease

Among all forms of glomerulonephritis IgG and IgM are the most common immunoglobulins seen and C3 the most usual component of complement (Fig. 9.12). If there are immune complexes the deposits have a granular pattern and mirror the distribution of those seen by electron microscopy in the basement membrane and mesangium (Fig. 9.13). In IgA nephropathy the predominant antibody is IgA and this is seen in the mesangial regions and may reflect trapping of immune complexes. Recognition of the antigen forming an immune complex is extremely uncommon. An increasing number of antigens (Table 9.3) are recognized but the occasions on which these are identified are few. The deposition pattern of the antigen is reflected by the antibody and is invariably granular. A similar pattern is seen with the components of complement and the individual component gives some insight into the complement pathway involved. C1q and C3 together show activation of the classical pathway while with C3 alone there is the possibility that the alternate pathway is involved.

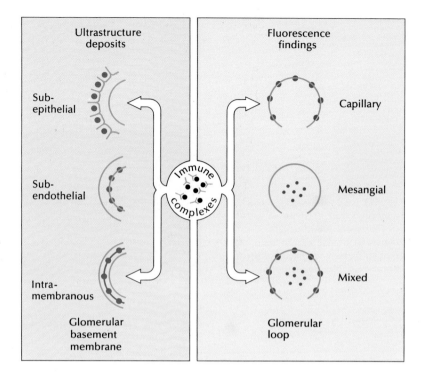

Fig. 9.13 Findings in immune complex glomerulonephritis.

Antibody disease

When the glomerular injury is via antibodies directed against the basement membrane their deposition is linear and smooth and confined to the basement membrane. IgG and C3 are found in these circumstances.

No immunoglobulin labelling may occur either because none is present as occurs in minimal change glomerulonephritis or because the immunoglobulin has been removed or masked during resolution or progression of the disorder. Technical faults can also contribute but rarely absence of serum immunoglobulins or complement.

Ancillary immunological studies

Immune complex disease

Circulating immune complexes can be demonstrated but this is technically difficult and does not distinguish between non-specific complexes and those implicated in the renal disorder. Similar difficulties apply to studies of immune complexes within the kidneys. These first necessitate removal or elution of the complexes, a process involving acid digestion of renal tissue.

Antibody disease

When renal damage follows circulating antibasement membrane antibody this can be demonstrated by exposing sections of normal human kidney to the patient's serum and labelling this with anti-human IgG. A smooth, linear pattern of fluorescence results along the glomerular basement membrane.

Circulating immunoglobulin and complement levels as well as the numbers of T- and B-cells and their subsets are all affected by renal disease but not in any specific patterns. A partial exception is membranoproliferative glomerulonephritis which is often but not invariably related with a persistently low circulating level of C3. The cause of this is an auto-antibody, *C3 nephritic factor*, which activates the alternate complement pathway and thereby depletes C3. The role of this auto-antibody in membranoproliferative glomerulonephritis is unclear, since it is neither the cause nor related with the course or prognosis.

Mechanisms of injury

The mechanisms of glomerular injury in glomerulonephritis is not understood but immune factors are strongly implicated. These revolve around immune complexes and in a much smaller group antibodies to the glomerular basement membrane (Table 9.2). A further group including minimal change glomerulonephritis, the focal forms of the disorder and some chronic patterns have little evidence for any immune injury. Different HLA patterns are evident among some of these forms and may indicate potential susceptibility to the disorder rather than an inevitable immune response.

Immune complex injury

The latent period of one to four weeks intervening between infection with the beta-haemolytic streptococcus, Lansfield Group A and Griffiths type 12, and glomerulonephritis provides the firmest evidence for immune complex injury. Experimentally Dixon and colleagues showed that immune complex production led to glomerulonephritis in rabbits and extrapolation of their observations has led to the acceptance that up to 90% of human glomerulonephritis is due to this mechanism. The size, dose and solubility of the complex are all factors influencing deposition as well as the complement and fibrinolytic systems, platelets and neutrophil polymorphs. Complexes may form in antigen or antibody excess or in equilibrium and result in small, large and intermediate sized complexes, respectively. Evidence for these claims often applies only in carefully controlled conditions and mainly to the acute experimental disorder. Proof of a role for immune complexes in renal disease requires:
● recognition within the glomerulus of granular antibody deposits;
● antigen demonstration at the same sites as the antibody. Elution of this antigen is alternatively possible but gives no indication of the site of deposition;
● finding the same antigen either within complexes or intermittently within the serum;

These criteria are difficult to achieve in human glomerulonephritis, principally because the antigen is rarely known.

Observations that undermine an association between immune complexes and glomerulonephritis include:

1   Only a minority of rabbits given bovine serum albumen as the stimulus to complex formation developed glomerular injury.

2   Direct inoculation of *in vitro* formed complexes results in almost no glomerular injury unless the capillary permeability is also increased.

3   Circulating immune complexes accompanying a range of human disorders, most without glomerular lesions.

4   Circulating immune complexes occur with minimal change glomerulonephritis but none are deposited in glomeruli.

5   In most glomerulonephritides there are either no circulating complexes or the levels present fail to correlate with the extent of the disorder. Glomerulonephritis following streptococcal infection is an exception.

6   The antigenic stimulus to the complex formation is rarely identified including that for post-streptococcal glomerulonephritis.

7   Immune complexes within non-renal tissues are not related with ultrastructural basement membrane deposits.

Despite these reservations it is highly probable that immune complex deposition has a role in disease following streptococcal infection and in membranous glomerulonephritis. Post-streptococcal glomerulonephritis mirrors closely the acute disease model and membranous glomerulonephritis the chronic. Also in each disorder, recognized antigens are often either strongly implicated or demonstrated (Table 9.3) and in both the variable clinical course may be attributed to differences in immune complexes and their fate.

Alternatively, injury may arise not from immune complexes from the circulation but from those formed in the glomerular basement membrane. This could occur either from a local build-up of small complexes into larger ones or from circulating antibody combining with trapped antigen and in situ complex formation. The attraction of this concept is that complexes and antigen are passing through the basement membrane and local phenomena could influence the random distribution of the trapped complexes, including their subepithelial and subendothelial localization. Even so, the exact mechanism of glomerular damage whether from immune complexes or other agencies (complement, fibrinogen, platelets, neutrophil polymorphs and cell mediated immunity) still remains to be clarified.

Anti-glomerular basement membrane antibody injury

Circulating antibody against the basement membrane causes glomerulonephritis. The antibody is found in 5% of patients and is directed against the basement membrane of the glomerulus and lung alveoli. Within the lung mild to massive intra-alveolar haemorrhage may result, sometimes precipitated by cigarette smoking and sometimes with renal involvement. The combination of haemoptysis and glomerulonephritis seen in 60% of patients forms *Goodpasture's syndrome*. The glomerulonephritis is a diffuse proliferative one with crescent formation. Upper respiratory tract infection is often described 24–48 h before the clinical symptoms. Evidence relating the auto-antibody and glomerulonephritis rests upon:

1 Showing the auto-antibody in the serum or eluates of the kidney by immunofluorescence on normal human kidney.

2 Transferring the antibody from the serum or kidney eluates to other species, particularly sheep and horses, and producing the same pattern of glomerulonephritis. In man the disorder develops within a transplanted kidney in recipients with circulating auto-antibody.

3 Finding a continuous linear deposit of IgG and C3 in the glomeruli of affected kidneys unrelated to ultrastructural deposits.

Experimentally comparable glomerulonephritis can be produced after immunization with heterologous basement membrane. It is also apparent that the complement and coagulation systems as well as neutrophil polymorphs are involved. The stimulus for the auto-antibody is unknown and the titre is unrelated to the course or severity of the disease. With time the antibody disappears. Plasmaphoresis lowers the titre and hastens the speed of the antibody's disappearance. There is no association with other auto-immune disorders and nor is their HLA pattern shared.

Fig. 9.14 Acute glomerulonephritis. (*Right*) Enlarged pale kidneys from a child of 3 years with nephrotic syndrome and minimal change glomerulonephritis. The change is seen equally in both kidneys and the cortices are substantially widened; (*left*) a similar kidney but with finely dispersed petechiae on the surface.

APPEARANCES

These depend upon the stage in the natural history that the glomerulonephritis has reached. Acute forms, especially the rapidly progressive types, will have equal enlargement of both kidneys affecting all parts (Fig. 9.14). The kidneys will be pale from oedema and cellular infiltration and there can be widespread petechial

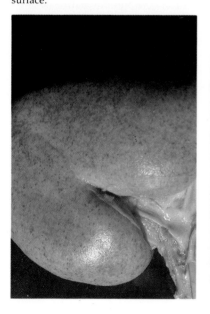
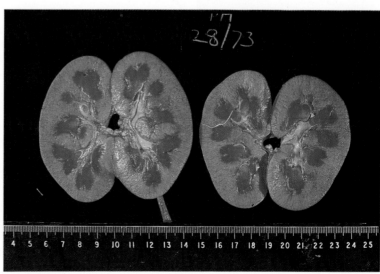

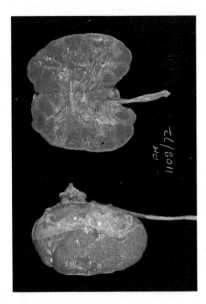

Fig. 9.15 Shrunken kidneys from an adult with chronic renal failure and rapidly progressive glomerulon-ephritis. There is equal involvement of both kidneys and the cortex is reduced to a thin ribbon.

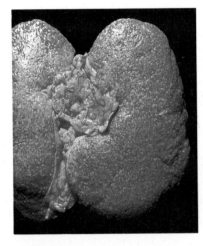

Fig. 9.16 Kidney from a man with end-stage renal failure and membranoproliferative glomerulonephritis. The diffusely distributed fine scarring on the surface is typical of glomerulonephritis and illustrates the uniformity of the glomerular involvement.

haemorrhages in the cortex. The glomeruli may be recognized as discrete grey-white nodules. The early stages of most of the other types of glomerulonephritis include similar features but generally without the petechial haemorrhages. As the disorder progresses both kidneys undergo an equal and uniform reduction which is most conspicuous in the even narrowing of the cortices (Fig. 9.15). Underlying this is a progressive loss of the tubules, mainly the proximal convoluted tubules, and fibrosis. The proximal tubules form the bulk of the cortex and are metabolically highly active and consequently very prone to anoxia and atrophy. Fibrosis contributes to the parenchyma becoming firmer and paler and the capsular surface finely granular (Fig. 9.16). The intrarenal arteries are thickened and the pericalyceal fat is increased.

Dialysis or transplantation can lead to further atrophy. Theoretically in these non-functional kidneys, infection and infarction might be anticipated but both are exceedingly rare. Cysts develop in some kidneys, especially if ancillary renal support is used, and also benign and malignant tumours. Amyloid formation has recently been described.

Glomerular changes and systemic disease

A dilemma faced by clinicians and histopathologists is to decide if a patient has glomerulonephritis or glomerular involvement as a part of a systemic disorder (Table 9.4, Fig. 9.17). The segmental and focal forms of glomerulonephritis most often cause confusion but even with proliferative patterns there is the possibility of a systemic disorder. The greatest help for the histopathologist is unquestionably the clinician's findings, particularly evidence of other organ involvement. A proliferative or segmental 'glomerulonephritis' in a setting of bacterial endocarditis is immediately explained as is 'IgA nephropathy' in a patient with liver disease. The organism underlying the endocarditis provokes immune complex formation and in many forms of liver disease there are raised levels of IgA. Glomerular features that can lead to a diagnosis of a systemic disorder are:
- lack of uniformity of the changes with some glomeruli totally uninvolved;
- segmental changes within abnormal glomeruli;
- changes in the pattern of the glomerular injury in consecutive biopsies;
- features in other parts of the nephron and most especially blood vessels.

Vascular disorders

Anatomy

The kidney receives about one-quarter of the cardiac output which is distributed by a complex arterial tree. A single vessel enters the hilum and subdivides into five main branches, each further subdividing and terminating as afferent glomerular arterioles, one

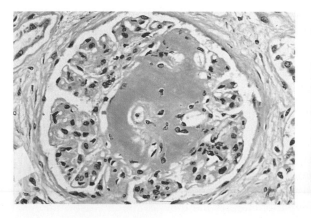 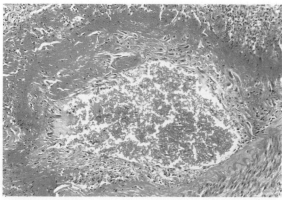

Fig. 9.17 Examples of systemic disorders involving the kidney. (*Above left*) Amyloid deposited within a glomerulus; (*above right*) acute fibrinoid necrosis of an intrarenal artery as part of polyarteritis nodosa.

Table 9.4 Systemic and extrarenal disorders producing glomerular injury

Systemic lupus erythematosus
Henoch−Schonlein purpura
Polyarteritis nodosa
Wegner's granulomatosis
Amyloidosis
Sickle cell disease
Eclampsia of pregnancy
Diabetes mellitus
Multiple myelomatosis
Bacterial endocarditis
Liver disease

million to each kidney (Fig. 9.18). There are no arterial shunts amongst the subdivisions and no collateral supplies. Most vessels are in the cortex, the site of maximal nephron activity, and the effects of any vascular impairment will be reflected in this area. The small arterial supply from the renal capsule is insufficient to counter any ischaemia. None of these observations applies to venous impairment, since multiple shunts exist between the subdivisions of the venous tree which parallel those of the arterial tree.

Vascular impairment

The effects are either none, renal failure or hypertension depending on the extent, degree and speed of the injury. In some instances it may be difficult to distinguish cause and effect. Acute renal failure from drugs and poisons may induce vascular spasm or directly poison the nephron but microthrombi are also invariably found. These reflect disseminated intravascular coagulation and may have developed at the inception of the renal damage or at a later stage. A similar interpretive dilemma arises with hypertension.

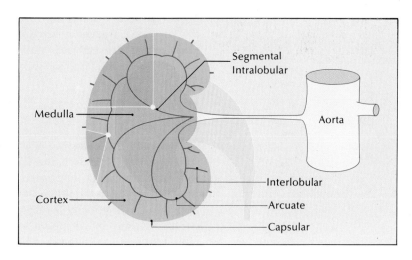

Fig. 9.18 Renal arteries and infarcts.

Hypertension has renal and extrarenal causes but with both there can be either renal changes or, even when the hypertension is renal initally, none.

Disorders

Vascular impairment may arise from disorders of the lumen of the vessel, the wall or the extramural tissues or combinations of these.
1 Many blood disorders cause thrombo-embolism and these, as well as other causes of emboli and disseminated intravascular coagulation, can occlude large and small renal vessels.
2 Arteriosclerosis, affecting the vessel wall, with or without superimposed hypertension, is the most common reason for renal ischaemia. Its effects are on the intrarenal vessels or via stenosis of the main renal vessels. Renal allograft rejection leads to both endo-thelial and intramural changes upon which thrombus may be formed.
3 Vascular injury from extramural causes is less common but may stem from compression, e.g., tumour or idiopathic retroperitoneal fibrosis.

Focal infarcts, cortical necrosis and total renal infarction are the potential morphological consequences of all of these events.

Hypertension

Hypertension implies a level of blood pressure greater than normal. The disorder has two clinical patterns, a rare acute or malignant variant and a common benign or essential variant. *Malignant hypertension* includes evidence of systemic disease with blindness, strokes, left ventricular failure and acute renal failure. The common de-nominator to these is fibrinoid vasculitis, seen clinically in the retinal vessels. *Essential hypertension* can be asymptomatic or ac-companied by symptoms and disorders common to the patient's age group. Essential hypertension is hence not defined by a level of blood pressure but by a level above that of the spectrum for the individual and for the population, both increasing with age.

Unusually, in 6% of patients, causes for hypertension are found. Extrarenal causes range from intracerebral disease and coarctation of the aorta to adrenal tumours, while intrarenal causes include renal artery disease and almost all types of renal parenchymal disease both unilateral and bilateral.

Mechanism

How hypertension is produced and maintained remains unclear but it may be multifactorial. Following the observations of Goldblatt, who produced hypertension by clipping the main renal artery, it was believed that an important precursor was renal artery stenosis and stimulation of the renin angiotensin axis. Angiotensin from the juxtaglomerular apparatus may produce vasoconstriction and a tem-porary increase in peripheral resistance. However, many patients without hypertension have renal artery stenosis and raised levels of angiotensin are not found in all hypertensives. Experience with renal dialysis shows that salt and fluid retention are fundamental since correcting these relieves any hypertension. Sodium, together with calcium, may affect vascular contractility. Other patients with space-occupying intracerebral disorders are relieved of their hypertension by correcting the disorder, as are some patients with increased renal perfusion, indicating both neurogenic control and the influence of cardiac output. It is also believed that the kidney possesses an antihypertensive factor.

APPEARANCES

Essential hypertension results in macroscopic and microscopic features indistinguishable from those of arteriosclerosis and ageing. There is equal reduction in size of both kidneys. The surface is diffusely granular with deeper scarred areas and patchy adherence of the capsule. The cortex is irregularly narrowed and vessels at and radiating from the corticomedullary junction are prominent. Arteriosclerosis underlies the prominence of the vessels and atrophy of nephrons, the cortical changes. The pericalyceal pattern is normal.

Malignant hypertension in the early phases causes enlarged and 'flea-bitten' kidneys, a description given to the scattered petechial haemorrhages on the surface and in the parenchyma. These reflect fibrinoid necrosis of arterioles and glomeruli and focal interstitial haemorrhage. The enlargement is contributed to by oedema. These changes are indistinguishable from some acute glomerulonephrities and acute renal involvement during some systemic disorders. If, with antihypertensive therapy, the patient survives, the kidneys become indistinguishable from those of essential hypertension. A characteristic cellular mucoid endarterial fibrosis of large intrarenal arteries, often compared with the cut surface of an onion, may nonetheless persist (Fig. 9.19).

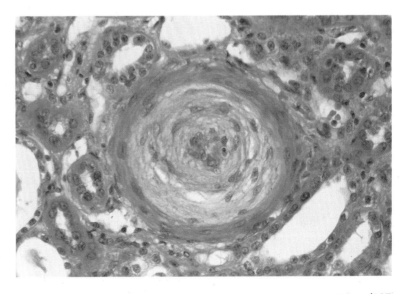

Fig. 9.19 A small intrarenal artery with concentric cellular proliferation of the media associated with malignant hypertension.

Complications of hypertension include cardiac and renal failure and atherosclerosis. The basis of the cardiac failure is reflected by an increase in the size of the left ventricle. Renal failure results from the progressive ischaemic loss of nephrons.

Renal artery stenosis

This is a cause of renovascular hypertension but it is also found radiologically and at autopsy unrelated with hypertension. The main renal artery to one or both kidneys is most often affected but stenosis can also appear in the segmental branches. There are numerous causes including thrombosis but arteriosclerosis is the most common. Varying degrees of fibromuscular hyperplasia of the vessel wall are a rare basis. Removal of the stenotic lesion or of the affected kidney can relieve the hypertension but only if this is done before the uninvolved kidney develops severe hypertensive damage. Paradoxically the kidney associated with the stenosis does not suffer similar injury but does undergo atrophy which, initially, is reversible.

APPEARANCES

The stenotic lesion may be focal or widely dispersed. Arteriosclerosis or thrombus are easily recognized but other causes require light microscopy. The kidney behind the stenotic region is uniformly atrophied and provides one cause of unequally sized kidneys (Fig. 9.20). Microscopically there is an apparent abundance of glomeruli due to atrophy of the proximal convoluted tubules and secondary crowding of glomeruli.

Ischaemic lesions

Ischaemic lesions include infarcts, cortical necrosis, acute tubular

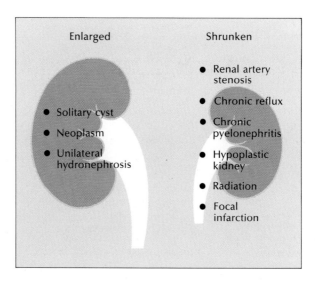

Fig. 9.20 Unequally sized kidneys.

necrosis and poorly defined conditions such as micro-angiopathic haemolytic anaemia and the haemolytic uraemia syndrome. Common to all these is vascular occlusion, from either thrombo-embolic disease or disseminated intravascular coagulation. The latter may be precipitated by immune mechanisms or infections, especially viral, but this is rarely proven.

Infarcts. The site of infarction is governed by the site of the blockage since no collateral arterial supply exists. The level of the blockage depends upon the size of the thrombo-embolism and the diameter of the artery. The renal arterial pattern ensures that any infarct is rhomboid with the apex towards the kidney hilum and the base at the capsular surface (Fig. 9.18).

Embolus from the heart arising from infarction, left-sided valvular endocarditis or atrial fibrillation is the most frequent cause but arteriosclerosis and focal renal artery disorders can lead to the same result. Multiple main renal arteries with small lumina are especially prone to these complications and since the smallest vessel often supplies one pole, polar infarcts result. Infarcts also occur in acutely and chronically rejected renal transplants and micro-infarcts as part of any form of vasculitis.

Early infarcts are dark red and sharply demarcated from the surrounding parenchyma. As the entrapped red cells haemolyse the area becomes paler and yellowish and undergoes necrosis and shrinkage.

Cortical necrosis. This is a naturally fatal condition. The underlying mechanism is unclear but vasospasm and disseminated intravascular coagulation are implicated, in part precipitated by severe hypo-volaemia. It follows haemorrhagic and hypertensive complications of pregnancy, severe infection, burns and shock from any cause. Both kidneys are involved although not all the cortex may be affected. Cortical necrosis also develops in the acutely rejected renal transplant.

The cortex is anaemic and yellow and may be widened or narrowed depending upon the interval between necrosis and examination (Fig. 9.21). A thin surviving zone, representing the area supplied by the capsular vessels, separates the capsule and necrotic tissue. The uninvolved medulla is engorged and bright red.

Acute tubular necrosis. This condition is comparable to cortical necrosis but the injury centres upon the tubules rather than all elements of the nephron within the cortex. The causes are similar but also include crush injuries as a cause of shock and direct poisoning of the proximal convoluted tubules by substances including antibiotics, mercury and gold. The important difference from cortical necrosis is that renal failure is potentially reversible. Vascular injury may thus be less significant than direct injury to the tubular cells. These cells are metabolically highly active with an immense regenerative capacity.

Patients dying with acute tubular necrosis have enlarged,

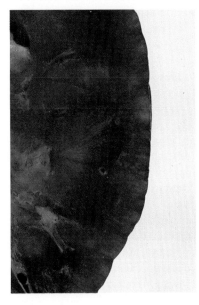

Fig. 9.21 Cortical necrosis. The cortex includes blotchy yellow zones and is congested. The patient had survived for some days following a ruptured aneurysm.

oedematous, pale kidneys. Oedema and a mixture of tubular necrosis and regeneration are the essential microscopic features but these may not be as severe as the functional impairment might infer.

Cystic disease

Simple cysts. One or more renal cysts of varying size are found in approximately 50% of autopsies. The incidence and number increase with age and most are symptomless. There is an increased incidence in end-stage non-functional kidneys in patients on dialysis or given renal transplants. Rarely cysts are large enough to cause clinical or radiological confusion with a neoplasm.

Adult polycystic disease. In contrast to simple cysts this disorder causes renal failure and, in many centres, forms the third most common cause of end-stage renal failure. The disease is autosomal dominant and expresses itself from 30 years of age onwards but only in about 30% of patients. The reasons for this variable outcome are unknown. The classical presentation is chronic renal failure which is extremely insidious in its development. The recognition of grossly enlarged kidneys, abdominal pain secondary to infection or haemorrhage within the cysts, or hypertension and haematuria are other presentations. Ten per cent of patients have berry aneurysms and some develop subarachnoid haemorrhage.

Juvenile cystic disease. A range of cystic disorders present with renal impairment in the neonate or early childhood. The cystic dysplastic kidney is the most important. Others are autosomal recessive disorders and accompany organ disorders, most often hepatic fibrosis.

Development

The basis for cyst formation is unknown. Clearly occurrence in the neonate implies a developmental abnormality, probably during nephron formation. Genetic and environmental factors may encourage the aberration both in the neonate and the adult. The proposition that certain metabolites excreted by the kidney lead to cyst formation is unsubstantiated, partly by the failure of the development of cysts in kidney transplants to these patients. Cysts in the native kidneys of transplant patients are probably analogous to those found incidentally in normal kidneys, possibly arising from blockage of the nephron and subsequent dilatation. Any blockage could come from the contents but nephron dissection suggests that parenchymal scarring is the main cause. Ischaemia associated with age, hypertension and infection contribute to interstitial fibrosis as well as coincidental renal disease.

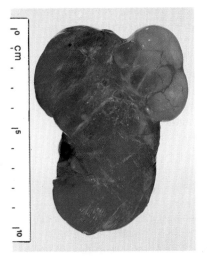

Fig. 9.22 Large simple cyst projecting from the upper pole and a smaller cyst in the centre within the kidney substance.

APPEARANCES

1 *Simple cysts* may be unilateral or bilateral and single or multiple (Fig. 9.22). Their size varies from millimetres to several centimetres

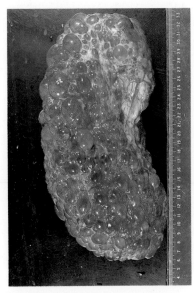

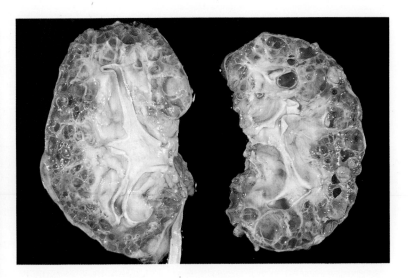

Fig. 9.23 Adult polycystic disease; (*left*) external and (*right*) cut surface appearance. The kidneys are hugely enlarged but the calyceal and pelvic pattern is maintained.

and they may project from the surface or remain confined within the parenchyma. The contents are generally clear or yellow/orange. There is no communication with the calyceal pelvic system.

2   *Adult polycystic disease* can be unilateral but is usually bilateral. The kidneys are always enlarged and may reach massive proportions with each weighing 5 kg or more (Fig. 9.23). Their shape is maintained and there is a normal unenlarged calyceal–pelvic system and ureter. The entire parenchyma is replaced by cysts which bulge from the surface. The cysts differ in size from a few millimetres to several centimetres and their contents include clear yellow-to-orange fluid, blood clot and brownish semifluid. The cysts have no direct communication with one another nor with the calyceal–pelvic system. Between the cysts, often scarcely discernible, are the remnants of parenchyma and invariably, with careful microscopic examination, some normal glomeruli. Similar cysts but in much smaller numbers and without clinical features are found in the liver (Fig. 9.24) in 40% of patients and less often in the pancreas, lungs and ovaries. Berry aneurysms in the circle of Willis are a complication in 10% of patients.

3   *Juvenile cystic disease.* The kidneys are small and scarred. The cysts are small and randomly scattered within the parenchyma. The calyceal–pelvic system is dilated and often like that of reflux nephropathy.

Interstitial nephritis

This condition provides a popular diagnosis but is frequently inappropriately applied. The term should be confined to inflammation of the renal parenchyma that, importantly, is not due to glomerular or vascular changes. The features include oedema, mononuclear cell infiltrates and later fibrosis, all of which can accompany most renal disorders. The changes can also, as a secondary phenomenon, provoke glomerular and vascular lesions and since a wide range of

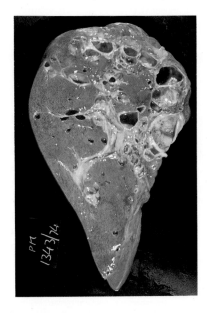

Fig. 9.24 Multiple cysts in the liver accompanying adult polycystic disease.

drugs including penicillin produce interstitial nephritis it is possible for this and other renal disorders to coexist. There is no unique clinical feature but aids to the diagnosis are eosinophilia and other systemic disorders, most frequently a rash, all of which remit if the cause is withdrawn and re-occur with its re-introduction.

Development

The mechanism underlying the interstitial inflammation is probably different for different causes and for many it is unknown. Potential mechanisms include direct toxic injury and immune injury (Fig. 9.1). The latter very rarely centres upon antibasement membrane antibodies to renal tubules, immune complex deposition and hypersensitivity Type IV reactions. The last presents an attractive hypothesis because of the substantial mononuclear cell infiltrate but there is little positive supportive evidence. An immune basis would, nonetheless, explain the extrarenal features.

APPEARANCES

These mimic very closely those of arteriosclerosis and reflux nephritis although without the latter's calyceal features and supracalyceal localization.

Analgesic nephropathy and papillary necrosis

Long-term ingestion of substantial quantities of phenacetin and phenacetin-containing compounds including salicylates will lead to end-stage renal failure. The basic morphological lesion is necrosis of the renal papillae. Analgesic abuse is seen particularly in women and if stopped early normal renal function is restored. The disorder is an important cause of renal failure in some countries, especially Australia and Scandinavia. Papillary necrosis also occurs in diabetics, those with sickle cell disease and in hypotensive neonatal shock.

Development

The mechanism of analgesic injury has yet to be fully explained. The analgesics concentrate in the papillae and medulla and one of the earliest changes is damage to the tubular epithelial cells. Vascular changes are the logical explanation for the necrosis but whether this arises from toxic injury or as a secondary effect of the interstitial inflammation is unclear. The other causes of papillary necrosis also reflect a vascular role.

APPEARANCES

The necrotic papillae may break off and pass per urethra with or without obstructive symptoms. The denuded area is bowed and confusion with reflux nephropathy can follow. If the necrotic papillae

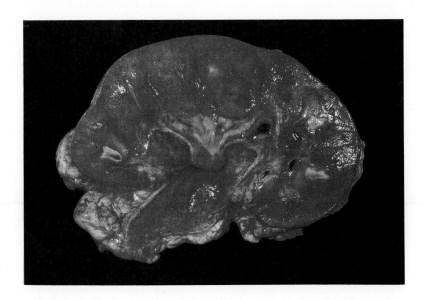

Fig. 9.25 Papillary necrosis affecting renal papillae at the upper and lower poles of the kidney.

are in situ these are dark red and are sharply demarcated from the overlying parenchyma (Fig. 9.25). One or several papillae in one or both kidneys may be involved. Shrinkage and fibrosis with calcification and rarely bone formation are longer term changes. Once end-stage renal failure is reached it may be extremely difficult to differentiate the features from those in end-stage reflux nephropathy or interstitial nephritis.

Transplant kidney

Renal transplantation is widely practised in the treatment of end-stage renal failure and is applicable to all but a very small group of patients. Those excluded are principally those whose disease will be transmitted to the graft (Table 9.5). Animal experimentation, however, has strongly indicated that failure would be much higher because of the natural immune responses that destroy the graft. By narrowing the relationship between the donor and recipient the reaction is diminished but because humans are antigenically complex perfect tissue matching is rare. Antigenic matching involves ABO blood grouping and HLA (human leucocyte antigen) typing but an absolute match rarely occurs except with identical twins. Rejection primarily involves T-lymphocytes and macrophages and to a lesser degree B-cells and humoral antibody. These responses can be counteracted by immunosuppressive therapy. By the use of tissue typing and immunosuppression, graft rejection can be substantially suppressed and long-term graft survival achieved. Unfortunately the immunosuppression is not specific and an important side effect is that other parameters of the immune response are affected. Infection and tumours are then potential consequences and both, but especially infection, occur, most notably in the early stages of the therapy when the largest doses are given. Currently, graft biopsy is the only certain method for the diagnosis of rejection. On occasions

Table 9.5 Some disorders transmitted to renal transplants

Commonly recurrent	Focal glomerulonephritis Mesangiocapillary (dense deposit) glomerulonephritis IgA nephropathy Oxalosis Cystinosis
Uncertain frequency	Mesangiocapillary (Type 1) glomerulonephritis Anti-basement membrane (glomerular and tubular) disease Amyloid Diabetic glomerulonephropathy Progressive systemic sclerosis
Rarely recurrent	Membranous glomerulonephritis Idiopathic crescentic glomerulonephritis Henoch−Schonlein purpura Haemolytic uraemic syndrome Malignant hypertension Renal Fanconi syndrome

this gives indications that allow one to anticipate this reaction and thereby act before the tissue is damaged.

Graft rejection

Rejection is sited initially around vessels where a mononuclear cell infiltrate develops (Fig. 9.26). Unchecked this increases and randomly dispersed vascular changes occur. Fibrinoid necrosis is the most important of these since this is unresponsive to immunosuppression and inevitably progresses to graft destruction. Similar but more protracted destruction can follow from intimal and medial changes arising from chronic rejection processes and resulting in arterial narrowing and ischaemic fibrosis. These all depend upon mononuclear cells which are continuously perfusing through the graft,

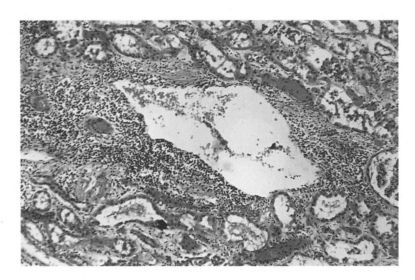

Fig. 9.26 Early appearances of rejection in a renal allograft. There are mononuclear cells around a vein together with oedema.

recognizing foreign antigen expressed either by dendritic messenger cells or by the graft's endothelial or interstitial cells. The host lymphocytes, once sensitized to the graft antigens, proliferate and produce antibody with or without central involvement and initiate graft destruction. Important contributors to the process are the complement and clotting cascades and ischaemia.

A few patients have circulating cytotoxic antibodies either from blood transfusions or pregnancies or following rejection of previous grafts. These antibodies result in fulminant rejection, *hyperacute rejection*, which occurs soon after the vascular clamps are released.

Non-immune graft failure

Graft failure is not inevitably due to rejection although this is the main cause (Fig. 9.27). Shortly after transplantation tubular necrosis following ischaemic damage developing between death of the donor and the completion of the transplant procedure occurs. Cyclosporine A can also contribute to tubular necrosis and this is probably part of the nephrotoxicity arising from this immunosuppressive. Diffuse disorders present prior to tansplantation will embarrass function as does any primary renal disease, particularly glomerulonephritis. Distinction has to be made between glomerulonephritis established within the graft before transplantation and that developing after. Glomerulonephritis transmitted from the recipient must match exactly that of the native kidneys and that developing as a primary disease may form part of the rejection process. Any of these events are unusual and many of the glomerular changes are probably primarily ischaemic.

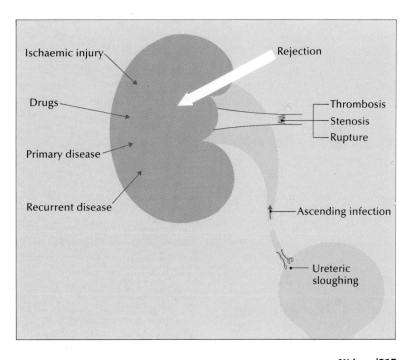

Fig. 9.27 Renal transplant failure.

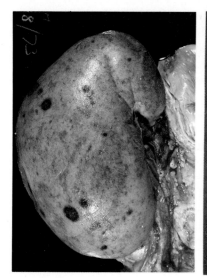

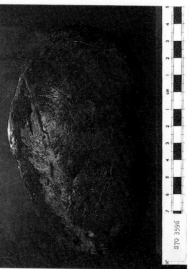

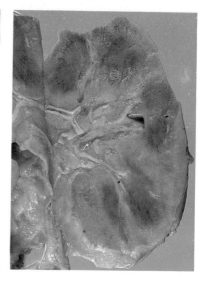

Fig. 9.28 Transplant kidney that is enlarged, pale and includes haemorrhagic areas on the surface overlying areas of infarction.

Fig. 9.29 Transplant kidney with more florid changes than in Fig. 9.28 and manifesting severe acute rejection.

Fig. 9.30 Chronically rejected transplant kidney. This, in contrast to those in Fig. 9.28 and 9.29, is small and pale. The parenchyma was very tough and fibrotic and the intrarenal vessels severely narrowed.

APPEARANCES

These depend upon the type of rejection and the time at which the graft is examined. Any successfully grafted kidney enlarges, mainly due to hypertrophy. Rejection contributes to enlargement with the cellular infiltrate and oedema and early rejecting kidneys are consequently large, pale and moist (Fig. 9.28). If fibrinoid necrosis is present focal areas of haemorrhage, localized infarcts, cortical necrosis and even papillary necrosis are potential additional features (Fig. 9.29).

Longer term grafts with chronic obliterative arterial lesions undergo ischaemic damage and shrink (Fig. 9.30). The random vascular involvement ensures that this is uneven and irregular scarring results. Since acute vascular lesions may be superimposed upon these changes infarcts, cortical and papillary necrosis and focal haemorrhages may also be found.

Tumours

A variety occur within the kidney but, in adults, adenocarcinoma is the most common. Renal carcinoma forms between 1–2% of all adult malignancies and up to 80% of renal tumours. Wilms' tumour is confined to children and forms 20% of all childhood malignancies.

Adenocarcinoma

The tumour arises from the epithelium of the proximal tubules and in its early stages is confined to the cortex. Previous uncertainty of the origin, notably from the adrenals, led to the terms *Grawitz tumour, hypernephroma* and *clear cell carcinoma*. The tumour has been related to smoking, especially pipe and cigar, and to the use of Thorotrast for retrograde pyelography. Other associations are congenital and acquired cystic disease, horseshoe kidneys and the inherited *von Hippel—Lindau disease* (multiple systemic angiomas and cysts within the brain and spinal cord).

Men are affected slightly over twice as often as women and the maximum incidence is between 50—60 years. The classical presentation, by which time metastatic lesions are invariably established, is seen in only 10—15% of patients. This is the triad of haematuria, loin pain and an abdominal mass. Haematuria is the more common symptom but a variety of other presentations are recognized, including many with a hormonal basis. The best known is a form of polycythaemia attributed to an erythropoetin substance but others include Cushing's syndrome and hypercalcaemia related with ACTH and parathormone-like substances. All of these may remit if the tumour is removed, a phenomenon also met with in other patients with associated hypertension and renin secretion.

The tumour is an adenocarcinoma with potential for a range of cytological appearances. The most common of these are the clear, granular cell types but mixed patterns are often found. There is no prognostic significance for any of the patterns except that in which the entire cell population is oncocytic when this can be excellent.

Prognosis

This is determined by the size of the tumour and spread beyond the kidney. Tumours larger than 5 cm diameter are most likely to have metastasized and the 5-year survival is 20% as opposed to 60% for tumours of less than 5 cm diameter. When metastases are recognized at nephrectomy survival rarely extends more than 3 years but if there is a solitary metastasis it should be removed, since long-term survival can then occur. Spontaneous regression of renal carcinomas is also recorded.

APPEARANCES

Tumours vary from less than 3 cm diameter to massive diameters and weights. The smallest are confined to the renal cortex and are nodular and yellow/orange. Larger lesions include areas of haemorrhage, necrosis, calcification and cyst formation (Fig. 9.31). Tumours may remain in the renal parenchyma or extend beyond this, restricted by a pseudocapsule of compressed perirenal tissues. Enlargement into the pelvis results in calyceal and pelvic deformities complicated by obstruction.

Metastases

Less than 5% of renal carcinomas are multiple and even smaller numbers bilateral. The difficulty, virtually impossible to resolve, is

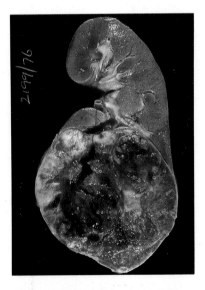

Fig. 9.31 Adenocarcinoma replacing the upper pole of the kidney. There is extensive necrosis and haemorrhage.

whether these examples represent primary growths or metastatic spread. The carcinoma can be clinically silent for years and the size gives no indication of the metastatic potential. Metastases are more common with tumours over 5 cm diameter but have been recorded with those of less than 3 cm diameter, hence the disuse of the term adenoma for renal cell tumours.

Venous spread is recognized in at least one-third of patients at nephrectomy and in substantially more after microscopic examination. The tumour may spread into the vena cava with further dissemination during surgery. Metastases from blood spread develop, especially in the lung but also in the liver and bone and even the opposite kidney. Others are via lymphatics, principally to the para-aortic lymph nodes and by local invasion. The latter must be distinguished from the common passive expansion and local compression of perirenal structures.

Wilms' tumour (nephroblastoma)

This tumour is virtually confined to children between 1–5 years. An abdominal mass is recognized by the parents and clinically this must be distinguished from the slightly more common neuroblastoma.

The tumour includes immature and mature mesenchymal tissues intermingled with abortive glomeruli and tubules. It is hence assumed that it has originated during differentiation of the metanephric blastema. With modern therapy the life expectancy for some patients may be normal. Widespread extrarenal tumour, poor histological differentiation and a patient of over 2 years all adversely affect the prognosis.

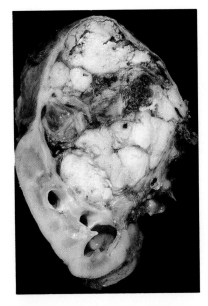

Fig. 9.32 Nephroblastoma almost replacing the kidney in a 2-year-old child.

APPEARANCES

The tumour may reach huge proportions, 500 g or more, and consequently compresses adjacent structures (Fig. 9.32). A rounded mass, often filling one pole of the kidney, is seen with a firm greyish-white rubbery parenchyma containing foci of haemorrhage, necrosis and cyst formation. Approximately 10% of patients have bilateral tumours.

Direct spread can occur into the liver and other organs as well as down the ureter. Lymph node involvement and venous spread, invariably to the lungs but also the liver, skeleton and brain, have often occurred by diagnosis.

Other tumours

Metastases

Metastatic tumour is generally bilateral and is seen with approximately 5% of malignant tumours. The most common primary sources of carcinoma are the lung, breast, stomach and ovary. Leukaemias and lymphomas are other important sources of metastases.

Further reading

Heptinstall, R.H. (1983). *Pathology of the Kidney* (3rd Edition). Little, Brown and Co: Boston.

Klahr, S., Schreiner, G. and Ichikawa, I. (1988). The progression of renal disease. *New Eng. J. Med.* **318**, 1657–66.

Risdon, R.A. and Turner, D.R. (1980). *Atlas of Renal Pathology*. MTP Press Ltd: Lancaster.

Jones, N.F. and Peters, D.K. (1982) (Editors). *Recent Advances in Renal Medicine 2*. Churchill Livingstone: London and Edinburgh.

Cameron J.S. and Glassock R.J. (1988) (Editors). *Kidney Disease Volume 2*. Marcel Dekker: New York.

10   Male genital tract

The male genital tract includes the testes and supporting scrotum, vas deferens, prostate, seminal vesicles and penis. Disorders of the scrotum and penis largely mirror those of the skin although eponyms are sometimes used. *Balanitis* is a term applied to inflammation of the prepuce and glans penis and *erythroplasia of Queyrat* that given to carcinoma in situ of the prepuce. Specific infections of the penis include warts and primary chancres while the most common tumour is squamous cell carcinoma. Infections and tumours can involve the vas deferens and seminal vesicles but rarely do so in the absence of concurrent disorders of the testes and prostate. The virtually benign adenomatoid tumour of the epididymis and malignant rhabdomyosarcoma in this site in the child are notable exceptions.

Testis

Inflammation of the testis is called *orchitis* and since this invariably involves the epididymis, it is generally referred to as *epididymoorchitis*. Infection reaches the testis via the bloodstream but can also spread in a retrograde manner from the epididymis and urethra. Bladder infections and Gram-negative organisms are the causes, especially when complicating abnormalities of the urinary tract and surgical procedures. Mumps virus, *Chlamydia*, tuberculosis and syphilis are other causes (Fig. 10.1). A long-term effect can be infertility contributed to by destruction and atrophy of the testis.

Infertility

Male infertility is becoming increasingly recognized and may require testicular biopsy. The only patients in whom this can provide diagnostic aid are those with a testicular basis for their infertility. The procedure will not be contributory in men with pretesticular causes for infertility which are predominantly endocrine or those with posttesticular causes which include obstructive lesions and impaired sperm mobility. Testicular biopsy, even in those in whom these causes have been eliminated, will show nothing abnormal in over a quarter of the patients. Positive findings in 50% of the remaining include some interruption of the normal maturation pathway of the spermatozoa, *spermatocytic arrest*, which in some with gonad dysgenesis syndromes will be complete. The other finding is of generalized fibrosis.

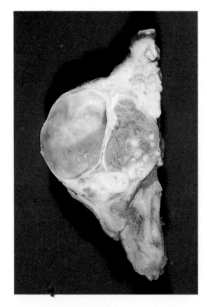

Fig. 10.1 Tuberculous involvement of the testis with replacement of the epididymis and cyst formation. Much of the testis is atrophic and miliary type tuberculous lesions lie in the remaining parenchyma.

Tumours

Testicular tumours are rare with some 600 examples occurring annually within England and Wales. This incidence is, however, increasing although no cause has been identified. These tumours are the most common neoplasms amongst men of 25–34 years and most are malignant. Men in the higher socio-economic groups in Scandinavia and Europe are predominantly affected but blacks rarely so. Nevertheless, recent advances in therapy, principally chemotherapy, have dramatically altered the outlook. Cure is now a distinct possibility for 90% of those with a tumour either confined to the testis or with extratesticular spread restricted to beneath the diaphragm.

The epithelium of the seminiferous tubes is the site of spermatogenesis but it also includes the supporting Sertoli cells. These cells may produce hormones but the main source of hormones is the Leydig or interstitial cells which lie between the seminiferous tubules. They produce 95% of the circulating testosterone which is under control of the leutinizing hormone of the pituitary. Smaller amounts of testosterone come from the prostate where active conversion of adrenal precursors occurs. The tubular epithelium, Sertoli and Leydig cells are all foci for testicular tumours but only those from the Sertoli and especially the Leydig cells produce endocrine changes. Gynaecomastia and precocious puberty depending upon the patient's age are the main features. The majority of tumours are recognized as testicular masses which in young boys must be differentiated from hernias and torsion of the testis but in older patients, hydrocoeles and epididymo-orchitis are further possibilities. Hydrocoeles only very rarely accompany testicular tumours; most are idiopathic although tuberculosis remains an important, although uncommon, cause (Fig. 10.2).

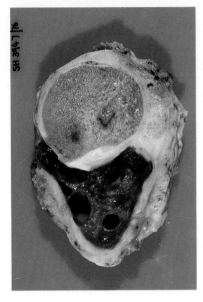

Fig. 10.2 Chronic hydrocoele in which haemorrhage has occurred. There is marked fibrosis of the tunica vaginalis and atrophy of the testis.

Cell of origin

The tumours are grouped into germ and non-germ cell tumours with the germ cell types contributing over 90%. The cell of origin of non-germ cell tumours is undisputed and a number of different cell types including interstitial and Sertoli cells are involved (Table 10.1).

Germ cell tumours fall into the two broad categories of seminoma and teratoma, or non-seminomatous tumours. Nevertheless, in a significant number of tumours both of these categories are represented, an observation inferring a common stem cell. Further evidence for common origin includes the development of both types of tumours within testes at risk of malignant change, most notably undescended testes, and the presence of alpha-fetoprotein and human chorionic gonadotrophin in the majority of teratomas, and also in some seminomas. (Placental alkaline phosphatase is more characteristic of seminomas.) The stem cell probably exists within the epithelium of the seminiferous tubules. This epithelium develops from the mesenchymal cells of the urogenital ridge and

Table 10.1 Testicular tumours

	%
Seminoma	39.5
Teratoma	31.7
Combined seminoma and teratoma	13.5
Lymphoma	6.7
Sertoli cell Interstitial (Leydig) cell Yolk sac Metastases	each <2

the coelomic epithelium and similar tumours can thus be anticipated within the descent pathway of the testis, so explaining the rare germ cell tumours in mid-line structures such as the third ventricle of the brain, the pineal gland, the anterior mediastinum and the retroperitoneal tissues. Nevertheless, with such tumours the presence of a primary testicular tumour must always be ruled out.

Comparisons with the germ cell tumours of the female genital tract, for which a similar stem cell is postulated, can be made. Seminomas are the male counterpart of dysgerminomas and within both sexes teratomas develop. What is not comparable is the age distribution and, more importantly, the behaviour of the teratomas. In males teratomas are invariably malignant while in females they are almost uniformly benign.

Associated factors (Fig. 10.3)

1 *Cryptorchidism.* Incomplete descent of the testis into the scrotum occurs in 0.5—1.6% of the male population. The discrepancy between these figures probably reflects a recent increase in incidence rather than improved diagnosis. The incidence of testicular tumours among these patients is 14—30 times greater than among other men and the tumours may occur within the undescended or the ipsilateral normally positioned testis. Both seminomas and teratomas develop although the former are the more usual and together they contribute 6—10% of all testicular tumours. The risk of neoplasia is greatest for the testis within the abdomen but this can be substantially reduced if orchiopexy is performed, provided this is done before 5 years of age.

2 *Infertility.* A consequence of cryptorchidism for almost 50% of affected men is infertility, which is also found in those with gonadal dysgenesis, including *Klinefelter's syndrome* (a mainly XXY karyotype accompanied by gynaecomastia). Among all other infertile men a small number develop testicular tumours. Infertility may be incidental but may reflect an epithelial deficit provoking germ cell tumours, possibly produced by temperature. Intrascrotal temperature is lower than the intra-abdominal temperature and provides that most favourable for spermatogenesis.

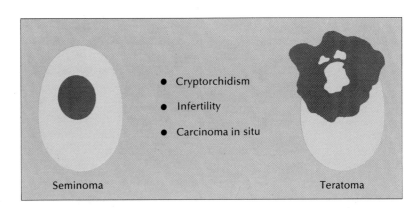

Fig. 10.3 Testicular germ cell tumours.

3 *Carcinoma in situ.* Large atypical cells can be found within the epithelium of the spermatic tubules and less often among the interstitial tissues. These changes are carcinoma in situ and are invariably recognized within the tubules adjacent to germ cell tumours and in dysgenetic gonads. They are also seen in testes of infertile men; in the contralateral testis to that with a teratoma and to that that is or was undescended; in undescended testes even when placed within the strotum; and in testes of patients with extragonadal germ cell tumours. The incidence among these conditions is 0.4–5.4%. Germ cell tumours also characterize these conditions and although progression from carcinoma in situ to germ cell tumours is not inevitable, the two are closely related. Further proof will come if chemotherapy for testicular tumours also halts the appearance of second tumours in the contralateral testis.

4 *Injury.* A history of injury, both physical and inflammatory, is commonly given but no firm evidence exists that this has any part in the tumour's development. It is often instrumental in bringing the patient's attention to his tumour.

Classification

A division between non-germ cell tumours and germ cell tumours is easily made. Distinguishing between different types of germ cell tumours is more contentious and for the teratomas involves three different classifications, one each from the USA, WHO and UK. Comparisons between these, although attempted, are often confusing and only that used by the British Testicular Tumour Panel is given (Table 10.2). The basis of these are the histological appearances and the aim is to define patterns of behaviour and prognosis. Chemotherapy has radically altered the prognosis and made these aims largely redundant. Moreover, marker studies, at present restricted to alpha-fetoprotein, human chorionic gonadotrophin and placental alkaline phosphatase, may ultimately provide a classification reflecting developmental and functional characteristics that is both more appropriate and therapeutically more useful. Whatever system is used it is extremely important that there is adequate sampling with examination of multiple sections since there can be

Table 10.2 British classification of testicular teratomas

Teratoma differentiated (TD)	
Malignant teratoma intermediate (MTI)	Either the tumour harbouring malignant epithelium or this is found in other regions
Malignant teratoma undifferentiated (MTU)	
Malignant teratoma trophoblastic (MTT)	Trophoblastic tissue present (choriocarcinoma)
Orchoblastoma or yolk sac tumour in children (MTU in adults)	Yolk sac elements

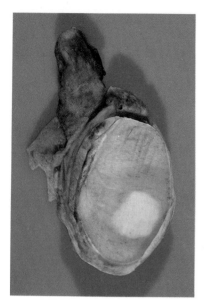

Fig. 10.4 Seminoma replacing part of the testis. The tumour is uniform and paler than the testicular parenchyma.

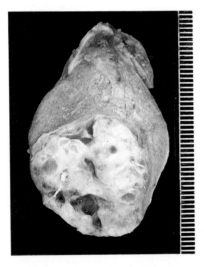

Fig. 10.5 Teratoma filling much of the normal testis. The tumour is partly cystic.

significant variation within an individual tumour, and classification depends upon the most malignant elements. At the same time it must be realized that teratomas at the most well differentiated end of the spectrum can metastasize and thus even in the prepubertal boy, in contrast to their appearances and their counterparts in women, are potentially, even if rarely, lethal.

Seminomas form a virtually homogeneous group but with a subgroup of less than 5% classified as *spermatocytic*. These seminomas include tumour cells that are less uniform than those in the majority of seminomas and are rarely associated with extra-testicular spread. They also have a better prognosis and occur particularly in elderly men.

APPEARANCES

All testicular tumours marginally involve the right testis more than the left and bilaterality is exceedingly rare except for lymphomas.
1 *Seminomas* result in uniform enlargement, often two to four times that of normal, and lie within the parenchyma. They are ovoid with a uniform, creamy white cut surface which only occasionally includes yellow necrotic foci (Fig. 10.4).
2 *Teratomas*, in contrast, enlarge and deform the testis, often projecting from the surface and have a variable stroma. This may include cystic areas as well as solid regions associated with cartilage, and necrotic haemorrhagic foci in the more malignant variants (Fig. 10.5). The hair, teeth and keratin characteristic of most dermoids in women do not regularly occur. Tumours combining teratomas and seminomas are generally recognizable macroscopically from the obvious contrast between the two appearances.

Spread. Seminomas metastasize to the para-aortic lymph nodes and tumour may be found in lymphatics in the resected cut end of the spermatic cord. Teratomas spread mainly by the bloodstream and secondary deposits may develop within the lungs, liver, brain and bone.
3 *Interstitial and Sertoli cell* tumours form well circumscribed nodules. Those of the interstitial cell tumours are usually less than 5 cm diameter and are brownish-yellow. The Sertoli cell tumours can reach 30 cm diameter when malignancy should be suspected, but most are smaller and are firm and creamy white, sometimes with a few small cystic spaces. Ten per cent of either tumour are malignant but apart from a large size there are no distinctive macroscopic features.
4 *Non-Hodgkin's lymphomas* are the most common testicular tumours in men over 50 years and, in 20%, are bilateral. The tumour can be primary or part of a widespread lymphoma. The testis is enlarged with a fairly uniform soft white parenchyma.
5 *Acute leukaemia* in children involves the testis and when irradiation therapy has been used leukaemic cells escape destruction and provide a centre for recurrence. If massive numbers of leukaemic cells are present the features mimic those of a lymphoma.

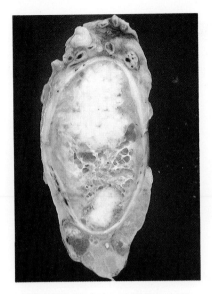

6 *Other metastatic tumours*, of which that from the prostate is the most common, invariably escape recognition macroscopically. They are usually incidental findings in orchidectomy specimens performed in the management of prostatic carcinoma (Fig. 10.6).

Prostate

The bulk of the gland is found between the urethra and the rectum and traditionally divided into an anterior, middle, posterior and two lateral lobes. All lobes have an endodermal origin apart from the posterior which originates from mesoderm. A study of the pattern of the mucous glands has suggested that the prostate should be regarded as an inner peri-urethral zone and an outer posterior peripheral zone (Fig. 10.7). This division is in keeping with the different distributions of hyperplasia (inner peri-urethral zone) and carcinoma (outer zone) as well as with the embryological origin of these areas and is thus increasingly used.

Fig. 10.6 Prostatic metastases found incidentally in an orchidectomy specimen. Prior to the operation hormone therapy had been given and the testis is consequently largely atrophic.

Nodular hyperplasia

This extremely common condition (Fig. 10.8) is seen with advancing age so that by the eighth decade 75% of men are affected. Hyperplasia develops mainly in the central zone and, by disrupting the integrity of the urethral sphincter, produce disturbances in micturition. The changes affect the glandular and the stromal elements which in individual prostates are involved to varying degrees.

Pituitary and gonadotrophin secretion is necessary for hyperplasia since castration before and after puberty halts the normal development, as does hypophysectomy secondary to oestrogen therapy. The exact sequence of events is, nevertheless, far from clear but is not comparable to the hyperplasia—adenoma—carcinoma sequence of endocrine glands since malignancy is unrelated.

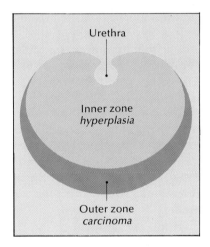

Fig. 10.7 Divisions of the prostate.

APPEARANCE

The involved gland can be hugely enlarged and weigh 300 g or more (normal 15−20 g). The parenchyma is white, firm and whorled or nodular and may produce distinct 'lateral' and 'median' lobes depending upon the areas involved. Calculi (Fig. 10.9), abscesses and infarcts are all occasional complications.

Carcinoma

These tumours are uncommon under 50 years of age but thereafter show an increasing incidence and form the fourth most common malignancy amongst men in the UK. They can be subdivided into clinical or active, occult and latent, indicating that the primary lesion, despite metastases, can be symptomless (the *occult tumour*) or occur as an incidental finding either at autopsy or prostatectomy (the *latent tumour*). The prognosis is worse for those with clinical

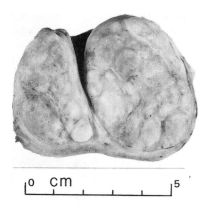

Fig. 10.8 Prostatic hyperplasia.

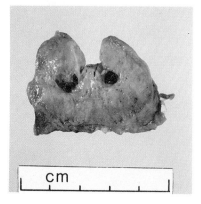

Fig. 10.9 Prostatic calculi complicating slight hypertrophy.

and occult tumours but, because of the age of the population affected, the tumour may not cause the patient's death.

The age incidence and the detrimental effects on growth of oestrogen therapy and orchidectomy suggest a hormonal influence. The prostate can metabolize testosterone precursors to active testosterone and in prostatic carcinomas this may contribute 40% of the circulating testosterone. Medical and surgical castration both dramatically reduce this synthesis supporting the hypothesis that the local accumulation and persistence of testosterone provide a stimulus for carcinoma. The tumour is not related to prostatic hyperplasia.

The tumour is an adenocarcinoma arising from the acini of the peripheral or posterior zone of the gland. Much of this region remains intact after a transurethral resection and tumour may arise later or be missed at the time of the resection. Perineal needle biopsies reduce the incidence of this complication. A further difficulty can be in distinguishing metastatic tumour, principally from the rectum, bladder and urethra, from a primary prostatic tumour. Labelled antibody to prostatic acid phosphatase and, better, prostatic specific antigen, help solve this dilemma, although neither is absolutely specific for prostatic tissue or always positive for prostatic carcinomas.

APPEARANCES

With the advent of transurethral resection, the intact prostate is rarely removed and the opportunity of seeing prostatic carcinomas macroscopically is drastically reduced. Occult tumours at autopsy invariably remain unrecognized until histology sections are examined. The features include a yellow gritty stroma, principally in the peripheral zones and often multifocal (Fig. 10.10). The gland may or may not be enlarged depending upon the bulk of tumour and the extent of any accompanying fibrosis or hyperplasia.

Perineural invasion and spread between muscle bundles are common but neither have any prognostic importance. More distant spread develops because of the proximity of the tumour to the

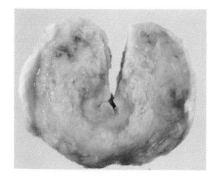

Fig. 10.10 Carcinoma of the prostate with sparing of the peri-urethral tissue.

capsule via lymphatic and venous channels. Metastases appear in local lymph nodes and especially bones of the axial skeleton where they may be recognized long before the primary growth. Other sites for metastases include the skin, testes and breasts (mimicking gynaecomastia), but ultimately any organ may be involved.

Further reading

Ansell, I.D. (1985). *Atlas of Male Reproductive Pathology*. M.T.P. Press Ltd.: Lancaster and Boston.

Chisholm, G.D. and Williams, D.I. (1982) (Editors). *Scientific Foundations of Urology* (2nd Edition). William Heinemann Medical Books Ltd: London.

Lancet Leader (1987). Carcinoma-in-situ of the testis. *Lancet* **ii** 545−6.

Pugh, R.C.B. (1976). *Pathology of the Testis*. Blackwell Scientific Publications: Oxford and London.

Van der Maase, H., Rorth, M., Walbom-Jorgensen, S., Sorensen, B.L., Christophersen, I.S., Hald, T., Jacobsen, G.K., Berthelsen, J.G. and Skakkebaek, N.E. (1986). Carcinoma in situ of contralateral testis in patients with testicular germ cell cancer: study of 27 cases in 500 patients. *Br. Med. J.* **293**, 1398−401.

11 Female genital tract

Cervix
 Squamous cell carcinoma
 Adenocarcinoma

Uterus
 Endometrial carcinoma

Ovary
 Ovarian neoplasms

Other Tumours
 Leiomyomas
 Trophoblastic tumours

A substantial number of the tissues examined by histopathologists are from gynaecologists and these often form the basis for their clinical diagnosis. The main phases of the menstrual cycle are recognized by light microscopy but exact dating is not possible. The microscopic observations must be interpreted by a clinician with some knowledge of the patient's endocrine profile and of any hormones she is receiving. Deviations from the normal pattern require similar knowledge, although hyperplastic, dysplastic and neoplastic changes as well as some localized infections including tuberculosis are primarily microscopic diagnoses. Support is also provided by the histopathologist in identifying conception products whether from the uterus or the fallopian tube (*ectopic pregnancy*) (Fig. 11.1) and much less commonly tubal infections (*salpingitis*). A comparable role occurs with the diagnosis of *endometriosis*. This requires the recognition of endometrial glands and stroma in sites other than the lining of the uterine cavity (Fig. 11.2), and when in the wall of the uterus this is called *adenomyosis* (Fig. 11.3). Endometriosis is a condition of unknown cause with hypothesis for an origin from coelomic metaplasia (see ovarian tumours) or for endometrial spread via the fallopian tubes, lymphatics, or bloodstream. There is also no clear reason for the relationship with infertility; over one-third of women with endometriosis are infertile.

The most common tumours within the genital tract in women

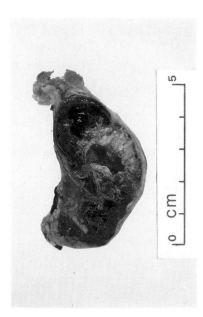

Fig. 11.1 Ectopic pregnancy within the fallopian tube.

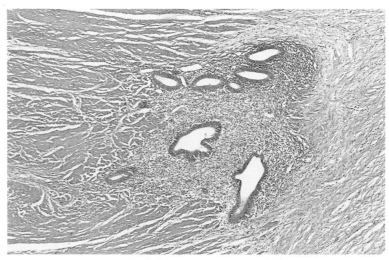

Fig. 11.2 Endometriosis. Endometrial glands and surrounding stroma lying within the submucosa of the colon.

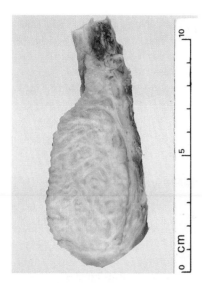

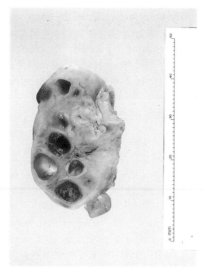

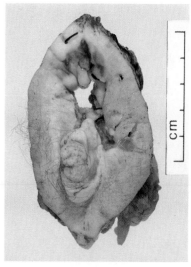

Fig. 11.3 Adenomyosis. The tumour within the myometrium is superficially similar to a fibroid. Light microscopy revealed endometrial glands and stroma.

Fig. 11.4 Cystic ovary. Luteal cysts with a yellow coat and thin-walled follicular cysts within an ovary removed as part of a hysterectomy.

Fig. 11.5 Squamous cell carcinoma of the vulva. The tumour is partly exophytic but is also infiltrating into the underlying tissues.

are probably the follicular and luteal cysts of the ovaries arising during normal oocyte maturation, but rarely symptomatic (Fig. 11.4). Another very common tumour is the fibroid or leiomyoma, found mainly in the uterus. The tumours that dominate gynaecological pathology are the malignancies of the cervix, uterus and ovaries. All have a substantial morbidity and mortality and the incidence of those in the cervix and ovaries continues to change. In contrast benign and malignant neoplasms within the vagina and vulva (Fig. 11.5) form a much smaller group and mirror, in their type and behaviour, counterparts in the skin.

Cervix

Squamous cell carcinoma is the most important disorder of the cervix. Other disorders including viral infections and changes related to intra-uterine devices can mimic some of its earliest histological changes although venereal infection is morphologically distinct. Non-specific inflammatory lesions and endocervical polyps are other benign entities.

Squamous cell carcinoma

This is the most common gynaecological malignancy under 50 years of age and is increasing among women of 35 years and less. The disease relates closely with sexual intercourse and progresses through a series of epithelial changes that can be observed cytologically, histologically and by direct vision of the cervix (colposcopy). Initially the lesion is confined to the epithelium but later it invades beyond this and widespread disease can follow. Progression is, nonetheless, not inevitable and the tumour may halt spontaneously, regress or be halted by therapy. Screening with cervical smears and appropriate treatment in the early stages offer the principal ways of recognizing and preventing progression and thereby reducing mortality. Within England and Wales there are over 2000 deaths annually from cervical cancer of which 70 affect women under 35 years.

Causes

The tumour is described as venereally and sexually transmitted (Table 11.1).

Intercourse. The cancer is almost unknown in the virgin. Women with multiple partners and especially if sexually promiscuous are at high risk with prostitutes, some divorcees and some women with multiple marriages numbered amongst these. The important denominator for all is an early age of first intercourse.

Role of the male. Some observations indicate that the male can act as a vector, giving rise to the concept of the high-risk male. There is an increased risk for the second and subsequent wives of men whose first wife had the disease and males have also been implicated in spreading the disease between different consorts. Circumcision was believed to reduce this risk and to protect Jewish women until it was appreciated that it was their sexual practices that were more relevant. Irrespective of religion, monogamous women with cervical cancer more often have polygomous rather than monogamous husbands but it is unresolved whether the male or the female is the source of the disease.

Viruses. Herpes simplex Type 2 was for many years associated with cervical cancer. The evidence hinged on the presence of serum antibodies, but also the knowledge that these viruses produce lymphoproliferative disease in chickens and an adenocarcinoma in frogs. The widespread nature of the virus means that raised antibody

Table 11.1 Factors involved with cervical carcinoma

Intercourse	Age started
	Number of partners
	Age at first pregnancy
	Socio-economic status
High risk male	
Viruses	Human papilloma virus
Other	Cigarette smoking
	? Immune response
	? Venereal infections
	? Non-barrier contraception

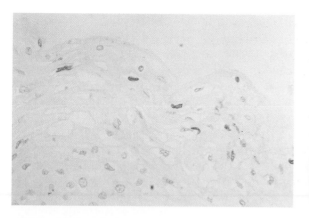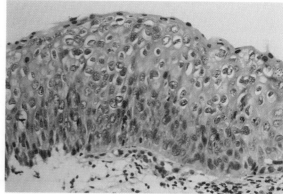

Fig. 11.6 Human papilloma virus; (*above left*) labelled with an antibody; (*above right*) within cells at the surface of the cervix.

titres are common and extensive controlled studies, involving 10 000 women with cervical cancer, have revealed no correlation between the neoplasm and herpes simplex antibodies. Hybridization techniques have also failed to consistently demonstrate herpes simplex virus-specific DNA within cells from cervical carcinoma. The role for this virus, if any, in cervical cancer is uncertain and similar comments apply to the Epstein—Barr virus, recently found in the cervix.

Papilloma viruses are species-specific and those infecting rabbits and cows are associated with squamous lesions. Over 30 human papilloma virus-types are described and all are related to proliferative disorders of squamous epithelium. Proving an association between these disorders and the papilloma virus depends upon demonstrating the virus in cells with specific human papilloma virus DNA probes. Most types are restricted to specific clinical disorders, although more than one type may be common to the same disorder. Types 1, 2 and 3 are seen with plantar, common and flat warts, respectively, but Type 4 is also found in plantar warts. Type 16, especially, and 18 are found in certainly over 60% and even in as many as 80% of invasive and pre-invasive cervical carcinomas but also in the normal cervix. The virus is not found in every cell and greater numbers occur with increasing age (Fig. 11.6). Multiple other types characterize many pre-invasive states and the possibility of predicting the infections most likely to proceed to carcinoma may exist.

Sexual transmission of cervical cancer is clearly compatible with viral infection but the exact role of the papilloma virus or other viruses remains unclear. Within some animal species these agents are oncogenic but in man, where spontaneous regression occurs and lesions may remain static, other factors must be necessary for malignant transformation.

Socio-economic factors. The wives of low income groups are affected more than those in high income groups, and women in deprived parts of the world, such as South America and India, rather than those in Western cultures. The disease is also uncommon among women of strict religious groups, including some orthodox Jewish, Mohammedan and Christian sects which disparage sexual promiscuity and demand rigid sexual hygiene.

Other factors. Smoking emerges as a factor unrelated to any social group or sexual activity and may affect local immune responses. Recipients of organ transplants, all of whom are immunosuppressed, have a 14-fold higher incidence of cervical neoplasia than expected and papilloma viruses are common among them. Infections superimposed upon papilloma virus infection may also be important and gonococcal, chlamydial and trichomonal infections are particularly implicated. Non-barrier contraception, including oral contraception, and poor personal hygiene are possible but less clearly defined factors.

Course of the disorder

Cervical carcinoma develops at the transformation zone of the cervix. This is the junction of the endocervix and ectocervix and the meeting place of columnar and squamous epithelium. From early foetal life, but especially during adolescence and first pregnancies, this junction is replaced by squamous epithelium which in time partly overlies the endocervical stroma and mucous glands (Fig. 11.7). The change is regarded as squamous metaplasia but its inevitability has led to the suggestion that it is a normal reaction. The replacement process can be followed by colposcopy allied with a solution of dilute iodine and sodium iodide, the iodide reacting with the glycogen in the squamous epithelium to produce a brown colour.

Established squamous cell carcinoma is usually preceded by a series of cellular changes within the squamous epithelium of the transformation zone. These changes affect the nuclei and cytoplasm and are reflected by alterations in the normal regular maturation

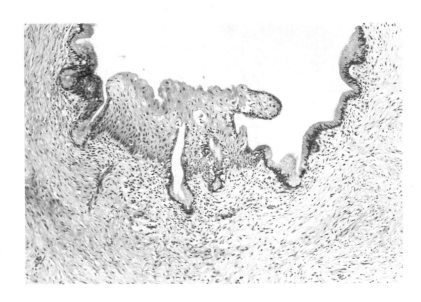

Fig. 11.7 Squamous metaplasia in the transformation zone of the cervix surrounded by a mucus secreting columnar epithelium.

pattern and can culminate in carcinoma in situ prior to an invasive carcinoma. The colposcopist, histopathologist and cytologist all recognize most of these phases and distinguish the early changes from the later ones but only the histopathologist is reliably able to diagnose the initial invasive stages. A common difficulty is distinguishing pre-invasive phases from viral changes, especially when both are present. Papilloma viral infection produces disordered squamous cell maturation characterized by cavitation of the cell cytoplasm and nuclear abnormalities (*koilocytosis*) (Fig. 11.6). This change, in contrast to the pre-invasive changes, is principally in the superficial parts of the epithelium and does not affect the basal cells.

Terminology

The epithelial changes antedating cervical cancer were referred to as dysplastic and were divided into mild, moderate and severe. Dysplasia that proceeded to carcinoma included a spectrum of potentially progressive events, possibly originating from reserve cells of the cervical epithelium and dependant upon many factors. Severe dysplasia differed from carcinoma in situ in that a superficial residue of maturation persisted. Critics of this nomenclature point out that it fails to distinguish between dysplasia potentially progressing to cervical carcinoma and that due to other processes, including some viral infections but unrelated with malignancy. The nearest approach at separating the two, at present, is by demonstrating the chromosome abnormalities peculiar to the neoplastic process. The term *cervical intra-epithelial neoplasia* (CIN) sidesteps these objections, although the three grades of CIN correspond with those of dysplasia (Fig. 11.8). CIN III, the most severe degree, also embraces carcinoma in situ, although not all authorities have totally discarded the use of this term. The common weakness to either classification is that distinguishing between the different grades is subjective and is open to observer error.

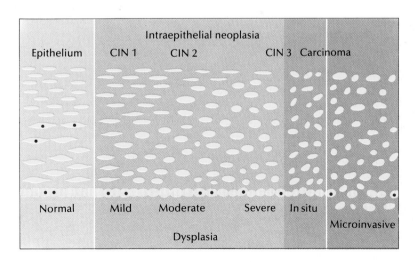

Fig. 11.8 Terminology of cervical precancerous features (CIN=cervical intraepithelial neoplasia).

Using the CIN terminology the following generalizations can be made:
- Progression from CIN I to invasive carcinoma occurs and can take up to 30 years.
- Approximately 50—60% of untreated CIN proceeds to invasive carcinoma.
- Approximately 22% of CIN at whatever stage can persist unchanged.
- Less than 10% of CIN will regress.
- Invasive cervical carcinoma can develop independently of CIN.

Role of cytology screening

CIN can be localized at colposcopy, the condition followed and treated and hopefully invasive carcinoma avoided. Detecting CIN, particularly in the early stages, is largely a random procedure since the disorder is invariably symptomless. Screening by cervical smearing and microscopic examination of the stained exfoliated cells offers a way of doing this and channelling affected women for therapy. The smear preparations are stained by the Papanicolaou method and the appearances of the cells correlate with any CIN present. Population screening of this type has been undertaken in a number of countries and within a 15-year period the occurrence of invasive carcinoma has in some been reduced. This claim is made in British Columbia as well as that cervical carcinoma is now seen only in new immigrants, or in women considered too old at the introduction of the screening programme to be included, and in a small number who have refused screening. False negative findings occur, representing laboratory and observer errors as well as errors in sampling. These constitute around 20% of all results in most centres but are guarded against by repeated smears and the usually slow natural history of the disease. False positive smears form 5% of all reported smears and are generally from non-neoplastic inflammatory disease. The cervical smear is therefore an acceptable way of screening a population provided that this can be done regularly. The factors governing the timing of cervical smears and the women examined are ultimately logistic and financial, involving decisions of central government and local health districts. The aim is to balance cost with maximum benefit for the individual and the community. Three-year intervals are used but ideally all women from their late teens should be examined annually. Practically this is not possible and regrettably those most at risk, because of their life-style, are those who least often present for cervical smears.

APPEARANCES

The pre-invasive phases can be recognized at colposcopy when changes in colour, capillary pattern and surface contours appear. The sites affected can be stained with iodine solutions or mapped and these areas then treated.

The histopathologist can recognize an early stage of invasion,

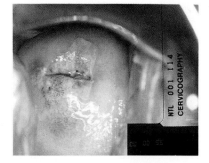

Colposcopy appearance of CIN III. The change is seen as a slightly elevated and roughened area above and below the os of the cervix.

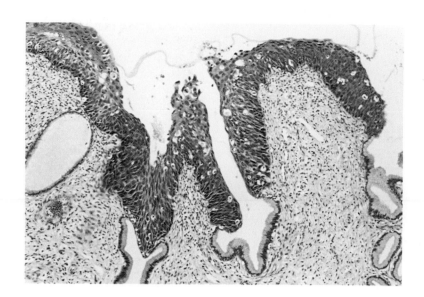

Fig. 11.9 Intra-epithelial neoplasia of the cervix. This extends through the full thickness of the epithelium (CIN III) to the surface and within the mouths of glands.

Table 11.2 Invasive cervical neoplasms

Squamous cell carcinoma	>90%
Adenocarcinoma	5–8%
Mixed adeno- and squamous carcinoma	2–3%
Undifferentiated tumours Carcinoid Malignant melanoma Sarcomas Lymphomas	0.5%

clinically indistinguishable from CIN III (Fig. 11.9) and called *micro-invasive carcinoma*. In addition to the cellular features of CIN III there are abnormal squamous cells limited to the immediate cervical stroma. According to most workers if this invasion is restricted to 3 mm in depth the risk of lymph node spread is less than 10%. Others regard the risk as identical for invasion of 4 and 5 mm and and yet others 1 mm, but the importance for the patient with any of these measurements is a virtually normal life expectancy. Measurement can, however, present problems for the histopathologist because of cross-sectioning arising from the angle at which the tissue is sectioned and from defining the tissue surface from which measurements are made.

Clinically invasive malignancy occurs as either an exophytic tumour projecting into the vaginal vault or as an endophytic growth infiltrating the cervix. Bleeding and offensive vaginal discharges are the usual presentations. With both patterns the cervix is often barrel-shaped, stony hard, irregular and ulcerated and simulates other cervical malignancies (Table 11.2). Underlying these appearances are a number of histological patterns. Well differentiated large cell carcinomas carry a better prognosis than the poorly differentiated small cell ones. These histological differences are, however, less important in the final outlook than the clinical stage of the disease.

Spread

This is mainly by direct local invasion and within lymphatics. Local invasion occurs upwards into the uterus and downwards to the vagina. Perineural and perivascular pathways contribute towards this and to that to the parametrium. Ultimately local spread affects the entire pelvic contents. This is preferentially anteroposteriorly rather than laterally and can involve the patient in great distress and discomfort including death from chronic renal failure secondary to ureteric blockage. Lymphatic spread is first to the external iliac, hypogastric and obturator lymph nodes and later to more distant nodes. Vascular spread affects a small minority of patients producing distant metastases to the lungs, liver and axial skeleton, particularly the lumbar vertebrae, although any tissue can be affected.

Adenocarcinoma

This tumour at one time formed around 4% of all cervical carcinomas but has now increased to nearly 10%. The reasons behind this are unclear but may reflect an absolute increase or improved recognition made possible by the early treatment of cervical squamous cell neoplasia. A contribution from oral contraceptives is also possible since more women with adenocarcinomas have used these than those with squamous cell carcinomas. There is no evidence for a role for venereal transmission.

Uterus

Endometrial carcinoma

This adenocarcinoma affects women during their reproductive and post-menopausal years. There is maximum impact between 55–60 years of age, although approximately one-quarter of diagnoses are made before the menopause. There has been a progressive increase in incidence for a number of decades although this is disputed when the figures are corrected for the concomitant rise in the age of the population. The tumour is the most common gynaecological malignancy if the intra-epithelial stages of cervical carcinoma are excluded and the number of new tumours annually is double that of cervical and ovarian malignancies. The mortality is low, especially for patients of 40 years or less, with a cure rate of 75–90% provided the tumour is confined to the endometrium or inner half of the myometrium. Affluent Western societies of North America and Western Europe are mainly at risk in contrast to the populations of Asia, Africa and South America. The common aetiological factor is oestrogen.

Causative factors

Oestrogen. Patients with endometrial carcinoma may have high oestrogen levels from endogenous or exogenous sources (Fig. 11.10).
1 Raised endogenous oestrogens are now the main association and are related to obesity. Obesity encourages oestrone production and availability since the site of conversion of androstenedione from the adrenals to oestrone is fat and muscle. The conversion occurs to the same degree in all obese women and no differences are recognized in the oestrone levels of obese subjects with and without endometrial carcinoma. The relationship is with the degree of obesity, in that there is a three-fold risk for women 21–50

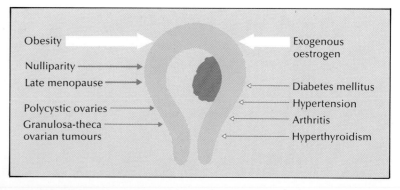

Fig. 11.10 Factors associated with endometrial carcinoma.

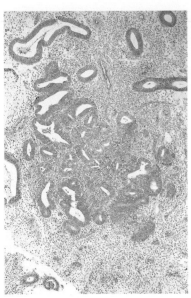

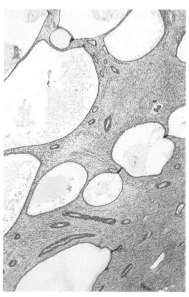

Fig. 11.11 Endometrial hyperplasia. (*Above*) Atypical hyperplasia; (*below*) cystic hyperplasia within an endometrial curettage sample.

pounds overweight and a 9–10-fold risk for those of 50 pounds or more overweight. An implication of these observations is that if all obese women were screened 50% of endometrial carcinomas could be detected. Endogenous oestrogen production also arises from polycystic ovaries where progesterone suppression is absent and oestrogen-producing ovarian tumours, particularly the feminizing granulosa–theca cell tumours. With either of these associations, as with obesity, the role of the hormone is unclear both in nulliparous women who form up to one-third of patients, and in women with a menopause developing between their late forties and early fifties.

2 Excessive use of exogenous oestrogens for menopausal symptoms was formerly a very significant factor in endometrial carcinoma. The recognition of this risk has resulted in more restrained usage of these hormones and the incorporation of progesterone. The risk was clearly demonstrated in patients with ovarian dysgenesis who, lacking endogenous oestrogens, were given oestrogens and later developed endometrial carcinoma. Oestrogens used in oral contraception, either alone or in combination, are not carcinogenic but possibly protect against endometrial carcinoma, an effect that persists for some years once they are discontinued.

Other factors. These include diabetes mellitus, hypertension, arthritis and hypothyroidism, all commonly accompanying obesity; they may contribute towards raised oestrogen levels but a clear sequence of events has not been demonstrated. A role for hypertension is discredited by some authorities.

Precursor states

The histopathologist recognizes a variety of patterns of endometrial hyperplasia (Figs 11.11 and 11.12) which may be premalignant and which are all associated with raised oestrogen levels similar to those of endometrial carcinoma. A spectrum of changes is acknowledged but the terminology describing these varies. The changes are not necessarily progressive and the risk factor for carcinoma corresponds with the atypicality of the hyperplasia. The most severely atypical hyperplasia is often indistinguishable from in situ carcinoma and

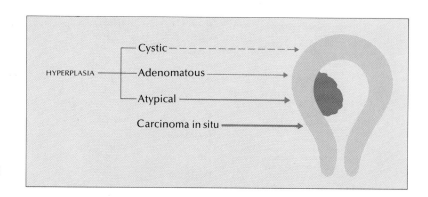

Fig. 11.12 Precursors of endometrial carcinoma.

may share similar chromosomal derangements to those of endometrial carcinoma. Relating hyperplasia and carcinoma is difficult since a diagnostic curettage or hysterectomy interrupts the natural history, but there are three linking pieces of evidence:

1 Atypical hyperplasia often accompanies endometrial carcinoma.

2 Retrospective studies of curettings from women with endometrial cancer often reveal atypical hyperplasia. This has been found in 72% of those over 60 years.

3 Prospective studies of women with hyperplasia, not subjected to hysterectomy, reveal a risk of endometrial carcinoma of 10−30% depending upon the atypicality present. The risk factor for cystic hyperplasia, the most benign end of the spectrum, is less than 0.4% and for all women the risk is greater after the menopause than before.

Despite these associations, in 20% of women, hyperplasia can revert to a benign state. When the hyperplasia is associated with exogenous oestrogens reversion can be encouraged by withdrawing these and giving progesterones.

APPEARANCES

The woman usually presents with an abnormal bleeding pattern and very frequently post-menopausal bleeding. Subsequent curettage may remove the tumour and any hyperplasia, as invariably happens, also, if local radiation is applied. The gynaecologist or histopathologist may suspect either hyperplasia or carcinoma from the gross appearances of the curettings but microscopic examination is essential for a firm diagnosis. Hyperplastic endometrium is generally abundant, soft and slightly mucoid while that including carcinoma, although also abundant, is friable, dry and granular and may include yellow necrotic areas. When a uterus is removed and incidentally includes endometrial hyperplasia or carcinoma, the endometrial features are similar (Fig. 11.13). The changes, however, are rarely diffuse but include polypoid masses and have a higher incidence on the posterior rather than the anterior wall of the cavity. The uterus can be enlarged but its size is often appropriate to the patient's age.

The depth of myometrial invasion clearly affects the patient's

Upside down

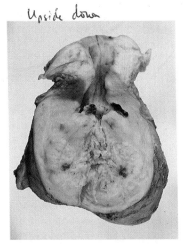

Fig. 11.13 Adenocarcinoma of the endometrium. Incidental finding in a hysterectomy specimen. The tumour is filling the endometrial cavity and invading much of the wall of the uterus.

Table 11.3 Some prognostic factors in endometrial carcinoma

5-year survival (%)	Spread	Histological differentiation	Clinical stage
90–70	Not beyond inner half of uterus	Good	1
60–30	Not beyond the uterus	Moderate	2 and 3
<10	Extra-uterine	Poor	4

prognosis. Without myometrial invasion 5-year survival is approximately 80%, with a slightly lower figure of 70% when the tumour spreads into the inner half of the myometrium. Beyond this level survival falls to a third but only if the tumour remains within the myometrium. Once the serosa is breached survival drops to below 10%. Other factors influencing the prognosis are the degree of histological differentiation, lymph node spread and, most importantly, the clinical stage (Table 11.3).

Spread. Spread beyond the uterus is unusual but may occur locally and via lymphatics and less often blood vessels. Vaginal involvement principally follows hysterectomy and is then most probably from implantation but can also be via the numerous lymphatics permeating the myometrium. More characteristically lymphatic spread involves the pelvic and inguinal lymph nodes. Para-aortic lymph node metastases radically reduce the patient's life expectancy. Despite the vascularity of the uterus blood-borne metastases are unusual. The sites of predilection are the lungs, liver, bones and brain although most organs can be involved. Intraperitoneal washings are taken at hysterectomy in some centres and any tumour cells found have probably spread along the fallopian tubes. Claims that these findings adversely affect the prognosis are controversial.

Ovary

Ovarian neoplasms

These occur mainly in perimenopausal and post-menopausal women although all ages can be affected. The majority are benign and have an epithelial origin but those that are malignant cause more deaths than equivalent cancers of the uterus and cervix, the mortality rate lying just below that of cancer of the lung, breast and gastrointestinal tract. Late presentation and lack of effective treatment are both important reasons behind this high mortality. It is also important that there is a follow-up period exceeding the usual 5- and 10-year intervals to unequivocally establish the benign nature of some ovarian tumours since in a few patients metastases develop 15 and 20 years or more after the initial growth.

Causes

There has been a continuous increase in incidence as well as a change in the pattern of the disease. Formerly, ovarian tumours were found more in social Group I than social Group V but a gradual increase has developed among women in Group V correlating with a diminishing size of families. Other factors implicating a protective influence from pregnancy are relative immunity amongst Roman Catholics and women in developing countries with high birth rates. A similar interpretation is given to the fall in incidence among first generation immigrants in the USA from Japan and Mexico, a period associated with increased birth rates. In contrast, unmarried women and those with few or no children are more susceptible to ovarian cancer. Similar susceptibility is evident in women with breast cancer raising the possibility of a shared hormone influence. The protective action of pregnancy may also be hormonal but is slightly dependent upon inhibition of ovulation, an action underlying the protective effect of oral contraception. Development of ovarian cancer in oophorectomized women and the rare familial incidence in those with congenital Peutz−Jegher and basal cell naevus syndromes show that factors other than pregnancy are involved.

Classification

Neither benign nor malignant ovarian tumours form a uniform morphological group. There are at least 22 different histological types each with benign and malignant variants and often also border-line and mixed subtypes. *Border-line tumours* are cytologically malignant but lack invasion and invariably have a better prognosis than unequivocal carcinomas. *Mixed tumours* include more than one tumour type and even admixtures of carcinomas and sarcomas. The basic classification is that of the WHO (1973) with modifications by individual workers. Common to all classifications are three main groups of tumours identified by their histological appearances, functional characteristics or behavioural patterns (Table 11.4).

Table 11.4 Main types of ovarian neoplasms

	Incidence (%)	Age group (years)	Endocrine changes	Tumour markers
Epithelial	70	50−60	None	None
Germ cell	20	<20	None	α-fetoprotein Human gonadotrophin
Gonadal stromal cell (sex-cord)	5	45−55	Present	None
Metastases	10−30	—	—	—

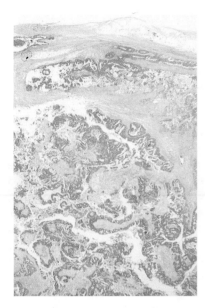

Fig. 11.14 Mucinous papillary cystadenocarcinoma.

Table 11.6 Examples of ovarian germ cell tumours

Dysgerminoma
Endodermal sinus tumour
Teratoma
   mature cystic (dermoid cyst)
   immature
   monodermal
Embryonal carcinoma
Malignant mixed germ cell
   (combination germ cell)

Table 11.5 Common examples of ovarian epithelial tumours

Serous	Cubical cells, some ciliated, lining to cysts
Mucinous	Columnar mucus cell lining to cysts
Endometrioid	Cytologically and architecturally simulating endometrium
Clear cell (mesonephroid)	Mainly cells with clear cytoplasm and hob-nail epithelium
Brenner tumour	Foci of epithelial cells in substantial fibrous stroma
Unclassified mixed	Combinations of the above

1 Epithelial tumours

These comprise the largest group of neoplasms and most are benign. Among all ovarian neoplasms approximately half will be benign epithelial tumours and these will form almost 90% of all malignant tumours, with 7−10% seen as border-line growths. Patients over 20 years are mostly affected with a maximum incidence between 50 and 60 years. Five main subtypes are described, each with benign and malignant variants, and each usually without functional effects (Table 11.5). Incidence of the subtypes differs in different series, depending mainly upon the age of the population studied, but serous and mucinous adenomas and carcinomas are the most common (Fig. 11.14).

Origin. This is envisaged as from the surface epithelium of the ovary. The epithelium is derived from the coelomic epithelium of the urogenital ridge and is capable of metaplasia, a property used to explain the variants among epithelial tumours. The pathway for tumour genesis originates from normal ceaseless ovulation and release of oocytes. The subsequent scar heals with collapse of the follicle, leakage of its contents and invagination of the surface epithelium into the parenchyma. This nidus of epithelial cells may then, under the influence of ovarian and placental steroids or pituitary gonadotrophins, develop from a simple inclusion cyst to an epithelial neoplasm. This hypothesis is consistent with the irregular pitted surface of the ovary, the protective effect of pregnancy and oral contraceptives, and the age of the patients. It may even be relevant to the high incidence of bilaterality. Their rarity in animals with infrequent ovulation and the converse in others such as the domestic hen with high ovulation rates is also supportive.

2 Germ cell tumours

About 20% of primary ovarian tumours have a germ cell origin but under 5% are malignant. Teenagers and those in their early 20s are involved and malignancy is more likely among the younger patients. There are five principal histological subtypes (Table 11.6)

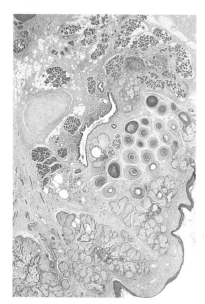

Table 11.7 Germ cell tumour cell markers

	Alpha-fetoprotein	Human gonadotrophin
Dysgerminoma	−	−
Endodermal sinus tumour	+	−
Teratoma	−	−
Embryonal carcinoma	+	+

Fig. 11.15 Dermoid cyst — epidermis, sebaceous glands, hair follicles, cartilage, sweat glands and columnar epithelium are all recognizable.

of which the benign cystic teratoma (dermoid cyst Fig. 11.15) is the best known and the most common. In marked contrast to testicular teratomas, virtually all ovarian ones have an excellent prognosis and, in common with most germ cell tumours, no functional effects. Precocious puberty may be a feature of some dysgerminomas and embryonal carcinomas.

Origin. The tumours in men and women all arise from the embryonic germ cells of the yolk sac. The dysgerminoma is the female counterpart of the seminoma but the other tumours share the same terminology. During embryonic development the germ cells migrate to the ovary but may become entrapped at other sites during this process. This explains the even more rare but similar tumours developing in mid-line structures including the third ventricle and pineal gland of the brain, the anterior mediastinum, the retroperitoneal tissues and the sacrococcogeal regions. The germ cells remain immature and some tumours consequently produce alpha-fetoprotein (AFP) and also human gonadotrophin (hCG). These products can be helpful in tissue diagnosis following antibody labelling (Table 11.7) as well as for detecting tumour recurrence by measuring serum levels.

3 Stromal tumours

Table 11.8 Examples of sex-cord stromal cell tumours

Granulosa
Theca-fibrous
Androblastomas (Sertoli−Leydig)
Gynandroblastomas
Lipoid

The stroma of the ovary forms 5% of all ovarian tumours. All age groups are involved, with patients of 1 year and 90 years, but most are seen in women early in their post-menopausal phase. Although there are five common variants (Table 11.8) there are a number of mixed examples and it is among stromal tumours, particularly, that considerable caution must be shown in predicting long-term behaviour. Any malignant potential is not always clear, either macroscopically or microscopically. Granulosa cell tumours (Fig. 11.16) are the largest group and, like many stromal tumours, produce systemic and uterine changes. Clinical manifestations vary with age but they are all expressions of excessive oestrogen. Thus, in the prepubertal, precocious puberty occurs while in the post-menopausal women there is uterine bleeding, breast enlargement and increased libido. A smaller number produce virilizing effects from androgen release. The endometrium becomes hyperplastic and, in some patients, will be associated with an adenocarcinoma.

Origin. Little is known or understood of the derivation and development of these tumours. They are easily induced in animals by

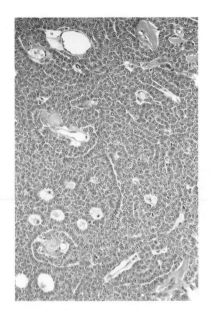

Fig. 11.16 Granulosa cell tumour — small dark staining cells in a follicle pattern. The larger paler cells surrounding spaces containing eosinophilic material are Call-Exner bodies.

dimethylbenzanthracine if a prior oophorectomy is performed. This can be done either surgically or by irradiation or by depressing the normal ovarian function by either intrasplenic grafting or parabiotic linking of a normal to an oophorectomized animal. An essential requisite for all of these experiments is a functioning pituitary gland which responds with excessive gonadotrophin production. The environment produced is potentially analogous to that in post-menopausal women but not to that in many younger patients. The massive oocyte degeneration that occurs prior to term in the foetus may, however, cause a similar environment in these younger patients.

Stromal cells are probably mesenchymal, developing from the embryonic ground substance, and have a potential for an ovarian or testicular cell type, although all include sex chromatin. This diversity of cell type is reflected by the hormonal content of stromal tumours with oestrogen predominating in the granulosa cell tumours and androgen in the androblastomas or Sertoli–Leydig tumours.

Other tumours. Metastases, sarcomas and undifferentiated tumours all occur. The metastatic tumours form 10–30% of all ovarian malignancies. The breast, gastrointestinal tract and endometrium are the usual primary sites and lymphatic spread the most important pathway. Other routes include direct, intraperitoneal and blood spread as well as spread along the fallopian tubes and iatrogenic implantation. Over three-quarters of the patients have bilateral ovarian metastases (*Kruckenberg tumours*).

Sarcomas may arise from the stromal cells but other sources are teratomas, ovarian leiomyomas (fibroids) and primary sites beyond the ovary. A separate variety, including mature connective tissue elements such as smooth muscle and cartilage, is the *mixed Müllerian sarcoma*.

Prognostic features

The outlook for the patient with a frankly malignant ovarian tumour is poor because, at diagnosis, most have spread beyond the ovary and because no effective treatment exists. The clinical stage provides the most important prognostic index but morphological factors closely influencing and worsening the prognosis include:
- a large mass of tumour;
- breeching of the capsule by tumour;
- the presence of ascites or tumour cells in cytological washings;
- a tumour that is not border-line;
- a poorly differentiated tumour. (This is the most subjective consideration and the one of least value.)

APPEARANCES

Ovarian neoplasms produce some of the largest tumours encountered but may also be recognized only by microscopy. The large tumours are those most often diagnosed clinically although some of the

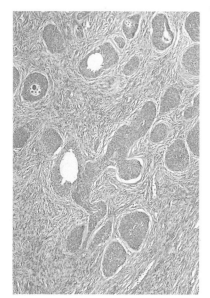

Fig. 11.17 Brenner tumour — characteristic islands of epithelial cells supported by a fibrous stroma.

smaller ones may be suspected from their hormonal effects. The largest tumours may weigh several kilogrammes and reach diameters of 20 cm or more and are generally malignant. Invariably in these circumstances no residual ovarian tissue remains.

The tumour may have a smooth or irregular surface with papillary excrescences, the latter being more common among malignant tumours (Fig. 11.18). The tumour's parenchyma can give some indication of its nature and type (Fig. 11.19). A useful but not infallible generalization is that cystic tumours are benign and solid ones malignant. This is true for many epithelial tumours but it is not applicable to the border-line types nor appropriate to germ and

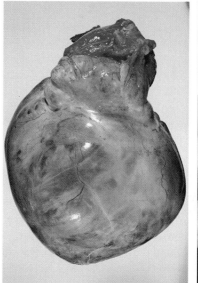 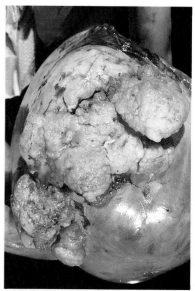

Fig. 11.18 Surface features of ovarian tumours; (*left*) smooth and uniform. This cyst was 500 g, filled with clear watery fluid and had a smooth lining. The tumour was a serous cyst adenoma; (*right*) papillary and smooth. A similarly sized tumour but this was a serous cyst adenocarcinoma.

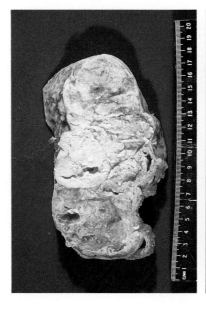 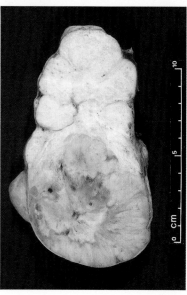

Fig. 11.19 Ovarian tumours with a solid and necrotic stroma; (*left*) mucinous cystadenocarcinoma; (*right*) endometrioid adenocarcinoma. These were categorized after examination of their light microscopy features.

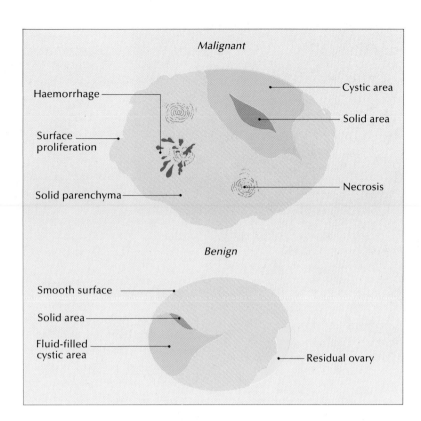

Fig. 11.20 Ovarian tumours.

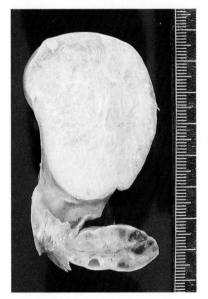

Fig. 11.21 Granulosa cell tumour. Much of the ovary is replaced but a residual focus is present on the left side. The typical yellow colour is evident.

stromal cell tumours. Mixed cystic and solid epithelial tumours also occur. Cystic epithelial tumours are often multilocular and have smooth or papillary linings. Solid areas within their walls must always be examined for malignant changes. Cystadenocarcinomas include many solid areas and also nodules of tumour obliterating the cysts (Fig. 11.20). Foci of old and recent haemorrhage and necrosis are other characteristics. Within the serocystic tumours there is clear watery fluid which after bleeding has an orange tinge, while in the mucinous types the contents are thick, tenacious and mucoid. This distinction is neither absolute nor clear cut since a substantial number of epithelial tumours include serous and mucinous epithelium.

From these criteria it is possible to recognize some cystadenomas and cystadenocarcinomas macroscopically but distinguishing primarily solid types from germ and stromal cell tumours may be impossible. These are solid but more uniformly so than the usual solid epithelial tumour and, in some, the consistency is rubbery and yellow or tan coloured (Fig. 11.21). The most distinctive of the germ cell types is the benign cystic dermoid. This encloses gliary, sticky yellow/green fluid, often with abundant hair and cheesy, offensive keratin debris. Teeth, bone and calcified tissue can all be found as well as mucin (Fig. 11.22).

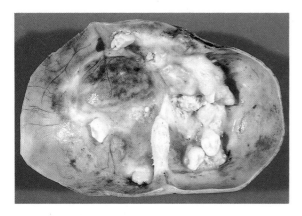

Fig. 11.22 Dermoid cyst. Hair and teeth are present. The yellow material is keratin.

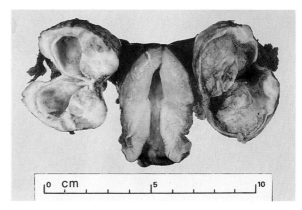

Synchronously occurring bilateral ovarian adenocarcinomas, each with the same histological features.

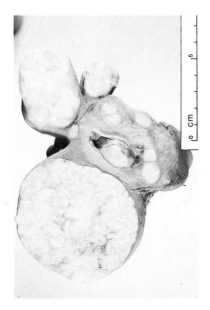

Fig. 11.23 Leiomyomas (fibroids). The tumours vary in size and are sharply demarcated from the compressed uterine muscle but not surrounded by capsules.

Bilateral tumours

Ten per cent of the serous and up to 20% of the mucinous epithelial tumours are bilateral, whether benign or malignant. Among other tumours this phenomenon is less common and even rare with the germ and stromal cell types. It is difficult to prove whether the bilaterality of the malignant tumours represents spontaneous synchronous primaries or metastatic spread. The similar distribution of bilaterality among benign and malignant tumours as well as the observation that both malignant tumours are of a comparable size, favours two primary growths.

Spread. Dissemination can involve all body cavities and is evident in most of the common epithelial types at diagnosis. Spread within the pelvis and abdomen is principally by seedling deposits and a malignant, often blood-stained ascites is the inevitable consequence. The deposits arise from surface papillary growths which break and implant on the peritoneum and within the omentum. In these sites the deposits may enlarge and obstruct but are not overtly destructive. Rupture of the primary tumour can produce similar results but this is rare as a spontaneous event although a hazard of surgery. *Pseudomyxoma peritonei* is the rare mucinous ascites seen when mucinous cystadenocarcinomas rupture. The phenomenon is most often spontaneous and is attributed to a persistent leakage of mucin with or without metaplasia of the peritoneum to a mucus-producing epithelium. This ascites is also found with a few cystadenomas as well as similar tumours of the appendix, intestine, common bile duct and urachus.

Lymphatics transport tumour cells and emboli to local lymph nodes in the pelvic, inguinal and para-aortic regions as well as more distantly to the parasternal, mediastinal and supraclavicular areas. Lymphatic permeation in the right diaphragm and pleural cavity is the cause of the unilateral right pleural effusion characteristic of ovarian malignancy.

Blood dissemination is a late event and produces widespread

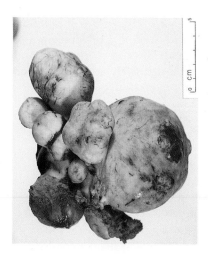

Fig. 11.24 Leiomyomas (fibroids). The uterus is deformed by multiple tumours of variable size; some are polypoid.

metastatic deposits, particularly to the liver and lung but rarely to bones. Central nervous system deposits are a feature in patients whose survival has been markedly prolonged.

Other tumours

Leiomyomas

Leiomyomas (fibroids) are among the most common tumours seen by most histopathologists (Fig. 11.23). A 40% incidence is claimed among women over 50 years and an incidence of 4–11% in the entire female population: they are thus tumours of older women and exceedingly rare among post-pubertal girls. Regression can occur after the menopause. Black women have a higher incidence than white women and among them there are greater numbers per patient although, in both groups, multiple tumours are the rule. The functional effects are numerous and can be manifest by changes in the menstrual flow and pattern, obstructive symptoms and effects on and during pregnancy. Even so some tumours remain silent. Any of these effects will be influenced by the patient's age and site together with their size and number and whether they are pedunculated. Despite the widespread distribution of leiomyomas and their frequency there is no substantial knowledge of their cause.

APPEARANCES

Any part of the genital tract can be involved but the uterus is the main site (Fig. 11.24) and within this leiomyomas may be found subserosally, intramurally and immediately beneath the endometrium, submucosal (Fig. 11.26). The subserosal and submucosal tumours may be with or without a stalk and, if a stalk is present, torsion is a potential complication. Submucosal tumours can undergo surface ulceration and depending on their site and location prolapse into the vagina.

Leiomyomas are grey to white oval masses varying from a few millimetres to many centimeters in diameter (Fig. 11.23). The more cellular ones are fleshy and somewhat rubbery and those with extensive hyalinization of their stroma tough and hard. Cystic change

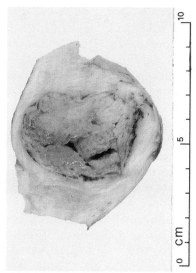

Fig. 11.25 Infarction of an intramural leiomyoma. This occurs as a complication during pregnancy and can present as an acute abdomen.

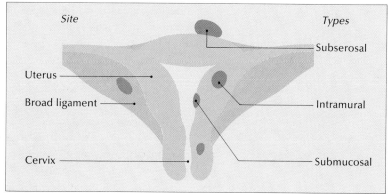

Fig. 11.26 Examples of leiomyomas.

is found within the larger examples as are yellow foci of necrosis. Haemorrhagic degeneration (*red degeneration*) is a phenomenon of pregnancy and oral contraceptives and leads to a dark red and slightly friable stroma (Fig. 11.25). The tumours are not encapsulated but compress the surrounding structures and can easily be shelled out.

Malignant potential

Leiomyosarcomas occur but evidence that they develop from pre-existing leiomyomas is not clear. In as much as most leiomyosarcomas are solitary it would seem that any relationship is unlikely. The leiomyosarcomas form in the region of 1% of all uterine malignancies but they do not behave in the aggressive fashion of most other sarcomas. Recurrence following removal is mainly confined to the pelvis and distant metastases, principally to the lungs, are unusual and lymphoid spread a rarity.

Diagnosis is often extremely difficult and ultimately comes from the tumour's behaviour. Initially it may be suspected histologically because of more than 10 mitotic figures per h.p.f. This observation is subjective and is also open to error from numerous technical factors arising during selection and preparation of the tissue.

Trophoblastic tumours

A range of tumours arise in relation to pregnancy from trophoblastic tissue. Pregnancy, normal or abnormal, may be coincidentally present or have preceded tumours even by many years and even with subsequent intervening normal pregnancies. Chromosome and HLA studies support these claims as well as illustrate that the great majority of tumours are paternal with an XX karyotype. The tumours embrace a spectrum of behaviour from malignant with metastatic potential to benign physiological overgrowths (Table 11.9). The best known malignancies are choriocarcinomas and hydatidyform moles, both of which, with the advent of methotrexate therapy, are, in experienced centres, now rarely fatal.

Primary growth is usually uterine but may also occur within any other part of the genital tract and, even more rarely, beyond this. Extragenital tumours have to be distinguished from metastatic deposits and the possibility of spontaneous regression of a primary genital tract focus is often difficult to rule out. The characteristic of

Table 11.9 Spectrum of trophoblastic tumours

Choriocarcinoma	Malignant with metastatic potential
Trophoblastic pseudotumour Atypical choriocarcinoma Invasive hydatidyform mole	Locally malignant with no metastatic potential
Non-invasive hydatidyform mole Syncytial endometritis	Non-invasive overgrowths comparable to hyperplasia
Benign chorionic invasion	Physiological overgrowth

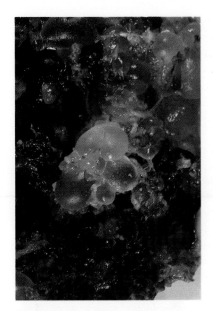

Fig. 11.27 Hydatidiform mole. The oedematous villi give an appearance often compared with a bunch of grapes.

all types of growth whatever the site is the synthesis and release of human chorionic gonadotrophin (hCG). This can be demonstrated by immunostaining within the tumour tissue and in the serum and CSF. Serum and CSF levels are used to monitor the extent of the disease, and its response and behaviour following treatment.

Trophoblastic tumours in the UK are, in comparison to tropical and subtropical regions, rarities. In tropical regions the incidence is probably 3—5 times that of other areas and within the UK the incidence approaches 1:70 000 live births. Accurate incidence figures are difficult to obtain, mainly because of variations in definitions, but also because of the use of hCG measurements; these can supersede tissue diagnosis as well as provide diagnosis without localizing the site of origin. The number of pregnancies is unrelated but pregnancy in older women does seem relevant, especially when between 40—50 years. Other factors affecting the appearance and subsequent behaviour are unclear.

APPEARANCES

A feature common to primary and metastatic lesions is their vascularity, leading to substantial bleeding following biopsy as well as haemorrhage into the tumour. The tumours are thus haemorrhagic, purple and friable and may vary from a few millimetres to several centimetres. Necrosis can either follow haemorrhage or arise as a sequel to rapid growth. The unique macroscopic feature, particularly of the hydatidyform mole, is the oedematous enlarged villi, often compared to a bunch of grapes (Fig. 11.27). The underlying histological features provide little help either in diagnosis or in distinguishing future behaviour and an absolute diagnosis is only possible from serum hCG levels. Raised levels provide the diagnosis unless there is coincidental AFP (alpha-fetoprotein) as occurs with some germ cell tumours. When metastatic spread develops this is blood-borne and the lungs, liver and brain are sites of common involvement. Deposits in lymph nodes are less often found.

Further reading

Barrasso, R., de Brux, J., Croissant, O. and Orth, G. (1987). High prevalence of papillomavirus-associated penile intra-epithelial neoplasia in sexual partners of women with cervical intra-epithelial neoplasia. *New Engl. J. Med.* **317**, 916—23.

Coppleson, M. (1981) (Editor). *Gynecologic Oncology: Fundamental Principles and Clinical Practice.* Volumes 1 and 2. Churchill Livingstone: Edinburgh.

Fox, H. (1985). Sex cord — stromal tumours of the ovary. *J. Path.* **145**, 127—48.

Fox, H. (1987) (Editor). *Haines and Taylor Obstetrical Pathology* (3rd Edition). Churchill Livingstone: Edinburgh.

Knapp, R.C. and Berkowitz, R.S. (1986) (Editors). *Gynecologic Oncology.* Macmillan Pub. Co.: London.

Lancet Leader (1987). Human papillomaviruses and cervical cancer: a fresh look at the evidence. *Lancet* **i**, 725—6.

Reid, B. and Coppleson, M. (1985). In: *Scientific Basis of Obstetrics and Gynaecology.* Ed. by R.R. Macdonald. William Heinemann Medical Books Ltd: London.

Vessey, M., Metcalfe, A., Wells, C., McPherson, K., Westhoff, C. and Yeates, D. (1987). Ovarian neoplasms, functional ovarian cysts, and oral contraceptives. *Br. Med. J.* **294**, 1518—20.

12   Endocrine system

The endocrine system is an integrated system, one part affecting the responses of the other parts. Thus in many endocrine disorders there are altered anterior pituitary responses, although the primary disorder does not lie within this gland. The system includes organs formed mainly from endocrine cells and others harbouring variable, but usually small, numbers of endocrine cells (Table 12.1). The thyroid and adrenals are endocrine organs while the neuro-endocrine cells within the alimentary and respiratory tracts illustrate the latter. Terms such as the *gastroenteropancreatic endocrine system* were introduced for the alimentary neuro-endocrine cells (*Kulchitsky cells*) but as further cells in other sites were discovered the wide dispersal of such cells was realized. They can be referred to as the *diffuse endocrine system* but they are best identified from their organ of origin such as gut or lung endocrine cells.

Development

There is no satisfactory explanation for the distribution of endocrine cells within the body or for the way that they sometimes form organs and in other circumstances exist as isolated cells. Studies on interactions between hormones may well clarify the issue. A concept advanced to explain the interaction of some hormones is that hormone-producing cells share an origin with the nervous system and have jointly developed from the neural crest. The foundation for this arose from the common histochemical reactions shared by endocrine and neural cells and gave rise to the concept of a common system, named the *APUD system* (Amine Precursor Uptake and Decarboxylation system). Hormones are present in the brain and positive immunolabelling of endocrine cells and neural tissue with neurospecific enolase and S100 is further support for this idea.

Table 12.1 Endocrine system

Diffuse endocrine cells	Endocrine organs
Thymus	Anterior pituitary
Alimentary tract	Thyroid
Pancreas	Parathyroids
Lungs	Adrenals
Breast	Extra-adrenal paraganglia
Gonads	

Animal transplant experiments, however, do not support the concept and nor does the monoclonality of many epithelial tumours that also include endocrine cells. However, an alternative explanation for these tumours is that there is a stem cell able to differentiate to either an epithelial or to an endocrine cell. *Ectopic hormone production*, i.e., hormone production from cells not normally producing hormones, is then intelligible, although strictly an invalid term. (Ectopic production must be distinguished from inappropriate secretion which refers to hormone production beyond the body requirements.)

Adaptations to function

The common feature to all endocrine cells is hormone secretion. Hormones are released directly into the surrounding tissues and are often transported via the blood and less often the nerves. To synthesize their hormones, the cells have within their cytoplasm abundant endoplasmic reticulum and mitochondria, as well as a well-developed Golgi apparatus. In addition many endocrine cells store their hormones in an inactive state as granules, so facilitating an immediate hormone supply. Other adaptations towards rapid responses are the close proximity of endocrine cells to vessels, often separated by only their basal lamina. Fenestration or multiple pores within the endothelial cells also encourages easy transport of hormones across the endothelium. When the action of a hormone is upon another endocrine cell (*paracrine function*) the proximity of the two cells is important as well as cell surface receptors. Membrane-bound receptors are common to all endocrine cells.

Recognition of endocrine cells

Endocrine organs, with the possible exception of the parathyroid glands, are easily recognized. Absolute identification of the parathyroids requires histological confirmation, especially when they are in abnormal sites such as the anterior mediastinum. Even with normally positioned glands confusion can occur with thyroid tissue and lymph nodes. It is for these reasons that surgeons require immediate examination, usually by frozen section, of all tissues removed during parathyroidectomy.

Endocrine cells in predominantly non-endocrine organs are not easily identified and light microscopy requires the support of ancillary investigations:

1 Silver stains react with many endocrine cells but are not specific.
2 Electron microscopy displays the cytoplasmic granules. These are membrane-bound and have dense cores which may be uniform, crystalline or surrounded by a clear halo (Fig. 12.1). The appearances are not unique for an individual hormone and are affected by tissue fixation and processing as well as the secretory activity. The plane of sectioning affects the granule's diameter and granules in tumours do not always correspond exactly with those of their non-tumorous counterpart.
3 Immunohistology and immuno-electronmicroscopy label a

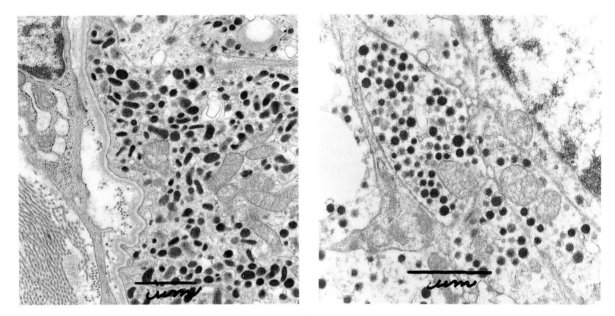

Fig. 12.1 Cytoplasmic granules as seen by electron microscopy within neuro-endocrine cells of the colon (*above left*) and in a paraganglioma (*above right*).

hormone and its granule and so unequivocally identify endocrine cells. These techniques show that endocrine cells are widely dispersed and present in most tissues, often with more than one hormone within any tissue. There are, for example, at least 35 hormones within the alimentary tract, although the cell types of only 15 have been found. These methods also show that with the possible exception of the anterior pituitary, any endocrine cell produces only one hormone; insulin-producing cells do not synthesize glucagon and vice versa. Some antibodies, however, will label more than one endocrine cell type and these can be used to screen tissues for endocrine cells rather than subjecting them to a battery of individually labelled hormone antibodies. *Neurone specific enolase* and *S100* are such antibodies but neither is specific to endocrine cells.

Auto-immunity relationship

An unexplained phenomenon is the frequency of endocrine disorders with auto-immunity. Clinical and subclinical hormonal changes often arise with auto-immune disorders and, in many patients, more than one endocrine cell is affected. Often unresolved is whether the endocrine component precedes or is the consequence of the auto-immune reaction. Auto-immune disorders have HLA-DR links and are common among women. Endocrine disorders unrelated with auto-immunity do not have any HLA-DR linkages but, overall, there are a greater number of women with endocrine disorders than men.

Disorders

The most common disorders are hyperplasia, atrophy and tumour formation, all of which may be seen with or without altered hor-

Table 12.2 Sites of oncocytic tumours

Pituitary	Stomach
Salivary gland	Lung
Thyroid	Kidney
Parathyroid	Breast

monal secretion. As a part of any of these specific hormone deficient cells, characterized by a granular cytoplasm, may appear. The granularity is due to abundant mitochondria and not to hormone granules. These cells are *oncocytes* and are also referred to, especially in the thyroid, as *Hurtle cells* and *Askanazy* cells; on occasion they can form the sole cell of an endocrine tumour (Table 12.2).

Hyperplasia and atrophy may be primary conditions or secondary to other disorders either within the altered tissue or within endocrine tissues elsewhere. When one of a pair of endocrine organs are disordered and their hormone secretion affected, compensatory changes invariably develop in the other gland. Adenomas are the predominant tumours, although carcinomas are occasionally seen. The distinction between adenomas, hyperplasia, and in the early stages, carcinoma is not always clear and histologically, is almost impossible to make.

Hyperplasia

This is clinically important in the thyroid, parathyroids and adrenals (Table 12.3). It occurs rarely in the interstitial cells of the testis and also the endocrine cells of the pancreas and gastrointestinal tract. Increased hormone release is not inevitable and in one of the most common manifestations, *nodular thyroid goitre* (Fig. 12.2), this does not occur. *Focal adrenal cortical hyperplasia*, often found at autopsy, is a further example. Parathyroid hyperplasia involves all the parathyroid glands and the primary disorder is only cured if all these are removed. A similar approach is necessary in primary adrenal hyperplasia.

Cells that are hyperplastic are the cause and the result of the circulating hormones (Table 12.4). Epithelial cells synthesizing thyroxine form the greater part of the thyroid gland but there is also a smaller population of cells producing calcitonin, *C-cells*. The more common manifestations of thyroid hyperplasia, *thyrotoxicosis* and *nodular goitre*, lead to hyperplastic changes confined to the follicular epithelium (Fig. 12.3) but in the much more rare multiple endocrine adenomatosis syndromes (MEA) with thyroid involvement it is only the C-cells that are hyperplastic (Fig. 12.4). Similarly

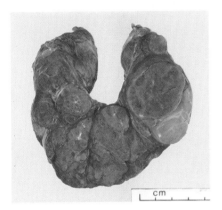

Fig. 12.2 Nodular thyroid goitre. The gland weighed 320 g, normal < 20 g.

Table 12.3 Hyperplastic conditions

Thyroid	Thyrotoxicosis; nodular goitre C (calcitonin)-cell hyperplasia
Parathyroids	1°, 2°, 3° hyperparathyroidism
Adrenal cortex	Cushing's disease Hyperaldosteronism (Conn's syndrome)
Testicular interstitial cells	Testicular dysgenesis syndromes (Klinefelter's syndrome) and cryptorchidism
Pancreatic endocrine cells	Nesidioblastosis
Gastric endocrine cells	Zollinger–Ellison's syndrome (gastrin-producing-cells)

Table 12.4 Causes of endocrine hyperplasia

Hyperthyroidism	Iodine deficiency; thyroid stimulating antibody and thyroid growth stimulating antibody
Secondary hyperparathyroidism	Chronic renal disease Metabolic bone diseases Malabsorption syndromes
Tertiary hyperparathyroidism	Autonomous functioning of one or more glands following correction of renal failure and secondary hyperparathyroidism
Secondary adrenal cortical hyperplasia	Protracted ACTH therapy Ectopic ACTH syndrome (e.g., tumours) Pituitary adenoma

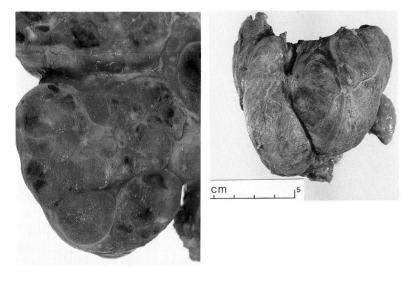

Fig. 12.3 (*Left*) Part of a nodular thyroid goitre. The variably sized follicles are filled with glistening reddish colloid and separated by thin strands of connective tissue. (*Right*) Subtotal thyroidectomy specimen for thyrotoxicosis. The gland weighed 130 g (normal < 20 g). Note the large vessels on the surface which contribute to the vascularity. The parenchyma appeared similar to the goitre on the left.

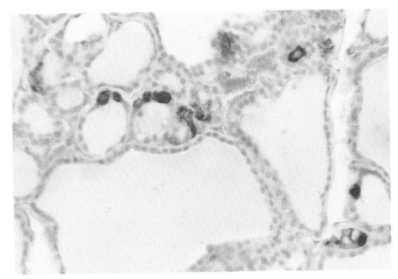

Fig. 12.4 Thyroid from a patient with the multiple endocrine adenomatosis syndrome and with raised serum calcitonin levels. The C-cells are red, labelled with an anti-calcitonin antibody, and more plentiful than in a thyroid from a normal individual.

in the adrenal gland, *Conn's syndrome* is associated with changes principally in the zone glomerulosa, the site of aldosterone formation, and *Cushing's syndrome* with changes in the zona fasciculata, the place of glucocorticoid synthesis. In neither of these disorders, in contrast to those in the thyroid, is this cytological division rigid and hyperplasia may affect any of the cortical regions in either syndrome. Parathyroid hyperplasia may also involve all three normal cell types or one cell type more than another but none of these variants have any significance in separating between the different forms of hyperparathyroidism. Distinguishing primary from other causes of hyperplasia is not usually possible histologically and must depend upon clinical data.

APPEARANCES

Macroscopically the affected glands are enlarged. The enlargement may affect the entire gland or be a focal phenomenon, sometimes with multiple areas of involvement. Multiple areas of hyperplasia are described as nodular hyperplasia. Hyperplasia is most easily recognized by comparing the weight of the gland against standard normal weights adjusted for age and sex when variations from a few milligrammes to many grammes may be found. The hyperplasia is associated with an increase in vascularity which leads to bleeding at operation and the dark colour and soft consistency of the affected glands.

Adenomas

These occur in nearly all endocrine glands. They may be functional with hormone secretion but many are incidental autopsy findings with no clinical associations. The functional adenomas give rise to well-recognized clinical syndromes (Table 12.5). A few non-functional adenomas produce palpable tumours and others, symptoms from compression of adjacent tissues. Palpable adenomas are almost confined to the neck, arising in the thyroid and parathyroids (Fig. 12.7). These can also lead to compression of the neck vessels

Table 12.5 Effects of some functional adenomas

Anterior pituitary	
Prolactin	Anovulation, menstrual abnormalities, galactorrhoea
Growth hormone	Acromegaly
Corticotrophin	Cushing's syndrome
Thyroid	Thyrotoxicosis
Parathyroid	1° hyperparathyroidism
Adrenal cortex	Conn's (70%), Cushing's and adreno-genital syndromes
Testicular interstitial tissue	Gonadal dysgenesis syndrome

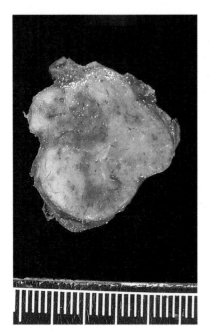

Fig. 12.5 Paraganglioma removed from the carotid bifurcation.

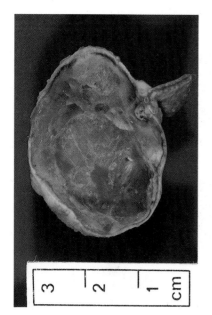

Fig. 12.6 Phaeochromocytoma filling the medulla of the adrenal with the yellow cortex stretched around it.

and trachea. Adenomas in the anterior pituitary, because of their confined surroundings, also produce compression symptoms; these involve the brain and optic nerves but awareness of these and improved methods of diagnosis have recently led to a remarkable reduction in their incidence.

Paragangliomas are tumours associated with adrenalin and noradrenalin release. They appear in many different sites corresponding with the distribution of the sympathetic and parasympathetic ganglia. Hormone synthesis does not occur in all of these tumours as some possess only chemoreceptors, and these can then be referred to as *chemodectomas* (Fig. 12.5). Morphologically it is impossible, even with immuno-electron microscopy, to distinguish between tumours producing adrenalin and/or noradrenalin and those not. It is mainly for this reason that all these tumours should be called paragangliomas rather than to confine this term to the hormone-secreting tumours. Paragangliomas of the adrenal medulla are popularly known as *phaeochromocytomas* (Fig. 12.6), drawing attention to their chromaffin—catecholamine-producing cells, and many others are referred to according to their anatomical site (Table 12.6). A useful mnemonic for paragangliomas is that 10% become malignant, 10% in the adrenal are bilateral, 10% are extra-adrenal and 10% occur in children.

Recognition of adenomas

The histopathologist can experience great difficulty in distinguishing these from hyperplasia and carcinoma. The adenoma should be well demarcated with a capsule and should include a fairly uniform population of cells. The cells are recognizable as glandular and do not include the pleomorphic features and abnormal mitotic forms characteristic of carcinomas. The surrounding tissue may be compressed and there is no local infiltration (Fig. 12.7). In practice these criteria are often not present. Sometimes this is because the lesion is shelled out and no normal tissue is included, and on other occasions because the lesion is functional and includes superimposed hyperplastic changes, cytologically merging with those of carcinoma. Multiple adenomas and nodular hyperplasia are further sources of confusion. To overcome these difficulties and clarify the patient's management the following guidelines are used:

1 Changes in one of a pair of glands or confined to the minority of the parathyroid glands are adenomatous rather than hyperplastic.

Table 12.6 Paragangliomas named by site

Tumour	Anatomical site
Carotid body	Bifurcation of the common carotid
Glomus jugulare	Internal jugular vein
Glomus tympanicium	Tympanic membrane of ear
Aortic bodies	Aortic arch
Organs of Zuckerkandl	Abdominal aorta

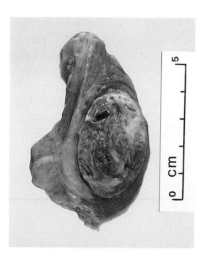

Fig. 12.7 Thyroid adenoma. The lesion was solitary and there is some compression of the surrounding gland but no infiltration.

2   Adrenal tumours greater than 5 cm diameter and pituitary tumours greater than 10 m diameter are potentially malignant.

3   Tumours in the thyroid with papillary formation are malignant.

4   Tumour thrombus incorporated into a vessel wall in any endocrine gland is indicative of malignancy (Fig. 12.8).

The cell population of adenomas is that of the parent tissue. Thyroid adenomas are epithelial and are all follicular although there is considerable variation in the size of the follicles. Parathyroid adenomas and adrenal cortical adenomas can include all the parent endocrine cell types. Anterior pituitary adenomas are characterized according to the hormones they include. Those storing prolactin form the largest group but there is wide variation among different series depending on the source of the patient (neurosurgery, endocrinology or gynaecology), and differences in the immunoperoxidase and electron microscopy techniques used. Rarely, adenomas in the anterior pituitary, thyroid and parathyroids may be formed entirely of oncocytic cells and these are referred to as *oncocytic adenomas*. Oncocytes more often form part of the population of the more common adenomas. Amyloid also occurs in some adenomas.

APPEARANCES

Macroscopically an isolated tumour can be recognized by a well demarcated capsule and some compression of the surrounding tissues (see above). The colour varies with the vascularity but most are brownish or tan coloured. Those in the adrenal cortex are yellow (Fig. 12.9). Haemorrhage and cyst formation are other features.

Carcinomas

Carcinomas do occur but they are uncommon and often present considerable difficulty in diagnosis. Their distinction from adenomas is discussed in the previous section but ultimately it is only

Fig. 12.8 Part of a follicular tumour of the thyroid with the larger acini of the uninvolved gland in the lower part of the figure. Separating the two is a vessel with tumour cells penetrating its wall and adherent to the endothelium, unequivocal evidence that this is a follicular carcinoma.

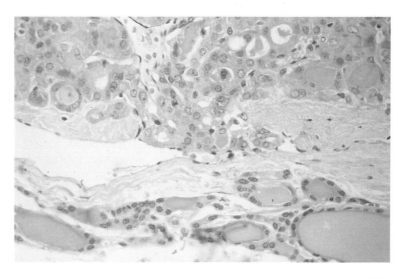

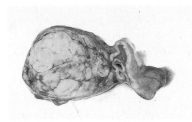

Fig. 12.9 Adrenal gland with an adenoma arising within the cortex. This was an incidental finding at autopsy and unrelated to any symptoms during life.

the appearance of metastases that provides unequivocal evidence of their development. Even when there are metastases it may not be possible to separate these from those of other primary endocrine tumours or from carcinoma elsewhere. This is because in the absence of hormone synthesis there are no cell markers for endocrine cells and because many common carcinomas include an endocrine component. The latter phenomenon is best known with lung tumours but is also encountered among carcinomas of the breast, alimentary tract, exocrine pancreas, ovary and prostate. Metastases within endocrine tissue are usually multiple and rarely stimulate hormone synthesis.

Clinical presentation

Most endocrine carcinomas are non-functional. Those that do release hormones can give rise to syndromes similar to those found with endocrine hyperplasia and some adenomas. The production of more than one hormone is common in tumours from the alimentary tract. Malignant *carcinoid tumours* (Fig. 12.10), which arise mainly in the small intestine Kulchitsky cells, lead to distinctive clinical features. These include diarrhoea, flushing attacks and asthma but they occur only if there are hepatic metastases. Carcinoid tumours of the appendix are rare, invariably benign and symptomless.

Other carcinomas present as palpable tumours, most easily recognized in the neck when the thyroid or parathyroids are involved. Compression of the trachea and neck vessels by thyroid, parathyroid and thymic tumours may also occur depending upon the size of the tumour as well as adhesions binding these to adjacent tissues (Fig. 12.11).

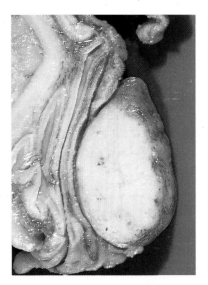

Fig. 12.10 Carcinoid tumour in the small intestine which had produced intestinal obstruction. Note the characteristic yellow colour.

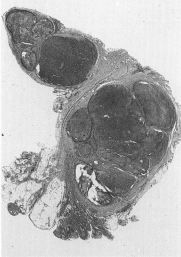

Fig. 12.11 Parathyroid carcinoma with marked fibrosis. The fibrous tissue bound the tumour to the surrounding structures in the neck.

Development

Progression to an endocrine carcinoma may be via hyperplasia and adenoma. This is most convincingly seen amongst families with *multiple endocrine adenomatosis* (MEA). These disorders run in families and multiple endocrine abnormalities appear with several distinct patterns. Other carcinomas arise without any preceding abnormality or recognized cause. A notable exception is some thyroid cancers where a relationship exists with radiation. Radiation was used to ablate the thymus in children and also in the management of tonsilitis and ankylosing spondylitis. Subsequently many of these patients developed thyroid carcinomas and a similar relationship has been recorded among survivors of the atomic bombing of Japan.

Classification

The histological features of endocrine carcinomas have led to various subclassifications. These may carry prognostic implications as illustrated by thyroid carcinomas (Table 12.7). The appearances range from well differentiated to frankly anaplastic tumours. Undifferentiated carcinomas may only be distinguished from lymphomas by immunocytochemistry but sometimes, even with these techniques, the distinction is not possible. Amyloid may be seen with any endocrine tumour but especially with the *medullary carcinomas* which arise from the C-cells of the thyroid (Fig. 12.12), thyroid papillary carcinomas and endocrine carcinomas of the pancreas.

APPEARANCES

The tumours are most often large in relation to their site of origin and have invariably grown rapidly. This is reflected in part by foci of haemorrhage and necrosis (Fig. 12.13). The neoplasms are poorly circumscribed from the normal tissue but notably firmer, often stony hard, and lighter in colour. Firm adhesions to surrounding structures are a common feature. Multifocal tumours are found with some papillary thyroid carcinomas, alimentary tract carcinoids and pancreatic endocrine tumours.

Table 12.7 Histological types of thyroid carcinoma

Histological type	%	Spread	Prognosis	10-year survival (%)
Papillary	46	Lymphatic	Good	80
Follicular	7	Vascular	Poor	60
Anaplastic giant cell } Anaplastic small cell }	13–24	Local/vascular	Bad	5
Medullary (C-cell)	—	Lymphatic	Good	50

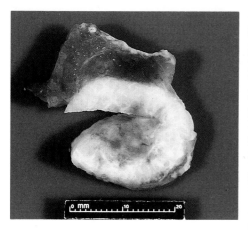

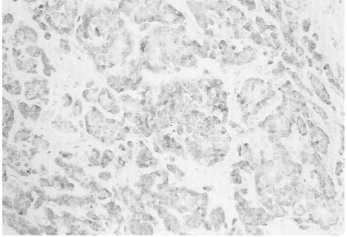

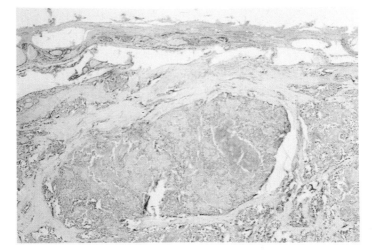

Fig. 12.12 Medullary carcinoma of the thyroid. (*Above left*) The tumour arises from calcitonin producing C-cells; (*above right*) labelled brown with an anticalcitonin antibody; amyloid (*right*), stained orange-pink, forms a part of these tumours.

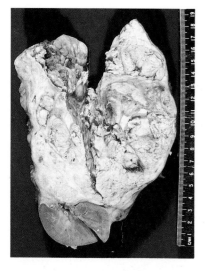

Fig. 12.13 Carcinoma of the adrenal with part of the adjacent kidney. Much of the tumour is necrotic.

Metastases spread locally and typically via the bloodstream to the lungs and skeleton. The normal vascularity of endocrine glands encourages haematogenesis spread. Lymphatic spread to regional lymph nodes is not uncommon and in the neck may be a cause of misdiagnosis. Foci of otherwise normal thyroid tissue in cervical lymph nodes was once regarded as a *lateral aberrant thyroid* gland but it is now realized that such tissue is metastatic from a thyroid carcinoma.

Atrophy

Atrophy of part or the whole of a gland may follow from a localized disorder or from hormonal replacement which is either from ectopic foci including neoplasms or from therapy. A functional adrenal cortical adenoma leads to atrophy of the uninvolved cortex and to that of the contralateral gland, and a similar effect is produced by corticosteroid therapy. Equivalent compression and functional atrophy is seen in parathyroid glands in association with non-functional and functional tumours confined to one or two other parathyroid glands. Within the thyroid, focal atrophy will also be produced by any localized tumour and diffuse atrophy by the persistent intake of thyroxin or more commonly thyroiditis. Auto-immunity has now replaced tuberculosis as the cause of the adrenal cortical loss underlying Addison's disease. Very rarely atrophy is idiopathic.

Miscellaneous conditions

Thyroiditis

As the name implies this is an inflammatory disorder. It may arise from a variety of infections including tuberculosis but all of these are rare. A granulomatous form, *De Quervan's thyroiditis*, has been ascribed to viral infection but this has yet to be proved. *Lymphocytic thyroiditis* in children or *Hashimoto's thyroiditis* in adults are auto-immune disorders and include substantial lymphocytic and plasma cell infiltrates. Other evidence of an auto-immune basis is
- the preponderance of female patients;
- the association with HLA B8/15 – DR 3/4;
- the circulating thyroid growth stimulating antibodies;
- the presence of other autoimmune disorders.

As in infective and granulomatous thyroiditis the cellular response in auto-immune thyroiditis compresses and destroys the thyroid epithelium (Fig. 12.14). If this destruction is extensive, as invariably occurs in the granulomatous type, the patient becomes hypothyroid. In other patients the euthyroid state is maintained and in a very small number hyperthyroidism develops.

APPEARANCES

The thyroid is initially enlarged, reflecting the cellular infiltrate,

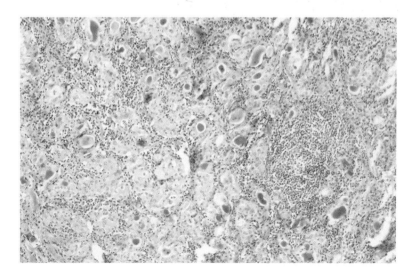

Fig. 12.14 Thyroiditis. There is a diffuse lymphocytic infiltrate with a lymphoid follicle and atrophy of the thyroid acini.

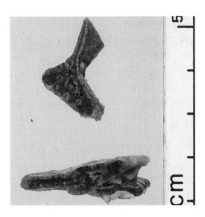

Fig. 12.15 Haemorrhage replacing much of the medulla and cortex of both adrenal glands. The patient died from a pneumococcal meningitis.

and later, partly or entirely, shrinks. There is some degree of fixation to the surrounding tissues and the gland is hard and often thought to harbour a carcinoma.

Bilateral adrenal haemorrhages

These underlie the *Waterhouse—Friderichsen syndrome*. There is destruction of the adrenal cortex leading to the collapse of the patient and death. The condition arises from septicaemias, especially with capsulate organisms and particularly the meningococci. Focal haemorrhages also occur in a wide range of other tissues. The mechanism may be immunologically mediated with the production of a vasculitis since no organisms are found in the lesions. Hypotension and 'stress' are also commonly but imprecisely implicated.

APPEARANCES

There are varying degrees of haemorrhage into both adrenals which microscopically involve both the cortex and medulla (Fig. 12.15). The adjacent cells are necrotic.

Developmental defects

Among the developmental defects that occur the best known involve the thyroid. These include persistence of the *thyroglossal duct* and enzyme pathway deficiencies resulting in *congenital goitres* and *hypothyroidism*. A persistent thyroglossal duct always lies in the mid-line of the neck and is clinically separated from the laterally placed *branchial cysts*, the developmental remnants of the first and second branchial clefts. Histologically unless there is thyroid tissue, a finding confined to the thyroglossal duct, the two can be indistinguishable.

Non-endocrine tumours

Craniopharyngiomas are pituitary tumours that develop from remnants of Rathke's pouch. They do not include endocrine cells and have no hormonal associations. There is squamous epithelium together with collagen and glial tissue. The patient will develop symptoms of an enlarging space-occupying lesion allied with compression of the optic chiasma.

Neuroblastomas are tumours predominantly of childhood with most appearing before 4 years of age (Fig. 12.16). They are often unilateral and most display metastatic spread at the time of presentation. The prognosis is not, however, always bad. The tumours arise from parasympathetic tissue and can occur in the adrenal medulla.

Lymphomas may involve the endocrine glands as part of a systemic disease or present confined to the endocrine glands. The lymphomas are usually of the non-Hodgkin's type and the thyroid is the gland most affected. Pre-existing lymphocytic Hashimoto's

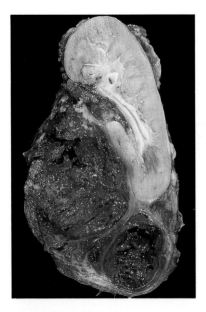

Fig. 12.16 Neuroblastoma arising in the adrenal in a child. There is extensive haemorrhage.

thyroiditis is almost invariable. A difficulty in diagnosis may arise in distinguishing lymphomas from anaplastic carcinomas but this can sometimes be resolved by immunocytochemical techniques. Clinically antilymphoma therapy will distinguish the two conditions by inducing prompt subsidence if the cause is a lymphoma. The prognosis for these lymphomas is better than that of anaplastic carcinomas.

Further reading

Bloodworth, J.M.B. (1982) (Editor). *Endocrine Pathology: General and Surgical* (2nd Edition). Williams and Wilkins: Baltimore and London.
McNicol, A.M. (1987). Pituitary adenomas. *Histopathology* **11**, 995–1011.
Polak, J.M. and Bloom, S.R. (1987). Some aspects of neuroendocrine pathology. *J. Clin. Path.* **40**, 1024–41.

13 Mononuclear cell system

Terminology

Lymphocytes and macrophages are mononuclear cells. They are widely dispersed throughout the body and share the common function of recognizing and inactivating foreign materials including antigens and micro-organisms. The cells circulate in the vascular and lymphatic systems and can also migrate through tissues. They form the major component of some organs such as the spleen and lymph nodes, and are a smaller part of most others, some referred to as the *mucosa associated lymphoid system* (Fig. 13.1). Other terms for the entire system include *lymphoreticular, lymphoproliferative, reticulo-endothelial* and *lymphoid*, all of which are derived from light microscopy features, before the development of modern immunology. Advances in immunology have revealed many of the functions of these cells and demonstrated the limitation of distinguishing them by their cytological appearances. Histochemistry and electron microscopy, and more especially immunohistochemistry incorporating polyclonal and monoclonal antibodies, have helped to define morphologically some of the functional subsets. New terms for the mononuclear cell sub-types are being introduced to histopathology and, although some of the old terms have fallen into disuse, others

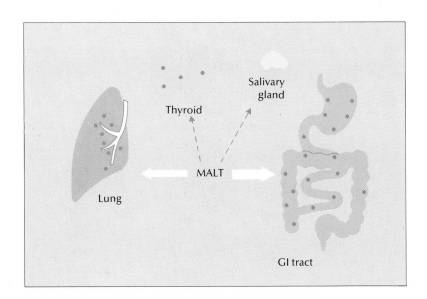

Fig. 13.1 Mucosa associated lymphoid system (MALT).

with an altered definition persist. The present terminology can thus be confusing and is in a state of flux.

Mononuclear cells

The basic mononuclear cells are lymphocytes, plasma cells and macrophages (Table 13.1).

Development

Lymphocytes and macrophages develop in the bone marrow (Fig. 13.2). They are then released to their end organs although some lymphocytes undergo further processing in the thymus. Lymphocytes homing directly from the bone marrow are *B-lymphocytes* and these are involved with antibody production, humoral immunity and defence. They pass through a series of stages with plasma cells as the end product. Lymphocytes processed by the thymus are *T-lymphocytes* and these are concerned with cellular immunity and defence as well as regulating some B-lymphocyte and macrophage responses. Specific T-lymphocyte subsets perform these functions through *T-suppressor* (Ts) and *T-helper* (Th) cells, respectively, which inhibit and promote some B-cell responses. Specific areas of B- and T-cells occur in the lymphoid organs and in regular patterns in other tissues (Figs 13.3 and 13.4).

Lymphocytes are round cells with uniform oval nuclei and a little clear cytoplasm. They vary in size from 6–12 μm. Antigenic stimulation results in cell division and change in their appearance. Variations in the nucleus include the assumption of a cleaved or bean shape and sometimes the development of a nucleolus. The ratio of nucleus to cytoplasm may alter and large and small cell forms appear. Proliferating B-lymphocytes are called large and small cleaved and uncleaved cells, centrocytic (including nucleolus) and centroblastic cells, terms which may be appropriate to the same cell. Alternatively, since B-cell division occurs in the follicle centres of the lymph nodes, these proliferating cells can be referred to as follicle centre cells.

Table 13.1 Mononuclear cells

Lymphoid cells	
Small lymphocytes	B-cells
	T-cells
	Non T-, Non B-cells
Medium/large lymphocytes	B-cells
	T-cells
Plasma cells	B-cells
Macrophages	
Monocytes	
Histiocytes	
Tingible body macrophages	
Veiled cells	
Interdigitating cells	
Follicular dendritic cells	

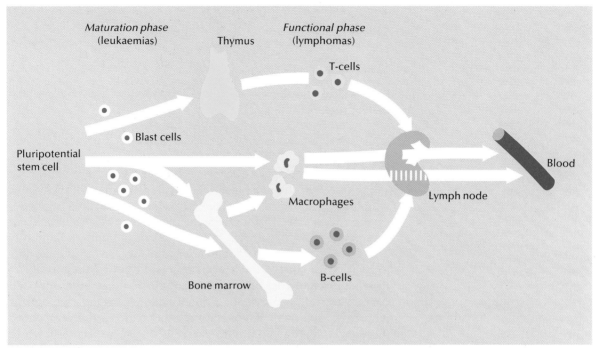

Fig. 13.2 Mononuclear cell development.

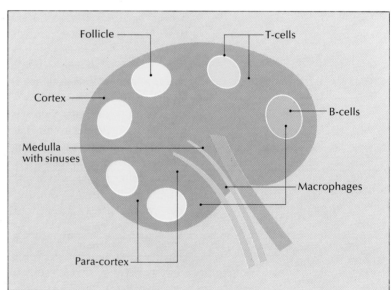

Fig. 13.3 Lymph node cell distribution.

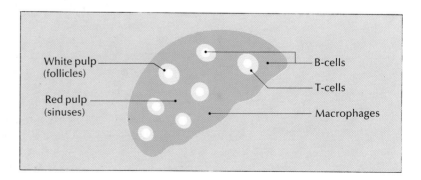

Fig. 13.4 Spleen cell distribution.

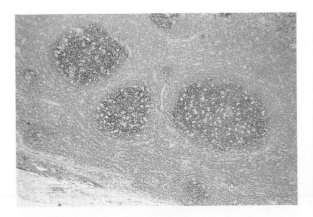 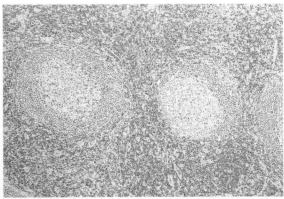

Fig. 13.5 Lymphocyte subtypes in a lymph node labelled with antibodies to B-cells (*above left*) and T-cells (*above right*). The distribution of the cell types compares with that in Fig. 13.3.

Lymphocyte subtypes

B- and T-cells cannot be differentiated from one another in routinely stained sections examined by light or electron microscopy, although plasma cells are easily distinguished. B-lymphocytes are identified by immunolabelling the immunoglobulin light and heavy chains they produce and T-cells by immunolabelling their membrane receptors. The technique involves monoclonal or polyclonal antibodies labelled with fluorescein or the enzymes peroxidase or alkaline phosphatase (Fig. 13.5). Most monoclonal antibodies can only be used on cryostat tissue sections and not on the routinely used formalin fixed and paraffin embedded tissues. Other ways of distinguishing B- and T-cells, such as rosette formation with red cells and the presence of complement receptors, necessitates separating the cells and preparing cell suspensions. The disadvantage of these methods is that location of the cells within the tissue is lost and separation of normal and abnormal cells is more difficult. Cell labelling is not done every time normal, reactive or neoplastic lymph nodes or spleen are examined. The cells are recognized by inference if the normal architectural pattern is maintained. These techniques are useful for distinguishing lymphoid neoplasms and for analysing these tumours in other sites. In any of these conditions some lymphocytes do not label and are known as *null cells*; their significance and origin is uncertain.

Plasma cells have abundant eosinophilic cytoplasm surrounded by a distinct cell membrane. The nucleus is often eccentric and its chromatin fragmented and aggregated peripherally, an appearance compared with a cart-wheel or hot cross bun. Electron microscopy reveals abundant rough endoplasmic reticulum (Fig. 13.6). Antibody studies demonstrate immunoglobulins in the cytoplasm with a specific type confined to each cell.

Macrophages are larger than small resting lymphocytes and have irregular cytoplasmic margins, variably shaped nucleoli and abundant cytoplasm. They are phagocytic and can be recognized from this property as well as from the use of labelled antibodies (Fig. 13.7). *In vivo* phagocytosed particles may be seen in the cytoplasm, while *in vitro* this activity can be stimulated by exposing the cell to

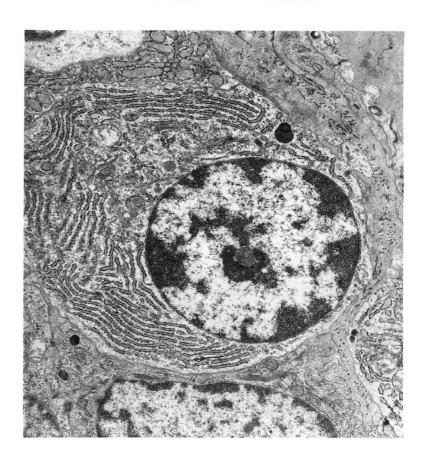

Fig. 13.6 Plasma cell: ultrastructural features. The nucleus is at one pole of the cell and the chromatin distributed around the nuclear membrane. The abundant rough endoplasmic reticulum filling the cytoplasm is evidence of the secretory function.

foreign material. Other features include a high lysosomal content demonstrated either by histochemical techniques or by electron microscopy. Histiocytes and blood monocytes are terms used for these cells in different tissues although the cells do not differ morphologically or functionally from macrophages. Macrophages are found in the lymphoid organs and include a variety of forms (Table 13.1).

Disorders

Disease may affect the entire system or remain confined to one facet. Diffuse involvement follows the suppression of mononuclear cell function, producing immune depression. This is seen either as a side effect of disease in other organs or in the course of antitumour therapy that inadvertently affects mononuclear cells. Immunosuppressive agents either to treat disease or to maintain transplants are another cause for immunodepression as is widespread replacement of lymph nodes by disease processes and the rare primary immune deficiency syndromes (Fig. 13.8). Immunodeficiency from any cause may result in infection and often with more than one micro-organism.

Localized disorders usually result in enlargement of the affected area and are due most commonly to reactive hyperplasia and less so to neoplasia. Lymph nodes are most often involved and, since the

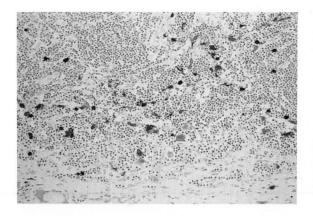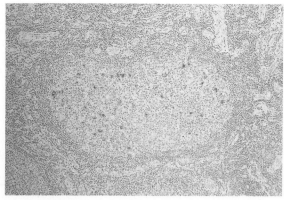

Fig. 13.7 Macrophages labelled with antibody in (*above left*) the medullary sinuses of a lymph node and (*above right*) a reactive lymphoid follicle.

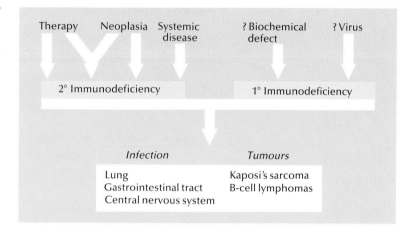

Fig. 13.8 Immunodeficiency.

majority of these are in the neck, cervical lymphadenopathy is a common presentation.

Reactive hyperplasia

Lymph nodes

Reactive hyperplasia in lymph nodes has been experienced by almost all individuals. Reaction may be local or widespread and may involve the entire node or only a part. The response may uniformly affect all lymph nodes in one region but more often individual lymph nodes vary in their involvement (Fig. 13.9). Causes of the reaction are legion and include micro-organisms, particularly viruses, drugs, local and systemic disease and tumours. The effect is to remove or inactivate the cause. Theoretically, if this requires humoral antibody, the response centres on the follicular regions, while if cellular immune responses are stimulated, the paracortical T-regions are involved, but very rarely are such pure responses observed. The reasons for this are complex but include:

1 The interrelationship of the humoral and cellular immune responses.

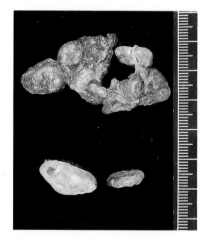

Fig. 13.9 Reactive lymph nodes. The variation is size reflects the differing involvement despite all the nodes coming from the same anatomical site.

2 The repetitive nature of the stimulus.
3 A concomitant inflammatory response.
4 The coexistence of other hyperplastic reactions.
5 Previous exposure to a similar antigenic stimulus.

The likelihood of identifying the cause of hyperplasia from lymph node morphology is therefore remote unless the antigen is present. Micro-organisms are most often recognized but occasionally other causes produce a distinct tissue pattern. Cat scratch disease with stellate abscesses and lymphangiogram changes with macrophages filled with lipid fall into this category.

APPEARANCES

The cellular proliferation may centre on the follicles or the sinuses or may present a mixed pattern. Within any example there can be an associated inflammatory response and in some nodes this predominates. When this is so multinucleate cells may appear and macrophages assume an epithelioid cell appearance. These cells may then form granulomas, displacing the normal lymphoid tissue. Lymph nodes affected by sarcoid (Fig. 13.10) and tuberculosis are good examples of this response. Any hyperplastic lymph node enlarges and can do so to a very considerable degree. It will, however, retain its shape and if several adjacent nodes are affected each node will also retain its identity and not become densely adherent to others. The cut surface is uniform and grey-white but on rare occasions includes foci of necrosis, haemorrhage and even abscess formation.

Spleen

Reactive hyperplasia probably occurs frequently in the spleen but generally escapes clinical recognition. A notable exception is hyperplasia accompanying infective mononucleosis (glandular fever). The

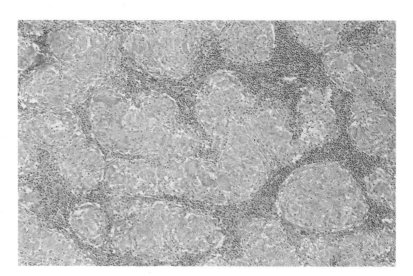

Fig. 13.10 Lymph node extensively replaced by discrete granulomas suggestive of sarcoid. The Kveim test was positive, confirming the diagnosis.

spleen is enlarged with changes in the white pulp mirroring those of reactive lymph nodes. The splenic enlargement often seen at autopsy may include hyperplastic changes but is mainly attributable to congestion secondary to heart failure and more rarely blood dyscrasias, particularly leukaemias.

Thymus

Hyperplasia is virtually confined to patients with *myasthenia gravis*. This disease is characterized by skeletal muscle weakness and circulating antibodies to the acetylcholine receptors and, in all but 10% of patients, the thymus is abnormal. Thymic hyperplasia is found in over two-thirds and may accompany a thymic tumour, thymoma. Thymomas are found in approximately 10% of such patients. The reactive changes are similar to those in reactive lymph nodes and are associated with the appearance of follicles. Gross enlargement does not necessarily result. The interrelationship between myasthenia gravis and thymic hyperplasia is unexplained and the disease is not always cured by thymectomy.

Following puberty the thymus undergoes steady involution so that from about 30 years of age thymic tissue is only found with considerable difficulty. The reason for this involution is unknown but it underlies the absence of hyperplastic changes in circumstances other than myasthenia gravis. Finding a thymus in the pre-pubescent child does not imply a hyperplastic response but simply reflects the normal.

Atrophy and immunodeficiency

Atrophy

Atrophy of the thymus, lymph nodes, spleen and even the more diffusely sited foci of mononuclear cells is a natural but unexplained phenomenon of increasing age. However, it may also be induced by any agent or disease which destroys or inhibits mononuclear cells and is then seen in a wide range of circumstances and in patients of all ages. The lymphocytes and macrophages disappear and the lymphoid organs become smaller. In the spleen, any reduction in size may be masked because there is no corresponding loss in the number and volume of blood sinuses.

Secondary immunodeficiency

The immune deficit arising from atrophy of lymphoid tissue is classified as secondary immunodeficiency and is the most common example of immunodeficiency met clinically. The severity reflects the degree and duration as well as the manner in which immunosuppression is induced. Elderly people are relatively immunodeficient but this is not a serious disability and only assumes importance when other conditions occur. Any patient with a transplant, in contrast, has a significant immune deficit which, in the

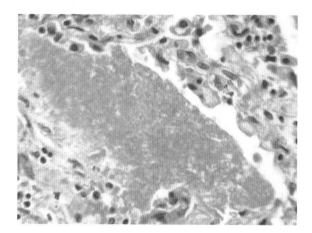 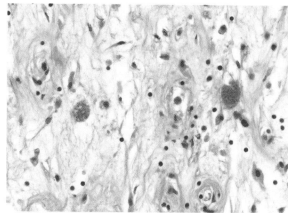

Fig. 13.11 Microbial infections highly suggestive of immunodeficiency. (*Above left*) *Pneumocystis carinii* — an organism, probably protozoa, which is restricted to the lungs. Multiple cysts fill the air sacs. (*Above right*) *Toxoplasma gondii* cysts within the brain. This protozoon can also occur in other sites.

early post-operative phases, can contribute to infection and death. Tumours may arise within the same patients and the immunodeficiency is again regarded as a contributory factor. Patients with AIDS (acquired immune deficiency syndrome) are another example where infection and tumours secondary to an immune deficit cause death. In any of these patients all the lymphoid components are affected. Immunodepression following splenectomy is not so profound. Nevertheless, in the short and the long term, there is low resistance to capsular organisms, especially *S. pneumoniae*, and such infections can then be fatal.

Types of infections

These involve all types of micro-organisms and often more than one form at the same time. In addition, organisms rarely causing clinical disease occur such as the protozoa *Pneumocytis carinii* and *Toxoplasma gondii* (Fig. 13.11). Other organisms are usually inactivated, but with severe immunodepression this reaction is not so effective and the infection progresses and death ensues. Common endemic viruses such as those of measles and chickenpox, as well as more unusual infections including that of the cytomegalovirus and atypical mycobacteria are examples (Fig. 13.12). It is often the practice to refer to these infections as *opportunist*. The disadvantage of this term is that it links certain organisms with specific disorders and modes of therapy which, with the increasing sophistication of medical practice, is no longer true. Any infection is the result of an imbalance between host resistance and the virulence of the organism and in all infections both responses are involved to varying degrees.

Tumours

Tumours related with secondary immunodeficiency are carcinomas, lymphomas and, rarely, sarcomas. Their incidence is greater than in matched populations but only in those with severe immunodepression. The carcinomas are mainly of the skin and cervix and

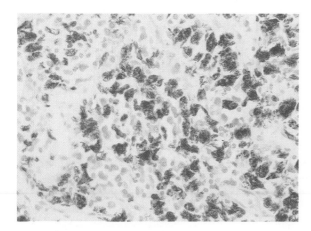
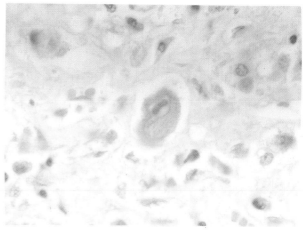

Fig. 13.12 (*Above left*) Atypical mycobacteria (red) lying in clumps in a lymph node from a patient with AIDS. (*Above right*) Characteristic owl's eye inclusion of a cell infected with the cytomegalovirus.

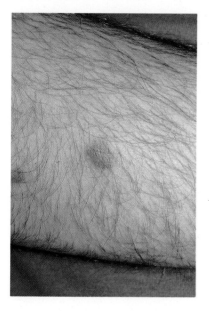

Fig. 13.13 Kaposi's sarcoma on the arm of a homosexual who was HIV positive.

thus readily accessible to treatment; they also share the malignant potential of similar tumours in other patients. The lymphomas are non-Hodgkin's B-lymphomas and have unusual features. They are found in sites such as the brain, and they behave more aggressively than their counterparts in non-immunodepressed subjects. Kaposi's sarcoma is the best known sarcoma (Fig. 13.13) and, although a characteristic of AIDS, is not unique to this form of secondary immunodeficiency. Neoplasia in any patient surviving for a sufficient period results in the development of a further tumour in 5–10%. The same phenomenon is observed with secondary immunodeficiency but with an infinitely higher incidence, reaching, for example, 20% among AIDS victims.

There is no satisfactory explanation for the association of neoplasia and immunodeficiency but several factors may be pertinent:

1 Tumours are often virus-related and there is circumstantial evidence of viral infection in many patients. Some lymphomas can be allied with the Epstein–Barr virus and Kaposi's sarcoma may be similarly associated with the cytomegalovirus. Some of the epithelial tumours may reflect papilloma virus infection.

2 Antigenic stimulation either from multiple infections and/or foreign grafts is present and might stimulate abnormal lymphocytic proliferation progressing to a lymphoma.

3 Immunosuppression will affect any immunosurveillance mechanism against neoplasia. A part of this is a decrease in the circulating *natural killer cells (NK cells)*, cells capable of destroying tumour cells.

4 Tumours, in some transplant recipients, have undergone remission. This has occurred either when the immunosuppressive therapy was stopped, or following removal of the graft and cessation of immunotherapy.

5 If a transplant recipient has an established malignancy or such a tumour is inadvertently transplanted with the graft, the tumour has invariably undergone rapid growth and widespread dissemination.

6 Suggestions that the immunosuppressants used in organ transplantation are directly oncogenic have not been proved.

Primary immunodeficiency

Primary immunodeficiency states were described by a variety of eponyms but are now classified according to the absent immune responses. They can be grouped broadly into those with a humoral deficit (50–75%), those with a cellular deficit (5–10%) and those with a mixed deficit (10–25%). They are not confined to children and many only declare themselves during adulthood. IgA deficiency, the most common form of primary immunodeficiency, is a notable example. Genetic defects may be the cause but most are unexplained. They are all extremely rare.

APPEARANCES

There are invariably abnormalities of the thymus or of the B-cell regions of the lymph nodes and spleen. The thymus may be absent as occurs with maldevelopment of the III and IV pharyngeal pouches, atrophic or undergo rapid involution soon after birth. In the spleen there can be diminution of the white pulp, absence of follicle formation and plasma cells. The lymph nodes may be absent but more commonly have no follicles or paracortical regions and are often without plasma cells (Fig. 13.14). Similar changes within the lymphoid tissues of the gut also occur. The findings within any patient depend upon the stage at which the tissues are examined and whether the principal deficit is cellular, humoral or a combination of both. Pure phagocytic disorders occur but these are very rare and hyperplasia of the lymph nodes and spleen result.

The potential effect for all patients is repeated infections, principally in the lungs. In some patients tumours, especially lymphomas, develop.

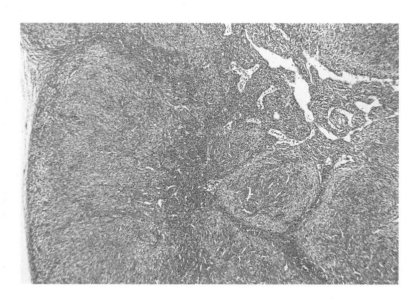

Fig. 13.14 Severe combined immunodeficiency. Lymph node from a three-month-old child who had failed to thrive. Although the node is cellular true follicles with reactive centres are not present. The majority of cells had no B- or T-cell markers and there were only small numbers of such cells circulating. A bone marrow transplant was curative.

Tumours

Metastases

Lymph nodes

Metastases are the most common tumours in lymph nodes. Carcinomas and melanomas predominate but deposits from any tumour occur. Regional nodes to the primary growth are generally involved but tumour can bypass these and appear in more distant nodes. Metastases may also present before the primary growth, a phenomenon often seen with nasopharyngeal carcinomas and occasionally with melanomas. Recognition of the origin usually requires knowledge of the primary growth.

Tumour reaches the lymph nodes either as isolated cells within the lymph or as thrombo-emboli propagating along the lymphatics and, in the early stages, is restricted to the subcapsular sinus. The parenchyma of the lymph node is later involved and may eventually be totally replaced.

APPEARANCES

The lymph nodes are enlarged and tumour areas firm to hard and greyish white (Fig. 13.15). Foci of necrosis and haemorrhage are sometimes seen. If the deposit is from a squamous carcinoma, soft greasy yellow material (keratin) may be evident while mucoid material or fluid within the tumour suggests an adenocarcinoma. A black tumour deposit is indicative of a melanoma metastasis (Fig. 13.16) and a bile-stained one of an hepatic cell carcinoma. Uninvolved nodes in the same region are often hyperplastic.

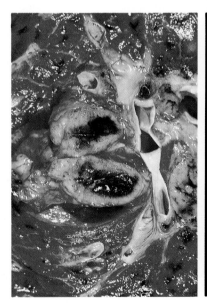 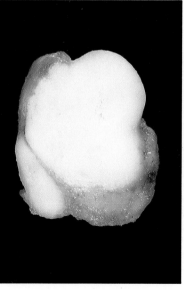

Fig. 13.15 Metastatic tumour in lymph nodes; (*left*) from a lung primary to the hilar lymph nodes. The black carbon identifies the uninvolved tissue; (*right*) from an adenocarcinoma in the colon.

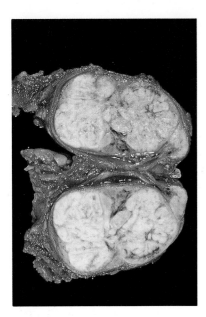

Fig. 13.16 Lymph node with a metastasis from a melanoma. The brown pigment associated with this primary is seen in parts of the metastasis.

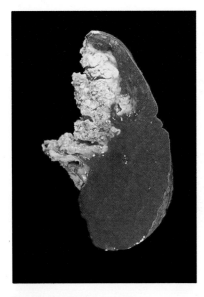

Fig. 13.17 Metastatic tumour spreading from a primary carcinoma of the kidney directly into the adjacent spleen.

Spleen

Metastatic tumour in the spleen is surprisingly uncommon. The substantial blood flow must include tumour cells and it is therefore possible that there is an inbuilt protective mechanism. This could arise from the macrophages but comparable numbers of these exist in the liver and the lungs which are among the most common sites for metastases. This suggestion also does not explain the equal rarity of spread of local tumour from the stomach, pancreas, colon and kidney.

Tumours producing splenic metastases are lung and breast carcinomas and less often melanomas. With the exception of melanomas, these probably reflect the high incidence of the primary growths and their greater opportunity to produce splenic metastases. Metastatic tumour occurs either as diffusely scattered cells which are only appreciated histologically, and less frequently as macroscopic greyish nodules (Fig. 13.17).

Thymus

The thymus is severely atrophic in adults and consequently metastatic tumour at this site is exceedingly uncommon.

Lymphomas

These are lymphomas, thymomas and macrophage proliferations, all of which manifest varying degrees of malignancy. The definition of each is disputed and their subclassifications are confused. These difficulties, principally the fault of histopathologists, have arisen from changes in cell nomenclature and from the modification and retention of discarded classifications.

Lymphomas

Definition. They arise from lymphocytes during their functional development phase and so result in immunodeficiency. This is in contrast to leukaemias which occur during the maturation phase of development. Confusion with leukaemias arises because although lymphomas are predominantly disorders of solid organs and leukaemias of the blood, each can spill into the other's territory. Lymphomas divide into two main groups, Hodgkin's disease or Hodgkin's lymphoma and the less common non-Hodgkin's lymphoma (NHL).

Hodgkin's lymphoma

This, world-wide, is the most common form of lymphoma but in the USA and Western Europe it contributes only 40% of all lymphomas. The prognosis has been radically altered by modern therapy and the tumour is now regarded as curable. If the disease is localized, 85% of patients will be alive after treatment in 5 years and, among all patients, 50% will be alive after 10 years. The hallmark and essential finding for the diagnosis is the *Reed—Sternberg cell* (Fig. 13.18). This cell is large with two prominent nuclei with each the mirror image of the other. The nuclei may be reneform or lobed and have distinct membranes and distinct nucleoli. Surrounding the nucleus is a variably sized halo beyond which there is abundant basophilic cytoplasm. The contour of the cell is irregular. Associated with the Reed—Sternberg cell are acute and chronic inflammatory cells including neutrophil and eosinophil polymorphs, plasma cells and lymphocytes, the last predominating (Fig. 13.19). Bands of collagen and fibrous tissue are characteristic of the nodular sclerosis subtype and divide the cells into nodules.

The importance of the Reed—Sternberg cell for diagnosis has led

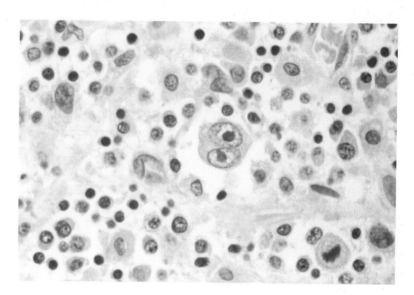

Fig. 13.18 Reed—Sternberg cell in an example of Hodgkin's disease.

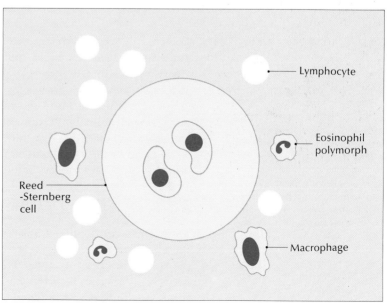

Fig. 13.19 Hodgkin's lymphoma cells.

Table 13.2 Classification of Hodgkin's lymphoma (as made before any treatment is given. Any change during the disease is towards a worse prognosis group)

Main group	Subclassification	Distribution (%) in two large series	
Lymphocyte predominant	Nodular and diffuse	17—20 82	Presenting at clinical I and II stages
Nodular sclerosis	Grade 1* and 2*	20—40 70	Young females. Mainly with mediastinal spread
Mixed cellularity	Nodular and diffuse	30—40 17	Most likely cause of abdominal involvement
Lymphocyte depletion	Nodular and diffuse	12—13 4	Presenting at clinical III and IV stages

* Grade 1 histology is predominantly similar to mixed cellularity and Grade 2 similar to lymphocyte depletion with poorer prognosis.

to suggestions that it is the basis of the disorder and not the lymphocyte. Lymphocyte function is, however, abnormal with a depression of cellular immune responses both *in vitro* and *in vivo*. Auto-immune disease, notably haemolytic anaemia, also occurs. Monoclonal antibody studies reveal that the tumour lymphocytes are T-cells and thus by displacing normal T-cells they may cause the impaired cellular immunity. The origin of the Reed—Sternberg cells is not clear. Positive labelling with T- and B-cell markers as well macrophages markers has been reported but others have failed to demonstrate any labelling.

Classification

Prior to modern treatment the prognosis and malignancy of the disease was equated with the number of lymphocytes and whether the cells were in a diffuse or a nodular pattern. Patients with tumours with large numbers of lymphocytes did well while those with few did badly. If the cells were arranged as nodules the outlook was better than when the pattern was diffuse. These observations led to the Rye classification (Table 13.2) which although still used is of less importance. The disease is staged clinically according to the number and position of sites involved and the presence or absence of symptoms (Table 13.3). Widely disseminated tumour with symptoms carries a poor prognosis while a good prognosis is associated with localized and asymptomatic tumour.

Aetiology

There are clinical and epidemiological findings which suggest that

Table 13.3 Clinical stages of Hodgkin's lymphoma — with or without symptoms

I	Single lymph node or focus of nodes
II	Tumour entirely above or below the diaphragm
III	Lymph node involvement only both above and below the diaphragm
IV	Widespread lymphoma both in nodes and extranodal

an important factor may be a low grade infection with a maximum impact in late adolescence.

1 Hodgkin's disease has epidemic characteristics in that patients have been linked, and family members and pupils from the same schools affected. With all these examples there was close and repeated contact between the sufferers.

2 Clinically the condition is often initially mistaken for an infection.

3 The Epstein—Barr virus causes infectious mononucleosis, (glandular fever) and can transform lymphocytes. Hodgkin's disease patients, although having the same incidence of antibody to the virus as control groups, have higher levels than controls. Reed—Sternberg cells occur in lymph nodes following infectious mononucleosis and among such patients there is a risk of developing Hodgkin's lymphoma.

Other findings that are less supportive are that the age of onset is bimodal with a peak at 20 years and a second at 45 years; males in either age group are afflicted more than women. Further, in affluent societies the disease is seen in adults whilst in deprived societies children are involved, observations that have also led to the suggestion that the disease has different causes in different age groups.

Against the infectious origin hypothesis are that many examples of Hodgkin's lymphoma do not have recognized contacts and that the Epstein—Barr antibody titres represent infection by a common virus. The higher levels in Hodgkin's lymphoma may also stem from the impairment of cellular immunity and coincidental upset in B-cell regulation.

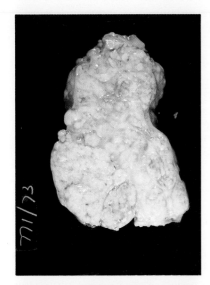

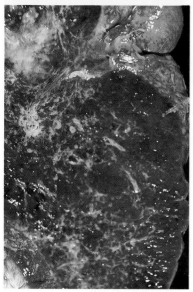

Fig. 13.20 Lymph node entirely replaced by Hodgkin's disease (*above*) and a spleen including similar tumour (*below*).

APPEARANCES

The disease generally starts in the lymph nodes, particularly those in the neck, and spreads to the contiguous regional lymph nodes irrelevant of the direction of lymph flow. The nodes become enlarged, rubbery and firmly matted with a white parenchyma, often compared to fish flesh (Fig. 13.20). Within some nodes a nodular pattern is recognized. Spread to extranodal sites is a late complication and results in similar lymphoma deposits within the spleen and liver which are probably blood-borne. Any other organ can be involved, invariably asymptomatically, but the lungs and urinary and gastrointestinal tracts are those most affected. Tumour within the bone marrow occurs but is less common and central nervous system and cutaneous involvement are both rare.

Complications

Infection is usually the cause of death and follows from the secondary cellular immunodeficiency. Impaired humoral immunity also contributes to these infections but this is principally the result of therapy. The patient, even when free of lymphoma, is prone to infection since the immune responses take several years to return to normal.

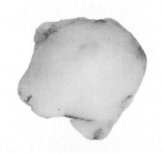

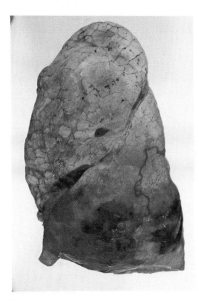

Fig. 13.21 (*Top*) Lymph node replaced by a non-Hodgkin's lymphoma. The parenchyma is rubbery and uniform. (*Bottom*) Vertebral marrow partly replaced by non-Hodgkin's lymphoma. The tumour was initially seen in lymph nodes.

Lymph node compression of vital structures, especially in the neck, is a further cause of death. Renal failure may develop following ureteric compression by para-aortic lymph nodes but is also caused by uric acid deposition, amyloid and immune complex formation. Other tumours, most particularly non-Hodgkin's lymphoma, leukaemias and gastric cancer may develop but are thought to be secondary to therapy rather than to the disease.

Non-Hodgkin's lymphoma (NHL)

Most NHL are B-cell in origin. They manifest some of the features of the follicle centre cells and have inflammatory mononuclear cells intermingled among the lymphoma cells. The macroscopic features are similar to those of Hodgkin's disease (Fig. 13.21). Humoral immunity is invariably depressed with hypogammaglobulinaemia and in a few patients hypergammaglobulinaemia. The hypergammaglobulinaemia can be light or heavy chain, monoclonal or polyclonal and even associated with cryoglobulins. The lymphoma spreads to B-cell areas, including the spleen and the marrow, in a centrifugal manner. The patient may thus present with complications of diffuse spread rather than local symptoms from enlarged lymph nodes.

Classification

This has justifiably been described as a 'semantic quagmire'. There are currently six complex main classifications and it is probably true that any histopathologist, although claiming to use any one of these, has modified it to his own usage. Nevertheless, within the 'system' used, crude prognoses for the different ends of the spectrum of NHL are both possible and consistent. A basic source of difficulty is that many NHL labelled as histiocytic are now clearly not. These lymphomas include 50–60% B-cell, 5–15% T-cell and 5% macrophage, making true histiocytic lymphomas extremely rare. Among these lymphomas there is also a high proportion that include no markers. The lack of markers may be because these are lost or do not develop or because these Null cells include markers not presently identifiable. Clearly morphological descriptions and functional correlations have not achieved an ideal classification. Such a classification should be simple and with clear prognostic information, thereby discriminating between different forms of treatment. Antibody cell markers provide the present focus of interest for this but no classification of other tumours relies upon such markers and for many the most useful prognostic index is an assessment of the bulk of the tumour.

Aetiology

There is no recognized cause for NHL although a number of risk factors are known. These include some forms of primary immunodeficiency and secondary immunodeficiency, most noticeably in

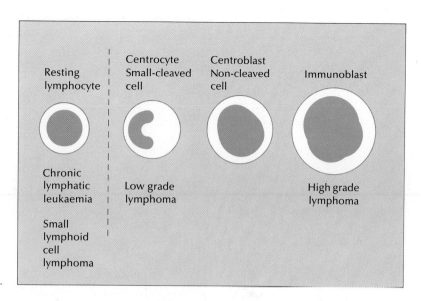

Fig. 13.22 B-cell lymphoma subtypes.

(figure labels:)
Resting lymphocyte
Centrocyte Small-cleaved cell
Centroblast Non-cleaved cell
Immunoblast

Chronic lymphatic leukaemia

Small lymphoid cell lymphoma

Low grade lymphoma

High grade lymphoma

allograft recipients, and as a complication of auto-immune disorders, Hodgkin's lymphoma, connective tissue disorders and anticonvulsant therapy. The common denominator among these is an aberration of the immune responses allied often with persistent antigen stimulation. Oncogenic viruses may form a part of this stimulus but evidence for this is only clear for the Epstein–Barr virus and Burkitt's lymphoma and the human T-cell leukaemia/lymphoma virus (HTLV I) and some T-cell lymphomas.

Prognostic features

A good prognosis can be expected for most follicle and nodular NHL and especially when the cells are at the mature end of the follicle centre cell spectrum (Fig. 13.22). A *low grade lymphoma* of this type is the tissue counterpart of chronic lymphatic leukaemia. Origin in extranodal sites, most especially the mucosal associated lymphoid sites, is also equated with a fair prognosis as is perhaps fibrosis within the lymphoma. Diffuse lymphoma with large lymphoblastic cells, in contrast, is a *high grade lymphoma* with a poor prognosis.

Complications

Lymphoma can extend beyond the lymphoid organs and can embarrass the function of the organs affected. Death is due to infection from the associated secondary immunodeficiency which is often aggravated by treatment.

T-cell lymphomas

These occur within the 'histiocytic' group of NHL and also in diffuse patterns and as mixed T- and B-cell lymphomas. They are,

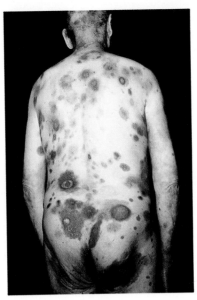

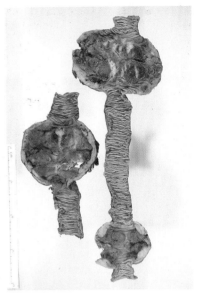

Fig. 13.23 Mycosis fungoides, a slowly evolving T-cell lymphoma restricted to the skin.

Fig. 13.24 Extranodal lymphoma in the small intestine. The multiple primary lesions are characteristic.

however, rare and in some patients are confined for many years to the skin and known as *mycosis fungoides* (Fig. 13.23).

Extranodal NHL

A diagnosis of extranodal NHL can only be made when it is clearly apparent that the lymphoma is confined to an organ and has not extended beyond its draining lymph nodes. Any organ can be affected but apart from the skin, the gastrointestinal (Fig. 13.24), respiratory and reproductive tracts are those most often involved. Brain involvement is almost confined to organ graft recipients and those with AIDS. Sjögren's syndrome, thyroiditis and atrophic gastritis are accepted precursors in the salivary gland, thyroid and stomach, respectively. Prognosis is often better than that for lymph node NHL except when the testis or breast are affected.

Thymic tumours

Thymomas are rare and arise from the epithelial cells of the thymus. They do not, despite their T-lymphocytic population and appearance, originate from lymphocytes. Their recognition depends on the demonstration in the tumour cells of cytokeratins by antibody labelling or of desmosomes and keratohyaline bundles by electron microscopy.

Classifications of thymomas were developed before the epithelial cell contribution was appreciated and were based on the lymphocyte population. These are now redundant. The tumour is associated

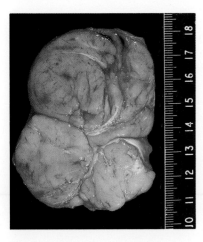

Fig. 13.25 Thymoma in an elderly patient who did not have myasthenia gravis.

with myasthenia gravis and, even less commonly, with red cell aplasia, pemphigus and hypogammaglobulinaemia.

APPEARANCES

The tumours are usually well circumscribed, varying in size from a few grammes to large masses (Fig. 13.25). A capsule may be evident but does not infer a benign tumour. The distinction between benign and malignant is not clear-cut and differentiation ultimately rests upon the patient's course.

Other primary thymic tumours include carcinoid tumours developing from the endosecretory (APUD) cells, which are a cause of Cushing's syndrome, and germ cell tumours. The origin of the latter is uncertain but a primary testicular tumour must be ruled out if a metastasis is not to be misdiagnosed. Lymphomas are also occasionally seen in the thymus and rarely metastases.

Tumours of macrophages

These are often not localized single masses but widely dispersed simultaneously appearing infiltrates, commonly termed *histiocytoses* (Table 13.4). Enzyme studies, monoclonal antibodies and electron microscopy all assist in their recognition but, in the most malignant examples, may fail to provide incontrovertible proof of a macrophage origin.

Among these conditions are those with an abnormal storage of either endogenous or exogenous matter in macrophages and others with proliferation and hyperplasia of macrophages. Because of the widespread nature of these cells, each condition is potentially diffuse but in practice some organs are more involved than others, thereby producing clinical variants. Nevertheless some, particularly the hyperplastic disorders, can be confined to a single organ. Within the neoplastic group, separation between benign and malignant examples may not be possible histologically and may even vary with the age of the patient. The diseases known as *Histiocytosis X*

Table 13.4 Forms of histiocytoses

Storage disorders	
Exogenous	Melanin (*melanosis coli*); paraffin (paraffin granuloma); mycobacteria; Whipple's disease
Endogenous	Lysosomal degradation defects (Gaucher's disease; Neimann–Pick's disease; gangliosidoses)
Proliferative disorders	Histiocytosis X (Letterer–Siwe disease; Hand–Schuller–Christian disease; eosinophilic granuloma of bone)
Neoplastic disorders	Malignant histiocytosis ? Histiocytic lymphoma of the intestine

fall into this group although the putative cell, Langerhan's cell, is not a true macrophage. Langerhan's cells, although sharing many of the macrophage cells markers, are characterized ultrastructurally by Birbeck or tennis racquet granules and are not phagocytic. Most examples of Histiocytosis X are not malignant.

Macroscopically tissues harbouring tumour are enlarged but the diagnosis hinges on the histological demonstration of collections of abnormal and bizarre macrophages.

Further reading

Basset, F., Nezelof, C. and Ferrans, V.J. (1983). The histiocytoses. In: *Pathology Annual, Part 2*. Ed. by S. Sommers and P.P. Sheldon. Appleton Century Crofts: Norwalk Connecticut.

Carr, I. and Hancock, B.W. (1984) (Editors). *Lymphoreticular Disease: an Introduction for the Pathologist and Oncologist* (2nd Edition).

Chu, T., D'Angio, G.J., Favara, B., Ladisch, S., Nesbit, M. and Pritchard, J. (1987). Histiocytosis syndromes in children. *Lancet* **i**, 208–9.

Isaacson, P.G. and Spencer, J. (1987). Malignant lymphoma of mucosa-associated lymphoid tissue. *Histopathology* **11**, 445–62.

Lee, F.D. (1987). Hodgkin's disease. *Histopathology* **11**, 1211–17.

Levine, G.D. and Rosai, J. (1978). Thymic hyperplasia and neoplasia: a review of current concepts. *Hum. Pathol.* **9**, 495–515.

Seminars on Oncology 7 (1980), Nos. 2 and 3. *Hodgkin's Disease: Non-Hodgkin's Lymphoma*.

Stansfeld, A.G. (1985) (Editor). *Lymph Node Biopsy Interpretation*. Churchill Livingstone: Edinburgh and London.

Suchi, T., Lennert, K., Tu, L-Y, Kikuchi, M., Sato, E., Stansfeld, A.G. and Feller, A.C. (1987). Histopathology and immunohistochemistry of peripheral T-cell lymphomas: a proposal for their classification *J. Clin. Pathol.* **40**, 995–1015.

14 Breast

Carcinoma of the breast is the most common cancer in women and is affecting an increasing number within Western societies. The mortality rate of 15 000 per annum in the UK remains constant and 1:200 women will develop the tumour. Early recognition, when the tumour load is small, offers the best way of reducing this mortality although no universal agreement exists on the ideal form of treatment and the cause is unknown. How to achieve early recognition is, however, unclear. Mass screening by mammography, programmes teaching self examination of the breast and the selection of women at risk for examination are all being assessed. Tissue examination is essential for diagnosis since clinically distinction between benign and malignant breast lumps is exceedingly difficult and often impossible. Biopsy, frozen section examination and fine needle aspiration all have their advocates but none is entirely devoid of error arising from either tissue selection or misinterpretation of the histological appearances. There is no specific cell marker for breast tissue and none that distinguishes benign from malignant breast disease.

Cancer of the male breast is a rarity and, as in women, less often encountered than benign disease, in the male referred to as *gynaecomastia*. Other breast malignancies in either sex are uncommon but include sarcoma and non-Hodgkin's lymphoma.

Benign disorders

These include a range of non-infectious changes, a small group of benign tumours and some uncommon inflammatory conditions.

Non-infectious benign disorders

Clinically, there are breast lumps of varying size which are often bilateral and which recur after surgery in about half the patients. The disorder has its main incidence between 25–45 years and is less often seen after the menopause. All these observations implicate a hormonal basis for the disorder but no clear pathogenesis has emerged. Some regard the disorder as a qualitative difference from the normal, a viewpoint supported by the frequency of minor forms of the condition found incidentally in breast tissue taken with other lesions and from autopsies. The occurrence with breast cancer makes it difficult to decide if the condition is a precursor of this, a dilemma made more difficult by the lack of a clear definition

Mammary dysplasia
Cystic disease
Fibrocystic disease
Chronic cystic mastitis
Cystic hyperplasia
Cystic mastopathia
Mastopathy
Chronic mastitis
Fibrous disease
Fibro-adenosis

of this form of benign breast disease. Numerous terms are used for the disease and its components, and among different authorities, the same terms may be used for different lesions (Table 14.1). The terms all apply to microscopic features and particularly to changes in the duct epithelium (Table 14.2). Since a number of these reflect hyperplasia and cyst formation combined with stromal reactions, and since these occur in numerous patterns, there is no consistent histological picture (Fig. 14.1).

APPEARANCES

Macroscopically no changes may be present and the lesion is an incidental finding. When there is a palpable mass this may be solid or include cysts of varying site distended with clear fluid (Fig. 14.2). These cysts often have a bluish tinge. The stroma may be tough and white and sufficiently hard to be mistaken for a carcinoma. There is poor demarcation from the surrounding breast tissue and no capsule. The left breast is involved more often than the right.

Benign tumours

Fibro-adenoma

This tumour of unknown aetiology is usually single and most often found in young women. There is no association with breast cancer

Table 14.2 Histological features of non-infectious benign breast disorders

Cysts	Variably sized epithelial lined spaces. The epithelium ranges from columnar to scarcely recognizable flattened cells or is apocrine (see below)
Adenosis	Proliferation of acini with persistence of a lobular pattern
Blunt duct adenosis	Enlarged terminal ducts without an increase in the number of acini
Sclerosing adenosis	Profuse adenosis with an irregular pattern mimicking carcinoma
Epithelial hyperplasia	American term equivalent to the British term, epitheliosis, and sometimes referred to as papillomatosis. Hyperplasia ranging from an orderly to an atypical pattern within the terminal ducts
Papillomatosis	Papillary proliferation of duct epithelium. Also used synonymously with epitheliosis when the proliferation fills the duct lumen. The term does not include intraduct papillomas
Apocrine metaplasia (pink cell change)	Large eosinophilic cells with luminal budding or snouting of their cytoplasm replace the duct epithelium. The cells resemble those of apocrine glands and may line entire ducts and cysts

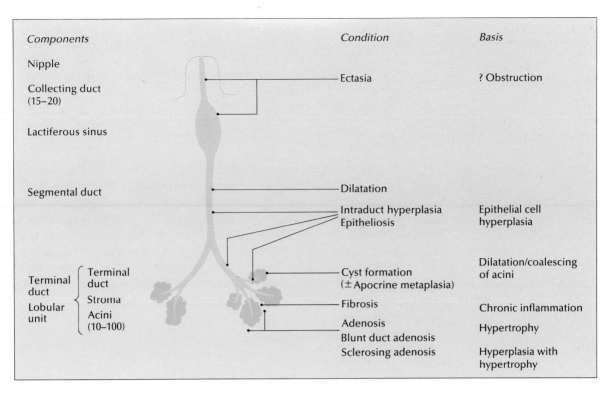

Components			Condition	Basis
Nipple			Ectasia	? Obstruction
Collecting duct (15–20)				
Lactiferous sinus				
Segmental duct			Dilatation	
			Intraduct hyperplasia Epitheliosis	Epithelial cell hyperplasia
Terminal duct	Terminal duct		Cyst formation (± Apocrine metaplasia)	Dilatation/coalescing of acini
Lobular unit	Stroma		Fibrosis	Chronic inflammation
	Acini (10–100)		Adenosis Blunt duct adenosis	Hypertrophy
			Sclerosing adenosis	Hyperplasia with hypertrophy

Fig. 14.1 Potential features of benign breast disorders.

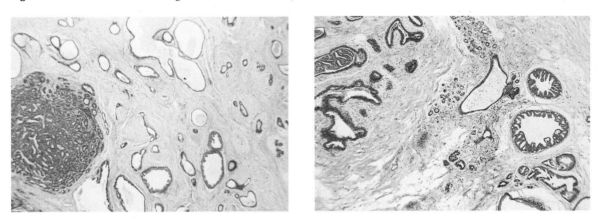

Fig. 14.2 Examples of benign breast disease. (*Above left*) On the left is sclerosing adenosis and in other parts ducts are dilated with those in centre bottom including apocrine metaplasia. The stroma is fibrosed; (*above right*) similar duct features to (a) and also, centre, adenosis.

and malignant change does not occur. The tumour increases in size during pregnancy and regresses with age. It is recognized as a firm, highly mobile mass and referred to as a breast mouse. Giant forms (1 kg or more) are occasionally seen in young girls.

APPEARANCES

The tumour is well circumscribed but has no capsule (Fig. 14.3). The surface is fleshy and white with a whorled and nodular parenchyma. A loose, moderately cellular stroma forms the bulk of the tumour and this is arranged around ducts (*pericanalicular type*) or is compressing and 'deforming ducts (*intracanalicular type*). Some tumours include both patterns (Fig. 14.4).

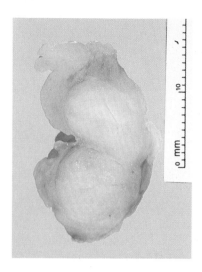

Fig. 14.3 Fibro-adenoma. There is a whorled pattern to the tumour.

Solitary intraduct papilloma

This lesion leads to a nipple discharge which is either serous or blood-stained. The papilloma develops in the large ducts beneath the nipple. Histological distinction from a malignant papillary tumour can be exceedingly difficult.

Phyllodes tumour

This is also known as *Cystosarcoma phyllodes* and has an unmerited reputation as a malignant tumour. The majority of these very uncommon tumours are benign, while others are locally recurrent and only a few metastasize. The main part of the tumour is the stroma although there is also a ductal epithelial element. Malignancy, if present, develops in the stromal part and can only be recognized histologically. Most tumours are less than 5 cm diameter but, if larger, they more often include haemorrhage and necrosis within the fleshy greyish stroma.

Inflammatory conditions

Abscesses

These can complicate lactation and, if incompletely treated, result in lesions clinically simulating carcinoma. Micro-organisms are the cause of the infection and milk, particularly if there is any stasis, the contributory factor. Tuberculous and mycotic abscesses are extremely unusual variants.

Fat necrosis

This occurs as a localized phenomenon, especially in adipose, pen-

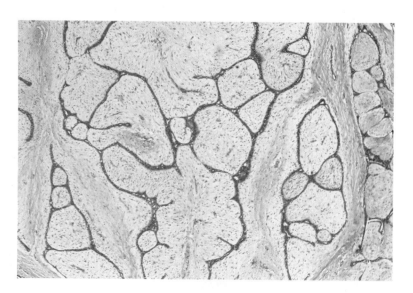

Fig. 14.4 Fibro-adenoma with a predominantly intracanalicular pattern.

dulous breasts but also after minor trauma including surgery. Clinically, confusion with malignancy occurs.

Mammary duct ectasia/plasma cell mastitis

The common denominator to these conditions is stasis within ducts. The appearances may be manifestations of the same disorder and are found principally in post-menopausal women, particularly the parous. The affected ducts are dilated and filled with grey/green contents.

Carcinoma

Women throughout the world are affected but despite an increasing incidence the mortality rate has remained constant for several decades. The natural history favours this as well as the mortality of untreated patients. There is improved survival with time and in untreated patients the mortality rate decreases from 20% after 5 years to 50% after 10 years. Variations in mortality are also found between countries. The highest incidence is in Western Europe, USA and Canada and the lowest in Costa Rica, Mexico and Japan. Treatment is at present unsatisfactory in that, although it may contain the mortality rate, it does not decrease it. Breast cancer is therefore the subject of innumerable therapy trials often producing unsubstantiated claims and equivocal results. The different populations studied, the varying stages of the disease and the different histological subtypes are all factors contributing to this unsatisfactory state but the fundamental problem is ignorance of the cause of breast cancer.

Aetiological factors

Although the cause of breast cancer is unknown the disorder is virtually exclusive to women. Other important genetic and hormonal associations recognized are (Fig. 14.5) as follows:

Family history

There are families with high incidence rates of breast cancer for both females and males and, in a number of these, the tumour is bilateral. The risk is probably 2–3 times that of women without affected relatives but greater if two first degree relatives have breast cancer. Inbreeding is not implicated and no HLA type has been recognized. Experimentally there are mouse strains in which almost 40% of the litter even when fostered develop mammary cancer.

Parity

The high rate of breast cancer among nuns, recognized for many centuries, reflects the risk for the nulliparous woman. The protecting factor with parity is the age at which pregnancy occurs but

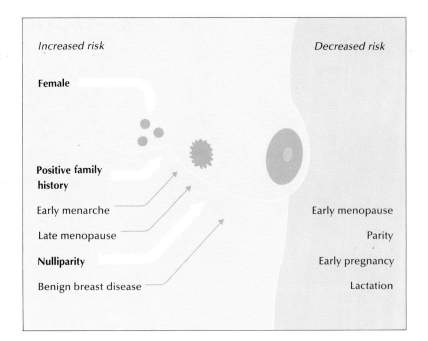

Fig. 14.5 Influences on risk of breast cancer.

Inside figure:

Increased risk | Decreased risk

Female

Positive family history

Early menarche

Late menopause

Nulliparity

Benign breast disease

Early menopause

Parity

Early pregnancy

Lactation

---

unresolved is whether this includes aborted pregnancies. With a first child before 20 years the risk of breast cancer is five times less than that with a first child at 35 years of age. The almost three-fold incidence of breast cancer amongst the Parsees as compared to that in the Hindu majority in India is similarly explained. The Parsees marry late and have small families in contrast to the early marriages of the Hindus and their large families.

Puberty

The age of puberty has constantly fallen in the West and in this interval breast cancer has increased. Any relationship is, however, unproven but an early menarche may be a risk factor.

Menopause

A trend exists in affected patients towards a late menopause (after 45 years). This is difficult to assess because of the possible influence of hormone therapy for menopausal symptoms and the patient's timing of the menopause. An artificially induced and early menopause appears protective, particularly if before 35 years.

Of more uncertain significance are:

Benign breast disease. A slight risk of breast cancer exists for women with benign breast disease, particularly if atypical epithelial hyperplasia is involved. The confusion in the histological categorization of this disorder makes any true assessment extremely difficult.

Breast feeding. It is often pointed out that the cow with almost constantly lactating mammary glands rarely develops breast cancer. Lactation, especially if prolonged, may protect against the disease. Among some Eskimo groups constant lactation provides nourishment for several decades and breast cancer is a rarity. In those Chinese who suckle only from one breast a quadruple incidence of cancer is seen in the unused breast. Western civilization has been associated with increasingly smaller families, a trend away from breast feeding and, when this is practised, only brief periods of suckling, all of which diminish the total lactation experienced.

Oral contraception. Oral contraceptives have had no or little effect on the disease. This is difficult to judge because of the variety of types and the changes in contraceptive composition that have been introduced. The different age intervals and time spans during which they have been used by the individual woman are other variables.

Racial groupings. The disease occurs world-wide but with geographical differences. These may be environmental rather than inherited since second generation immigrants manifest the same incidence of breast cancer as those in their adopted country. There is a higher incidence among American whites than the American black population which may be racial but can also be explained by social and cultural differences.

Age. Breast cancer has occurred in almost all age groups but is rare before 25 years. Thereafter there is a continuous increase in incidence.

All these observations imply that breast cancer, in common with many other malignancies, has a multifactorial basis. There is no clear evidence that viruses are involved, despite contrary experimental observations. In mice, the offspring of mammary cancer strains suckled by their mother all developed the cancer but fostered litter-mates did not. The factor concerned was isolated from the mother's milk and identified as a virus.

Prognosis

The behaviour of individual tumours is all too often idiosyncratic but certain prognostic features are accepted (Table 14.3). Variations in the importance of these occur when there is tumour necrosis or invasion of lymphatics, vessels or pectoral muscle, all of which are bad prognostic events.

Axillary lymph node involvement

Metastatic tumour in these nodes is the single most important prognostic guide. This must be assessed histologically since approximately one-third of clinical diagnoses are wrong. The total number of nodes involved is more important than the site since metastases can occasionally skip nodes in the lymphatic pathway.

Table 14.3 Favourable prognostic factors for breast cancer

Major	Minor
Absent lymph node spread	Rounded tumour edges
Small tumours	Abundant periductal elastic tissue
Good microscopic differentiation	Inflammatory response
	Large in situ component

Table 14.4 Variants of breast carcinoma

Carcinoma	% Among breast cancers
Invasive ductal/infiltrating duct	75
Intraductal/in situ duct	5
Infiltrating lobular	12
Lobular in situ	3
Tubular	2
Medullary	3
Mucoid/mucinous/colloid	2
Papillary	<1

Table 14.5 Rare variants of breast carcinoma

Carcinoid
Signet ring
Juvenile
Adenoid cystic
Squamous
Apocrine

Tumour size

As the size of the tumour increases the prognosis invariably worsens. Patients with a tumour 1 cm diameter or less have a 9% mortality at 5 years. This is in contrast to the 64% mortality at 5 years of those with tumours of 10 cm diameter.

Histological types

Breast cancer arises from the epithelium of the terminal ducts and/or lobules. There are several histological subtypes (Tables 14.4 and 14.5) and the frequencies of these are influenced by a number of factors, especially the patient source. Breast screening clinics invariably record the largest numbers of in situ duct carcinomas, some of which are related with a good prognosis. Other subtypes with a good prognosis are the medullary, tubular, mucoid and papillary carcinomas and carcinoma in situ but unfortunately none of these are common forms of breast cancer. Histological subtyping also identifies the risk of tumour occurring in the opposite breast, a phenomenon most marked with lobular carcinoma. Difficulties in subtyping arise from subjective variation amongst histopathologists, the failure to classify approximately 5% of invasive carcinomas and an increasing awareness of mixed patterns of breast cancer.

Factors that have gained less acceptance but may improve the prognosis include:
- Tumour within the outer rather than inner quadrants.
- Tumour with rounded rather than infiltrating edges.
- Tumour with large amounts of elastic tissue.
- Tumour with a substantial inflammatory cell response.

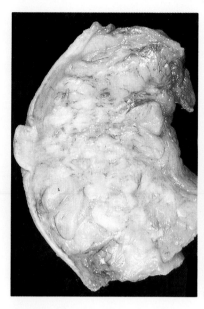

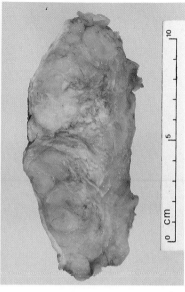

Fig. 14.6 Carcinoma that is poorly defined and spreading into the fat.

Fig. 14.7 Carcinoma causing inversion of the nipple. The hard and gritty nature is evident.

- Tumour with a major in situ component.
- Tumour oestrogen receptors *per se* are not beneficial but their presence may indicate a possibility of a response to hormone therapy.

APPEARANCES

The breast is mainly fat. The smaller component is epithelial and this is localized mainly in the upper outer quadrant and the central area around the nipple. Breast cancer occurs most often in these lateral and central sites and, for unknown reasons, slightly more often in the left breast than the right. The tumour is irregular and has no capsule (Fig. 14.6). The shape and the infiltration into the adjacent tissue can make assessment of the size difficult and cause confusion with some benign conditions. Many, but especially large tumours, more than 5 cm diameter, include necrosis, cysts and haemorrhage and the overlying skin may be ulcerated.

Most infiltrating ductal carcinomas (Fig. 14.7) with their substantial fibrous stroma are hard (*scirrhous carcinomas*) and worm-like yellowish grey material exudes from many cancers with in situ tumour (*comedo carcinoma*). A gritty consistency, appropriately compared to that of an unripe fresh pear, is noticed on sectioning most infiltrating carcinomas and is a macroscopic observation strongly suggestive of carcinoma. The consistency is also contributed to by the elastic tissue which, when marked, forms chalky yellowish streaks, often wrongly interpreted as necrosis. Mucoid tumours may be suspected macroscopically by their mucoid parenchyma, and like medullary carcinomas are soft (*encephaloid carcinoma*).

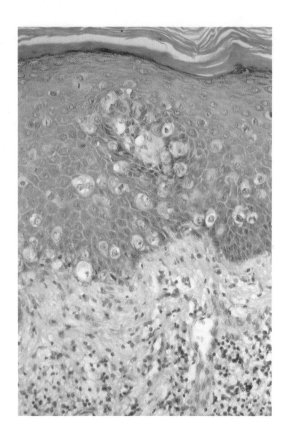

Fig. 14.8 Paget's disease of the nipple. The large vacuolated cells are carcinoma cells. A carcinoma was present in the underlying breast.

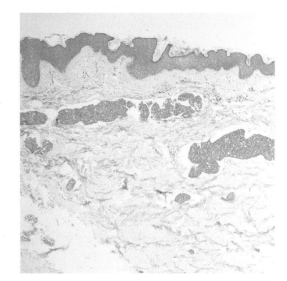

Fig. 14.9 Lymphatic channels in the skin dilated by masses of tumour cells from a primary carcinoma of the breast.

The uninvolved breast either immediately adjacent to or distant from the tumour may include benign breast disease. Multiple foci of carcinoma may also be found and are reported in 10–90% of

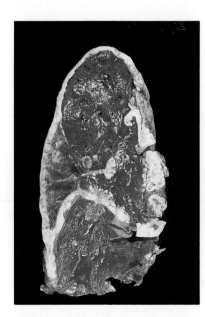

Fig. 14.10 Metastatic breast carcinoma encasing the lung and lying in lymphatics within the pleura. Macroscopically the appearances resemble those of a mesothelioma.

breasts with lobular carcinoma, depending upon the thoroughness of the investigation.

Spread. Metastases arise from local recurrence and lymphatic and vascular spread. Local recurrence is often confined to the surgical scar. An intriguing and still unexplained local appearance is *Paget's disease of the nipple.* Clinically Paget's disease is similar to eczema but histologically carcinoma cells are found in the epidermis (Fig. 14.8). The condition may precede a recognizable tumour but either eventually a tumour appears or with careful sectioning of the tissue beneath the nipple a carcinoma is found.

Lymphatic spread can involve the axillary nodes and the retrosternal lymph nodes, especially if the malignancy is in the medial half of the breast. Distant lymph node spread to sites such as the pelvic lymph nodes can cause diagnostic confusion. Permeation of lymphatic channels (*lymphangitis carcinomatosis*) is characteristic and is seen in the skin (Fig. 14.9) associated with dependant oedema and throughout the lungs (Fig. 14.10) when pleural effusions follow. This form of metastasis in the ovaries results in bilateral ovarian tumours (*Kruckenberg tumours*).

Blood-borne metastases are diffuse and can involve any organ. Bones, lung and liver are the usual sites but tumour in the brain, pituitary and adrenals is not an infrequent finding. When there are bone metastases these can be accompanied by either osteosclerosis and/or osteoporosis.

Further reading

Al-Sumidaie, A.M., Leinster, S.J., Hart, C.A., Green, C.D. and McCarthy, K. (1988). Particles with properties of retroviruses in monocytes from patients with breast cancer. *Lancet* **i**, 5−8.

Haagenser, C.K. (1987). *Diseases of the Breast* (3rd Edition). W.B. Saunders Co.

Hughes, L.E., Mansel, R.E. and Webster, D.J.T. (1987). Aberrations of normal development and involution (ANDI): a new perspective on pathogenesis and nomenclature of benign breast disorders. *Lancet* **ii**, 1316−19.

McPherson, K., Vessey, M.P., Neil, A., Doll, R., Jones, L. and Roberts, M. (1987). Early oral contraceptive use and breast cancer: results of another case-control study. *Br. J. Cancer* **56**, 653−60.

Millis, R.R. (1984). *Atlas of Breast Pathology*. M.T.P. Press Ltd.:Lancaster and Boston.

Sloan, J.P. (1985). *Biopsy Pathology of the Breast*. Chapman and Hall:London.

15　Brain

Nervous system

An intact nervous system is essential for the normal functioning and integration of most other systems. Cerebral disease may lead to intellectual and emotional changes and physical disabilities that profoundly affect the patient's role in society as well as impose severe burdens on that society. The study and management of such patients requires the specialized knowledge and skills of neurologists, neurosurgeons, neuropathologists and their many ancillary services. Nevertheless, many are never seen by these specialists and it is thus difficult to have a precise idea of the true incidence of some neurological disorders and equally, because of this extreme degree of specialization, false impressions of the incidence of other disorders arise. The neurological disorders referred directly to neurologists including epilepsy, Parkinson's disease, multiple sclerosis and other demyelinating disorders as well as the numerous neuropathies and myopathies, fall into this category. The histopathology of many of these is mainly limited to microscopic features which can sometimes be anticipated from their names. Multiple sclerosis as an example involves multiple plaques of sclerosis replacing central nervous tissue (Fig. 15.1) and hence neurological deficits corresponding to their site, while myopathies and neuropathies include inflammatory and degenerative changes restricted to the muscles,

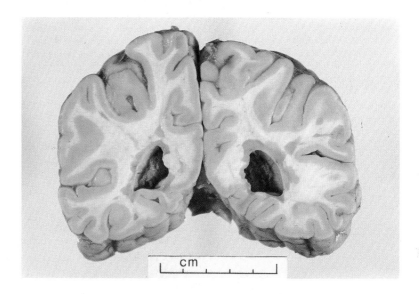

Fig. 15.1 Multiple sclerosis: TS of brain with several plaques of sclerosis in the white matter and around both ventricles. The ventricles are slightly dilated.

brain, spinal cord or the peripheral nervous systems. The histopathology of parasympathetic and sympathetic nervous systems is obscure and diagnosis hinges on clinical findings.

Neuropathological reactions

The basis for these is the same as in other tissues but the end results include important differences. These are affected by the following.

The neurones

These highly specialized cells, like other complex cells, have very limited responses to injury. They are also prone to injury especially from hypoxia and more so than any of the other components of nervous tissue. The natural loss of some neurones occurring with age may also aggravate the effects of disease.

Astrocytes

These and the cells of the microglia are phagocytic but their response compared to macrophages is less immediate or effective. Macrophages are invariably recruited from the circulation in many forms of cerebral injury. Focal collections (*microglial nodules*, Fig. 15.2) of cells, which probably include all three types of cell, are seen in a wide spectrum of disorders but they are only diagnostic if there are specific markers such as micro-organisms or viral inclusion bodies.

Cerebral oedema

Oedema exacerbates the effects of local or diffuse injury since:
1   It aids in the local spread of injury.
2   By permeating the brain tissue, it promotes further destruction.
3   Because the brain is confined within the skull, any oedema will raise the intracranial pressure and compress and further injure the brain, often to severe degrees. The oedema may arise from systemic and cerebral disorders. It involves altered vascular permeability and the release of plasma and fluids into the extravascular space as well as secondary osmotic changes in the cells of the nervous tissue.

Regeneration

This is only possible if the cell body of the neurone remains intact. Axonal regeneration is limited and dependent upon some residue of the basement membrane remaining to guide the newly formed axon along the correct course. Even when axon regeneration occurs function may not be fully restored since this requires a normal myelin sheath, which following injury or demyelinating disorders does not always result.

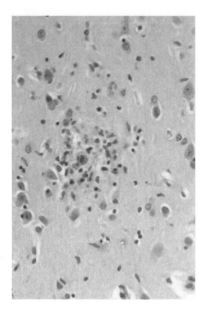

Fig. 15.2 Microglial nodule due to Cytomegalovirus infection. The cell in the centre has an inclusion typical of this virus.

Resolution and reparative processes

These are severely curtailed by the poor regenerative responses, the loose nature of the neuroglia and ground substance and the circulation of the CSF. Disorders are not effectively limited and infection, haemorrhage and neoplastic processes can easily spread from their initial focus both within the brain or via the CSF.

Glial tissue

This is analogous to fibrous tissue in other organs but because of its poorer tensile properties and the soft nature of the surrounding brain it is relatively ineffective in localizing disease and microorganisms. The tissue is formed by astrocytes.

Neurofibrillary tangles

This is a degenerative phenomenon within the cell bodies of neurones found with increasing age as well as in Alzheimer's disease and other types of senile dementia (Fig. 15.3).

Tissue specimens

These include cerebrospinal fluid (CSF) and biopsy of the brain, peripheral nerve or muscle.

Cerebrospinal fluid. Inflammatory cells within the CSF, organisms and increased protein content are all pointers to infective disorders, blood to intracranial haemorrhage and malignant cells to tumour.

Brain. The accuracy of modern radiological techniques in diagnosing tumours has diminished the use of brain biopsy although this can still be important in distinguishing chronic abscesses from neoplastic lesions. Autopsy examination of the brain, despite the most thorough investigations, still provides unexpected diagnoses and also the opportunity to delineate lesions and their effects. The brain is removed intact from the skull and the enveloping dura. It is soft because of the high water content and will, if examined in the fresh state, lose its shape and also be liable to physical injury. To overcome these difficulties the brain is fixed intact by suspending it for a minimum of three weeks in a formol saline solution. The areas selected for microscopy reflect macroscopic lesions and, in their absence, knowledge of neurological findings. In contrast to tissue from other organs, that taken from the brain includes much larger areas. This approach enables the neuropathologist to map the route of abnormal nerve fibres and tracts and their relationships to the cerebral nuclei and cortex, and thereby correlate abnormalities with the clinical findings. As a part of this, distinction must be made between the neurones, neuroglia and ground substance which together form the *brain substance*. Silver and gold impregnation methods are used to show the nerve cell fibres and myelin stains

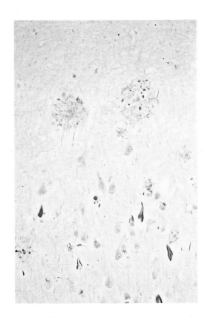

Fig. 15.3 High power of a silver stained section of brain from a patient with dementia. There are several neurones including neurofibrillary tangles (top) and two argyrophilic plaques (bottom). These appearances would support a diagnosis of Alzheimer's disease.

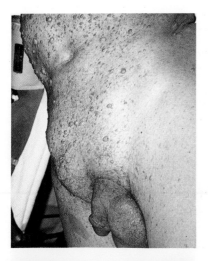

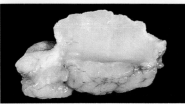

Fig. 15.4 (*Above*) Clinical appearance of neurofibromatosis. (*Below*) Half of bisected neurofibroma. The parenchyma is soft and gelatinous and the tumour clearly projecting from the skin surface.

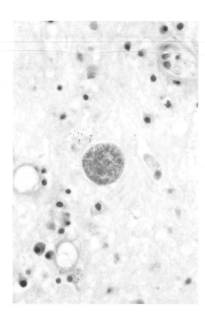

Fig. 15.5 Toxoplasma cyst in the brain of a patient with the acquired immune deficiency syndrome.

the presence or absence of their sheaths. Myelin is formed by the oligodendrocytes which with astrocytes form the *neuroglia*. Astrocytes can be demonstrated by silver and gold impregnation techniques and labelled antibodies. Recognition of the microglia cells which are cells with the potential of macrophages can now be made with labelled monoclonal antibodies.

Systemic disease

Disease of the nervous system can be part of a systemic disorder in which the nervous involvement is (1) incidental or (2) a main target.

1 Patients with bronchopneumonia, liver or kidney diseases may exhibit personality disorders and experience confusional states culminating from a combination of factors. These include metabolic changes, the formation and retention of toxins, anoxia and the development of cerebral oedema. Hypertension and other vascular disorders, such as polyarteritis nodosa and systemic lupus erythematosus, also incidentally involve the nervous system as do the storage disorders and the allied mucopolysaccharidoses in which abnormal lipids accumulate in macrophages.

2 In other conditions where nervous involvement is more integral to the disorder, systemic manifestations are present. Patients with *neurofibromatosis*, a condition characterized by multiple tumours of peripheral nerve sheaths, may have adrenal tumours, phaeochromocytomas (Fig. 15.4); whilst in *Epiloia* (tuberous sclerosis), in which there are cortical glial nodules, there may be a wide spectrum of tumours involving a variety of organs.

Infective disorders

Any infection in the brain can be fatal and even with antibiotics there is a high mortality and a substantial morbidity but, nevertheless, when compared with infection in other sites it is an uncommon event. All types of micro-organisms have been found and the incidence differs according to the type of patient, the geographical location and the reference source. *Toxoplasma gondii* infection in the UK was almost unknown until the onset of the acquired immune deficiency syndrome (AIDS) and is virtually confined to immunocompromised patients while meningococcal meningitis, recognized for many years, occurs among otherwise healthy patients. The number of *Toxoplasma gondii* infections among AIDS patients is well documented but the true incidence of meningococcal meningitis remains in doubt since many patients are not reported (Fig. 15.5).

Micro-organisms establish themselves once the natural defence barriers are broken. Virulent infections produce profound signs and symptoms because of the ease of spread whereas with less aggressive organisms, clinical features may be absent or minimal. For similar reasons, in acute disease histopathological changes can be entirely absent whereas in chronic infection there may be profound and widespread changes out of keeping with the clinical impression.

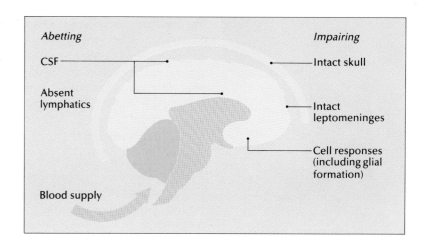

Fig. 15.6 The brain and infection.

Natural defences (Fig. 15.6)

The brain is protected principally by the limited access that organisms have. Both the skull and the meninges are difficult for them to penetrate and there are no direct pathways between the brain and the environment. The bloodstream is the most direct route of access with blood arriving via the carotid or vertebral arteries as well as draining through anastomotic venous channels from the scalp and face. Even these routes provide some protection since organisms have to cross capillaries, the blood–CSF barrier or the blood–brain barrier. The blood–brain barrier is normally impermeable to mononuclear cells and any intracellular organisms they contain.

Fewer protective mechanisms exist once organisms enter the brain and they are then free to proliferate and also more difficult to eradicate. CSF facilitates the spread of organisms both over the brain surface in the subarachnoid space and into its centre via the ventricular system. The virtual absence of inflammatory cells in the CSF and its low content of immunoglobulins and absence of complement encourage growth. Normal CSF includes low levels of IgG, traces of IgA and even smaller amounts of IgM. Immunoglobulins can diffuse from the blood into the brain but only when the blood barrier is altered as part of a disease state. They may also be produced within the parenchyma by B-cells but these, like T-cells, only appear in response to a stimulus and are not a normal component of the brain. The microglial cells function as macrophages but only when activated and then need the help of the circulating macrophages. The absence of lymphatics may embarrass all of these cellular responses.

Meningitis

This is mainly due to acute inflammation of the leptomeninges although chronic inflammation can develop. Organisms of low virulence cause the chronic disease but incompletely treated acute meningitis may become chronic. The organisms reach the meninges by:

1 Direct access from the environment as part of a fractured skull, penetrating injury, neurosurgery or mastoiditis. Streptococcal and staphylococcal organisms are mainly involved.

2 The bloodstream but without a systemic infection. *Streptococcus pneumonia, Neisseria meningococcus* and *Haemophilus influenzae* are the bacteria responsible with *Pneumococcal meningitis* characteristically developing in adults and *H. influenzae meningitis* in children.

3 The bloodstream from an infective focus. Examples and the type of organism are numerous but common sites of infection are the lungs (abscesses, empyema, and bronchiectasis) and the heart (congenital abnormalities with right to left shunts and bacterial endocarditis). Particular patients at risk are intravenous drug abusers, alcoholics and the immunocompromised. Viral meningitis in this group includes that related with the mumps virus and the enteroviruses.

4 Rupture of a brain abscess into the ventricular system or subarachnoid space.

Organisms

Bacteria are invariably the cause although meningitis from fungus and viral infections is found. All types of bacteria have produced meningitis but, in practice, only a small number are involved and infection is restricted to specific groups of patients.

Bacterial meningitis in the UK is predominantly due to *H. influenza, N. meningitidis* or *S. pneumoniae* and, with the first two organisms particularly, infection is often from symptomless carriers. Neonates are more at risk from Gram-negative organisms, most noticeably *E. coli* from the gut, and patients in any age group may present with tuberculous meningitis. Syphilitic meningitis, the precursor of many forms of neurosyphilis, is almost extinct compared with its impact in previous centuries.

Mumps viruses are the main cause of viral meningitis in Britain and the enteroviruses the main cause throughout the world.

Listeria monocytogenes, Candida and *Aspergillus* species and cryptococcus neoformans are the organisms especially likely to infect the meninges in patients with organ transplants, lymphomas or AIDS and chronic ECHO virus infection is a hazard peculiar to some patients with hypogammaglobulinaemia.

APPEARANCES

With an acute fulminating infection there may be no macroscopic abnormalities and only a very few at light microscopy. Inflammatory cells (Fig. 15.7) in the subarachnoid space both over the surface of the brain and within the deep recesses of the sulci are the important microscopic features. Potential clues to the possibility of meningitis are a macular-papular rash and adrenal haemorrhage but the diagnosis in these circumstances may only be established if cultures

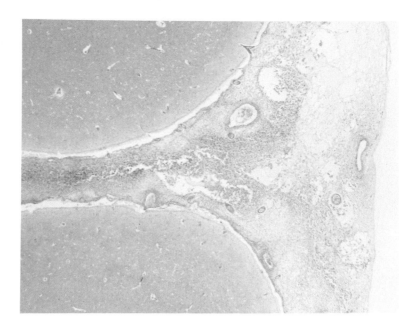

Fig. 15.7 Meningitis due to *S. pneumoniae*. Neutrophil polymorphs and pus fill the subarachnoid space and vessels are engorged and dilated.

are made of the blood, CSF or brain. With other patients, the meninges may obviously be congested and in yet others, pus may be recognized. This is greenish in *S. pneumoniae* infections and occurs over the entire surface of the brain (Fig. 15.8). Tuberculous infection provokes an opaque change and miliary lesions can be seen while with chronic inflammation the leptomeninges become thickened, most noticeably over the base (Fig. 15.9). Other features are less specific and attributed to increased intracranial pressure with flattening of the gyri and dilatation of the ventricles.

Examination of the CSF is an important diagnostic procedure. This is turbid and includes inflammatory cells and organisms. These may be identified in Gram smears but culture is essential and subtyping important for tracing the source. Tuberculosis produces a fibrin clot which provides a focus for the mycobacteria and so helps light microscopy recognition after Ziehl−Nielsen staining.

Encephalitis

Inflammation of the brain parenchyma is mainly caused by viral infections although there are also a wide range of non-infective causes. Encephalitis and meningitis imply precise clinical and ana-tomical distinctions. These, to the neuropathologist, are not always valid since infection in either site will inevitably impinge upon the adjacent tissue and the alternative term of *meningoencephalitis* may be used.

Viral encephalitis may be manifest as an acute disorder, a post-vaccinia phenomenon or as a subacute disease.

The acute disorder is the most common and is related mainly with Herpes simplex, rabies and arboviruses, both of the latter being rare in the UK.

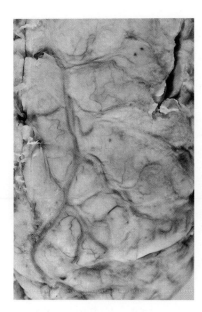

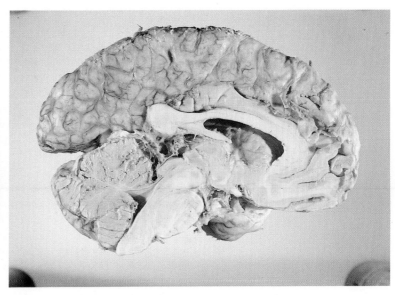

Fig. 15.8 *S. pneumoniae* meningitis. The greenish pus within the subarachnoid space discolours the brain surface and collects around vessels.

Fig. 15.9 Unsuspected *S. pneumoniae* meningitis in an old patient. The infection is apparent deep within the sulci and over the base of the brain.

Post-vaccinial encephalitis particularly followed smallpox vaccination but is now seen after measles, chickenpox, rubella and mumps inoculations. It may represent an immune reaction since cultures for viruses are negative.

The subacute disease was thought to be an immune related phenomenon but latent viruses have been identified. The disorders, which include subacute sclerosing panencephalitis due to measles, appear months or even years after the initial infection. Progressive multifocal leuco-encephalopathy (PML) related to papova viruses and Creutzfeldt—Jakob disease related to slow release viruses may also be subacute encephalitides, as may the dementia related to human immunodeficiency virus (HIV) but each with shorter latent intervals.

A wide spectrum of clinical manifestations can accompany these disorders including focal neurological signs together with mild to severe cerebral impairment. If the patient recovers from the acute disorder there may be lasting intellectual and emotional deficits as well as motor impairment. These sequelae are more likely with severe encephalitis which also has a very high mortality.

Route of infection

Viruses probably enter the brain via the bloodstream but the evidence for this is unclear and passage along axon cylinders and through the cribriform plate in the nose has been shown experimentally with Herpes simplex.

The majority of brains have little change macroscopically, and microscopically there may only be mononuclear cell cuffing of vessels. Herpes simplex encephalitis is an exception since with this there is focal, asymmetrical necrosis which is often concentrated within the temporal lobes. Inclusion bodies and the finding of viral particles, either by electron microscopy or through the use of labelled antibodies, provide positive support for the diagnosis.

Cerebral abscesses

These arise from circumstances similar to those causing meningitis but differ in that the main cause is long-standing middle ear disease or chronic sinusitis. The bacteria involved are those causing meningitis but mixed infections and infection with anaerobic organisms also occur. Abscesses from fungal and protozoal infection, notably *Toxoplasma gondii*, develop in immunocompromised patients, and in specific geographical locations, e.g., hydatid disease amongst sheep-rearing communities and Amoebiasis in tropical and subtropical climates.

The condition has a substantial mortality because it can be exceedingly difficult to diagnose and, unless suspected, may be entirely overlooked. There are often few symptoms and these are rarely very specific. Alternatively they may be masked by those of the middle ear or sinus infection or wrongly attributed to other neurological diseases.

Infection is established at the junction of the cortex and sub-cortex which is a region with a relatively poor blood supply, and most often in the temporal and frontal lobes. Abscesses below the tentorium are unusual. As the abscess enlarges a reactive gliosis develops and encompasses the lesion. This does not retain it effectively so that progressive destruction of the brain parenchyma follows and, sometimes, rupture into the ventricular system. The growth of some abscesses does, however, arrest spontaneously.

APPEARANCES

Unless rupture onto the brain surface has taken place or surgical drainage has been performed, no external abnormalities may be found but where there is either substantial oedema or raised intra-cranial pressure there will be evidence of these. There is usually a single abscess when the cause is local but, when there is haematogenous infection, multiple abscesses may be found. Abscesses occur slightly more often in the temporal than the frontal lobes but between them, these two sites account for just over 50% of brain abscesses. A firm area of gliosis surrounds a soft mushy centre into which haemorrhage may have developed. The micro-organism(s) can be identified by culture and serology but often, because the lesion is unsuspected, the brain is fixed and these are not then performed.

Vascular disorders

Cerebral vascular disorders are the cause of strokes and 80% affect patients over 65 years. The number of patients is uncertain because their management is not confined to a single clinical speciality and death certificates may not record the disorder. The motor and sensory disability imposes a considerable burden on both the patient, who at this age is not best equipped to cope, and on society. Prevention is the only effective treatment since rehabilitation cannot correct the neurological deficit and cerebral regeneration does not occur. Unfortunately, the factor precipitating most strokes is cerebral infarction secondary to arteriosclerosis for which there are no absolute preventative measures. Other contributing factors are hypertension, thrombosis and spontaneous intracranial haemorrhage which is mainly subarachnoid (Table 15.1).

Blood supply

The blood supply to the brain includes a good collateral system. The main arterial supply is from paired vertebral and internal carotid arteries which link at the Circle of Willis and give off branches to the cerebellar and cerebral hemispheres (Fig. 15.10). The main vessels on each side supply one half of the brain with no blood normally crossing the mid-line. Should occlusion occur in either of the main vessels on one side sufficient blood can reach the affected parenchyma via the posterior communicating arteries and occlusion of the internal carotid in the neck can be compensated for by reversed blood flow in the ophthalmic artery into the brain tissue. Profuse meningeal arterial anastomoses can also help in limiting infarction by supplying blood to the watershed zones at the edges of the areas fed by each of the main cerebral arteries. For any of these responses to maintain maximal cerebral blood flow, the vessels must be free of disease and a sufficient time span must elapse for the adaptive responses to develop. However, within the age group affected by cerebrovascular disease such circumstances are rarely present.

Cerebral hypoxia

An impaired blood supply to the brain produces cerebral ischaemia and brain damage. Experimentally irreversible anoxic damage occurs

Table 15.1 Causes of strokes

Vascular	Cardiac	Other
Atheroma	Infarction — embolus	Diabetes mellitus
Hypertension	Endocarditis — embolus	Obesity
Thrombus	Myxoma — embolus	Tumour—emboli
Carotid artery stenosis		
Subarachnoid haemorrhage		

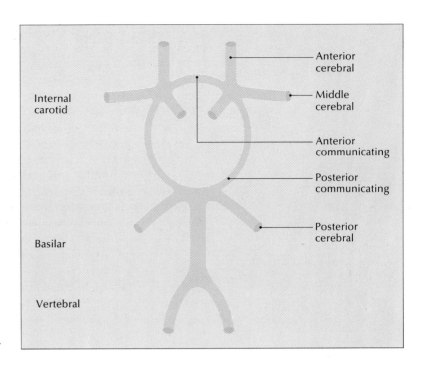

Fig. 15.10 Arteries of circles of Willis.

within 15 min and in man permanent changes are produced after
5—8 min. The combination of reduced blood flow and reduced
oxygen and glucose supply create these effects which are heightened
by the poor regenerative ability of nervous tissue. The brain receives
15% of the total cardiac output which is distributed at a higher rate
of flow to the grey than the white matter, where the metabolic
requirements are greater. This flow is maintained by an autoregula-
tory mechanism which balances vasodilatation with vasoconstriction
and is also affected by the blood volume, blood viscosity, integrity
of the vasculature and systemic blood pressure. An additional
factor is intracranial pressure which, when raised, inhibits cerebral
perfusion. Alterations in any of these parameters from either extracranial causes or cerebrovascular disease are more likely in elderly
individuals and may exacerbate the effects of any stroke and impair
any compensatory reactions. They are also relevant in perinatal
brain damage and the cause of spastic children.

Cerebral anoxia may lead to focal or diffuse changes depending
on the cause. Arterial disease, thrombo-embolism and intracranial
haemorrhage can all produce focal ischaemia and infarction, as can
vasospasm, a phenomenon demonstrable radiologically and seen at
craniotomy. Cardiac arrest, periods of severe hypotension and systemic haemorrhage are all causes of diffuse or global cerebral
ischaemia and 'brain death'.

APPEARANCES

The brain, following generalized hypoxia and brain death, may
include no gross abnormalities if it is examined between 36—48 h

after the precipitating event. Beyond this time there is progressive atrophy of all parts of the cerebral and cerebellar cortices allied with ventricular dilatation.

Cerebral infarction

Occlusion of either the anterior or the middle cerebral vessels underlies the majority of cerebral infarcts which occur predominantly in the basal ganglia and the frontal and parietal lobes. This is mainly from thrombosis superimposed upon arteriosclerosis and less often emboli, most arising from arteriosclerotic vessels within the skull or neck, but also from carotid artery stenosis. Emboli may also originate from the heart after infarcts or valvular disorders and may include tumour and septic emboli from other organs but, whatever their origin, the infarcts may be multiple. With either thrombosis or embolism many patients will also have hypertension, cardiac disease or diabetes mellitus and manifest other complications of arteriosclerosis. Clinically, the distinction between thrombosis and embolism and between cerebral infarction and intracerebral haemorrhage is not always easy.

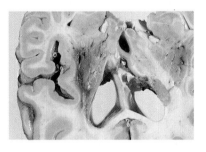

Fig. 15.11 Established infarct involving the basal ganglia. The patient had had a stroke some weeks previously.

Upside down.

APPEARANCES

The infarcted area(s) can be difficult to distinguish, especially in the early phases. The regions involved are swollen and soft and may be purplish compared with the adjacent brain but later they undergo shrinkage and become rubbery with some brownish iron pigmentation (Fig. 15.11). Some early infarcts are diffusely haemorrhagic and, in the acute stage, there may be evidence of raised intracranial pressure and cerebral compression. A longer term event is cyst formation. Thrombo-embolus, recent or organized, may be found but, especially with small infarcts, this is absent having lysed prior to examination. Arteriosclerosis is conspicuous in the larger vessels.

Spontaneous intracranial haemorrhage

This is seen in the subarachnoid space and the brain substance. Similar haemorrhage also occurs following head injuries and some space-occupying lesions and systemic disorders (Fig. 15.12). Subarachnoid haemorrhage may have an acute and fairly characteristic onset but other forms are, clinically, often very difficult to separate from thrombo-embolic episodes. The majority of patients are hypertensive and it is the improved control of this that has displaced intracranial haemorrhage as the main cause of strokes.

Whether intracranial haemorrhage develops within the brain substance or in the subarachnoid space a common denominator is a ruptured aneurysm.

1 The aneurysms within the brain parenchyma (*miliary, micro- or Charcot–Bouchard aneurysms*) develop in hypertensive elderly patients on striate and penetrating arteries, principally within the

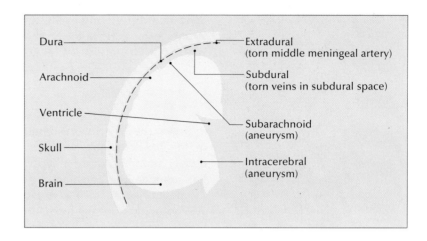

Dura — Extradural (torn middle meningeal artery)

Arachnoid — Subdural (torn veins in subdural space)

Ventricle — Subarachnoid (aneurysm)

Skull —

Brain — Intracerebral (aneurysm)

Fig. 15.12 Intracranial haemorrhage.

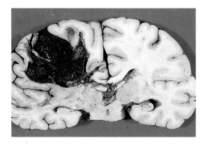

Fig. 15.13 Intracerebral haemorrhage associated with hypertension. The haemorrhage has replaced much of the parenchyma and ruptured onto the brain surface.

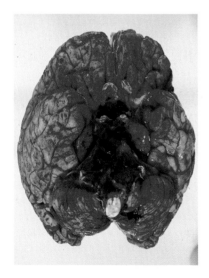

Fig. 15.14 Subarachnoid haemorrhage. No aneurysm was recognized.

basal ganglia and regions of the internal capsule. They are found in most examples of intracerebral haemorrhage and their rupture is associated with hypertension or arteriosclerosis.

2 Subarachnoid haemorrhage follows rupture of aneurysms on the circle of Willis (*Berry aneurysms*). These are found in over 50% of subarachnoid haemorrhages and occur at points of bifurcation where there is a gap in the media. The concept that they are congenital abnormalities is no longer tenable since there is a similar deficiency in the media of all arteries and aneurysmal dilatation and rupture rarely occurs in the brain in children or neonates. The cerebral arteries differ from systemic vessels in that they lack an external elastic lamina and are partly supported by the CSF as opposed to compact tissue. The increasing incidence with age and the frequent but not invariable presence of hypertension and arteriosclerosis imply that the aneurysms are age-related.

A small proportion of patients with subarachnoid haemorrhage have arteriovenous malformations and angiomas and, in an equal number, no cause is found.

APPEARANCES

Intracerebral haemorrhage presents a dramatic appearance with clotted and unclotted blood, replacing much of the cerebral cortex and basal ganglia (Fig. 15.13). Rupture into the ventricular system is often present and blood may have spread into the subarachnoid space. The underlying microaneurysms, which are multiple, can only be seen by light microscopy or perfusion studies.

Subarachnoid haemorrhage is recognized by unclotted and clotted blood in the subarachnoid space which is concentrated over the base of the brain (Fig. 15.14). This is discolored and compressed. A careful search for an aneurysm must be made and in most patients these lie at the bifurcation of the middle cerebral artery. The vertebrobasilar arteries are least involved and multiple aneurysms occur in 15% of patients. The aneurysms vary in size from a few millimetres to many centimetres (Fig. 15.15) and in the larger ones

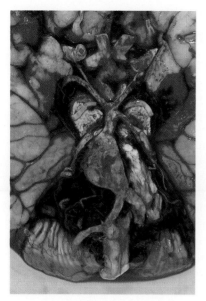

Fig. 15.15 Large aneurysm on the basilar artery. This had ruptured and resulted in a subarachnoid haemorrhage.

there may be thrombus. This is also found in smaller aneurysms that have ruptured and ceased bleeding spontaneously when vasospasm has probably closed the bleeding point and the thrombus provided the seal.

Head injury

One per cent of deaths in Britain are due to head injuries and the majority of these are from road traffic accidents with industrial accidents and sports, including horse riding and boxing, as other important causes. A substantial number, however, are not fatal nor associated with any apparent neurological deficit. The short- and long-term effects can range from none to persistent vegetative states, with periods of amnesia, fits and milder degrees of brain damage as other sequelae. No clear correlation exists between any pattern of external injury, and the neurological deficits can occur with and without severe facial and scalp lacerations and skull fractures. Nevertheless, it is probable that any head injury, and especially one associated with loss of consciousness or a period of amnesia, does produce changes in the brain.

APPEARANCES

The effects within the brain arise from a combination of acceleration and deceleration forces, often contributed to by compression and less often direct contact, in the form of local blows to the head or gunshot injury (missile head injury). Since the brain is suspended within the skull which in contrast is firm, missile or focal injury can injure the brain mainly on the opposite side, a type of injury referred to as *contrecoup*. Whatever the form of injury the potential effects, either singly or in combination, are as follows:

Diffuse axon damage

This arises from tension and sheering of axons and can only be recognized by light microscopy. The change probably occurs in all head injuries and may be the only one found. Patients who lose consciousness most certainly have axonal damage and it is most diffuse in those in vegetative states. Formerly such patients were thought to have a brain stem injury but it is now appreciated that this is not so and that the lesion is diffuse axon damage.

Cerebral contusion

Foci of punctate or linear haemorrhages are seen in the brain accompanied by oedema. Loss of consciousness will have occurred.

Cerebral laceration

Tears in the brain substance either on the side of the injury or the opposite side are found. Their severity reflects the force of the

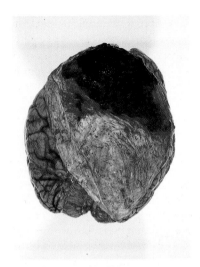

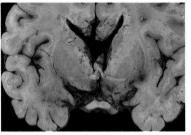

Fig. 15.16 (*Above*) Extradural haematoma complicating a fracture to the base of the skull following a road traffic accident. (*Below*) Brain from a patient who died some time after a road traffic accident and was maintained by artificial ventilation. There is softening and necrosis of the brain tissue around the ventricles and the parenchyma is swollen.

injury and the type and degree of any associated fracture, although they are not an inevitable complication of depressed fractures.

Intracranial haemorrhage

This may occur within the brain substance as well as within the extradural, subdural or subarachnoid spaces.

1 Haemorrhage in the brain substance is often multifocal and may lead to intraventricular haemorrhage and to rupture into the surrounding cerebral cortex, so bursting the affected lobe. For most patients this is associated with a bad prognosis and is diagnosed because of loss or deterioration in the level of consciousness following a lucid interval immediately after the injury. X-ray studies, however, suggest that haemorrhage is occurring from the time of the injury and thereby imply that the symptoms are precipitated by other events, most particularly oedema.

2 Other types of intracranial haemorrhage are invariably due to skull fractures. Extradural haemorrhage is the source in over 50% of patients and is caused by tearing of the middle meningeal artery (Fig. 15.16). Rupture of the veins bridging the subdural space and connecting the sagittal sinus and the superior surface of the brain account for subdural haemorrhage which once started spreads within the subdural space.

Subdural haematoma

Haematomas in the subdural space may be found after any head injury and arise from subdural haemorrhage. Common causes are minor falls and local injury in the elderly, alcoholics and battered babies when the head injury either passes unrecognized or is dismissed as trivial. Gradually symptoms of increased intracranial pressure develop which escape diagnosis because of their insidious onset and the interval since the head injury and its minor form. The haematoma is contained by a thin fibrous capsule and includes yellow fluid and altered blood invested by a wall of granulation tissue. In patients dying nearer the time of the injury only blood clot is present. Some haematomas resolve spontaneously but most enlarge, possibly from repeated episodes of bleeding, and lead to death with compression of the underlying brain.

Hypoxic brain damage

The immediate effect of a head injury is spasm of the cerebral vessels and a transient reduction in blood flow. This may also be reduced by either intracranial or extracranial haemorrhage, cardiac arrest or injury to the lungs or airways. Inhalation of vomit often causes the latter and the impaired oxygenation that results worsens the cerebral anoxia. The ischaemic injury is added to by any local injury as well as cerebral oedema and increased intracranial pressure (Fig. 15.17). The effects can either be diffuse, especially if there have been periods of cardiac arrest, or restricted to the boundary zones of the cerebral arteries, particularly the junction of the anterior and middle cerebral vessels. The macroscopic effects are largely influenced by the period elapsing between the onset of the injury and examination. Hypoxia produces degeneration and liquifactive necrosis with later repair and gliosis. If examined early after injury, the brain is soft with the areas of softening concentrated as outlined above. Later shrinkage may occur with palpable firm regions of gliosis.

Brain swelling

This may either be restricted to the site of injury or to one part of the brain, such as a cerebral hemisphere (Fig. 15.17), or involve the entire brain. The latter is seen most commonly in children. The reaction involves a combination of vasodilatation and oedema but the precise sequence is often unclear. The effects vary with the pattern present but the common manifestations are those of increased intracranial pressure and cerebral compression.

Complications

If the patient has a compound fracture, infection and meningitis or a cerebral abscess are hazards. Such fractures may escape recognition if the base of the skull is involved but with entry to the nasal sinuses they may be recognized by CSF rhinorrhoea. Fat emboli may follow from any extracranial fractures, notably those involving the long-bones. The boxer, from persistent head injury, is also liable to chronic traumatic encephalopathy (punch drunkenness).

Space-occupying lesions

The brain is fixed within the bony case of the skull. As a consequence a histologically benign lesion can destroy the vital centres and kill the patient and distinctions between benign and malignant processes are not always clear. These uncertainties are added to by the difficulty in gaining surgical access to some sites as well as the pointlessness in removing lesions in vital centres.

Any expanding lesion (a) displaces brain tissue and (b) very often increases the intracranial pressure. These effects produce either localizing neurological signs and symptoms and/or headache, vomiting and mental deterioration with late onset epilepsy and papilloedema. Lesions underlying these events include recent infarcts, haematomas, tumours, abscesses and rarely cysts arising from protozoal infection.

Brain compression and displacement

These depend on the size of the lesion and whether it continues to expand or remains static. If the latter circumstances prevail there may be only minimal local compression such as is seen with many subclinical meningiomas. Should the lesion expand, brain

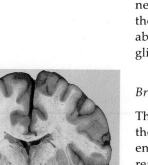

Fig. 15.17 Marked swelling and oedema of the left cerebral hemisphere following a road traffic accident and a blow to the head. The white matter on the left side appears increased when compared with that on the right side. There was no skull fracture.

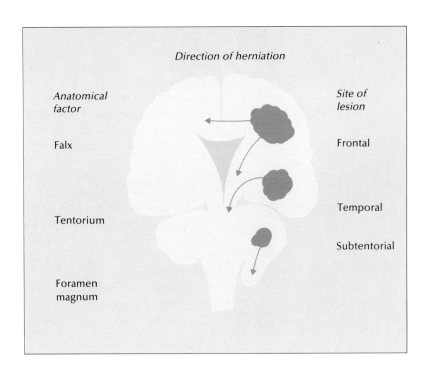

Fig. 15.18 Patterns of brain hernias.

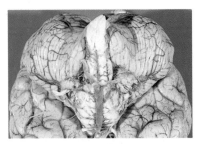

Fig. 15.19 Mild coning. There are compression groves around the cerebellum following herniation through the foramen magnum.

compression is more substantial with shift and distortion of the normal architecture including herniation from one compartment to another. Such hernias are restricted to a small number of sites where there are potential anatomical weaknesses but the pathway adopted also reflects the size of the lesion (Fig. 15.18). A lesion filling the frontal regions of one cerebral hemisphere can herniate brain from that site beneath the falx into the opposing cortex while a lesion associated with diffuse brain swelling induces cerebellar herniation into the foramen magnum around the brain stem and spinal cord, often referred to as *coning* (Fig. 15.19). A tentorial or uncinal hernia can also displace the brain stem and compress the III and VI cranial nerves.

Raised intracranial pressure

This is present if the intracranial pressure is sustained at 10 mmHg above normal. The normal pressure, ranging between 0–10 mm Hg, is usually zero in the upright position. Transient rises occur with respiration and coughing but produce no ill effects but the systemic blood pressure impairs the cerebral blood flow the nearer the two approach one another. All of the normal constituents of the brain, its coverings, vasculature, CSF and blood volume as well as the integrity of the skull, contribute to the intracranial pressure as will a space-occupying lesion. Initially with any increase there is a transitory compensatory phase which, if due to a tumour, is allied with some compression of the uninvolved brain but once this facility is exhausted a rise in pressure is inevitable and sustained.

Hydrocephalus

The newborn and young child initially escape brain compression because their cranial fontanelles are unfused and their skulls can enlarge, stretch and expand. The enlarged skull is hydrocephalus and as the term implies is produced by an increase in the volume of the CSF. The same term is applied to adults with an increased volume of CSF even though there is no skull expansion; their skulls on X-ray and at autopsy have thinning and flattening of the pituitary fossa and erosion of the clinoid processes. Hydrocephalus may arise from increases in secretion, decreases in absorption and obstruction to the circulation of the CSF. Obstruction can occur at any point in the circulation pathway and the effects will vary with the site, although usually above the obstruction the ventricular system will enlarge and the overlying brain undergo pressure atrophy. This response is more profound with an expanding lesion in the posterior fossa which obstructs the fourth ventricle than for a similar but larger lesion in a frontal lobe encroaching only upon the lateral ventricle. A secondary effect of obstruction at any site is impairment of the venous return which exacerbates the rise in the intracranial pressure.

Hydrocephalus is not always harmful and is seen more commonly as a compensatory phenomenon accompanying cerebral atrophy. The volume of CSF increases to fill the space previously occupied by the brain tissue but not to an extent sufficient to produce pressure atrophy (Fig. 15.20).

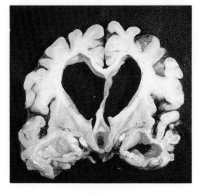

Fig. 15.20 TS of a brain from a patient with dementia. There is substantial dilatation of the ventricular system associated with thinning of the cortex, atrophy of the gyri and widening of the sulci. There was no evidence of any outflow obstruction. The features are in keeping with Alzheimer's disease, the cause of dementia in at least 70% of demented patients in the UK.

Tumours

There are 2250 deaths in the UK annually from brain tumours and these involve children and adults. Their aetiology is unknown. The incidence and pattern differs among the different age groups with brain tumours forming 19% of all childhood malignancies and less than 9% of those in adults (Fig. 15.21). Men are affected twice as often as women. The majority in children occur in the brain stem and cerebellum while in adults they are found in the cerebrum, particularly the frontal and temporal areas; tumours in the cerebellum are most often metastases. Primary tumours of the neuroglia are collectively known as gliomas and these form the bulk of brain tumours.

Astrocytomas

These are the main group of gliomas at any age and they arise from astrocytes. There are various subclassifications depending largely upon histological features and assessments of differentiation which in biopsy and smear preparations may be wrongly assessed when compared with the gross specimens. These differences can account for errors in prognosis, although in adults only those with better differentiated tumours live more than a few years. This poor prognosis is allied to inoperability and the associated brain destruction

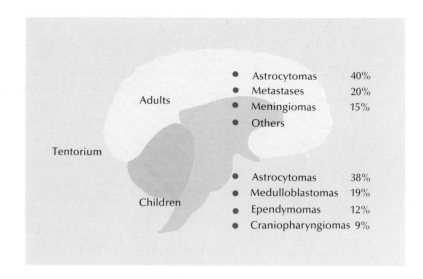

Adults		
• Astrocytomas	40%
• Metastases	20%
• Meningiomas	15%
• Others	

Children		
• Astrocytomas	38%
• Medulloblastomas	19%
• Ependymomas	12%
• Craniopharyngiomas	9%

Tentorium

Fig. 15.21 Brain tumours.

and compression. Most patients have probably had their tumour eighteen months to two years before diagnosis since careful questioning reveals symptoms extending over such periods. In practice metastatic spread outside the brain does not occur. It is rarely seen after surgical intervention.

APPEARANCES

The tumours are poorly demarcated and very difficult to recognize in the absence of destruction or deformity in the fixed brain (Fig. 15.22). In an unfixed brain the tumour is yellowish compared to the surrounding brain. Astrocytomas infiltrate rather than expand into the adjacent brain and provoke vascular proliferation at the tumour brain interface which is seen as a red halo. Necrosis, haemorrhage and cyst formation all develop in large tumours and infection either within the tumour or the meninges has also been described. Metastatic lesions in the brain are smaller than the primary.

Other features include focal and generalized brain swelling and signs of raised intracranial pressure with or without hydrocephalus.

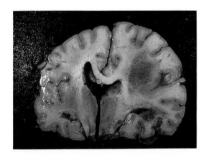

Fig. 15.22 Astrocytoma (on the right side). The tumour is ill defined and is expanding the involved hemisphere.

Meningiomas

These arise from the meninges and more precisely the arachnoid cap cells of the arachnoid granulations. Consequently over 50% develop near the vertex although tumour is also encountered in a wide range of other sites. Meningiomas can enlarge to reach a considerable size and can re-occur after removal. They can also occur in inoperable regions of the brain and for all these reasons, these histologically benign tumours may assume a malignant potential (Fig. 15.23). Nevertheless, many can be removed with no long-term effects and others may be incidental symptomless findings. The tumour in contrast to astrocytomas has a 2:1 predominance in women and does not appear in children.

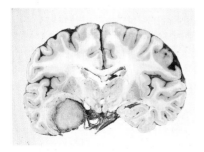

Fig. 15.23 Meningioma at the base of the cerebrum (left side). The tumour was unrecognized in an elderly woman and contributed towards death. The brain tissue is compressed but not infiltrated by this benign growth.

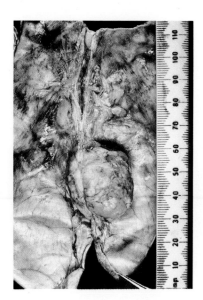

Fig. 15.24 Meningioma attached to the dura. The tumour has easily separated away from the brain.

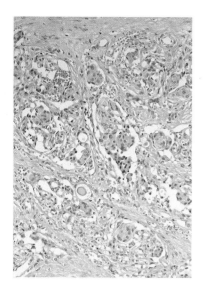

Fig. 15.25 High power of a meningioma. The cell clusters are associated with a few round eosinophilic masses, psammoma bodies.

APPEARANCES

Meningiomas are rubbery firm white nodules with a cut surface similar to fish flesh. Long-standing examples may be calcified. A stalk attaches the meningioma to the leptomeninges and the brain is pushed in front of the tumour and is separate from it so that it can be shelled out from the brain (Fig. 15.24). Thickening of the overlying skull (*hyperostosis*) and even erosion may be present. Among the variety of histological features *psammoma bodies*, round eosinophilic masses, are helpful diagnostically (Fig. 15.25).

Metastases

These are found more often than meningiomas and second to gliomas. They can involve any part of the brain but are especially prevalent in the cerebellum. With some primary breast and prostatic carcinomas and with lymphomas, metastases may be confined to the leptomeninges. Primary lung tumours are the most common source but carcinomas from any site, including melanomas, may lead to cerebral metastases. The lesions are usually multiple although occasionally single. The patients invariably but not always have other systemic metastases.

APPEARANCES

These are similar to those in other organs, and are pinkish and rounded, often lying at the junction of the grey and white matter. Melanoma metastases may be distinguished by their brown pigmentation.

Other neoplasms

A wide variety of other tumours develop in the brain but all are exceedingly rare. Currently there is interest in lymphomas. These are mostly non-Hodgkin's lymphomas and occur either as the primary tumour or more often as part of spread from an extracranial primary site. They form less than 1% of all brain tumours except in some immunocompromised patients where greater numbers are found. These patients include those with organ grafts, some forms of primary immunodeficiency and AIDS. Why lymphomas should be rare in the brain in most patients and equally why they should develop in immunocompromised individuals is unknown.

Further reading

Brain's Diseases of the Nervous System (1985) (9th Edition). Sir John Walton. Oxford University Press: Oxford.

Greenfield's Neuropathology (1984) (4th Edition). Ed. by J.H. Adams, Jan Corsellis and L.W. Duchen. Edward Arnold: London.

Utiley, D. (1978). Subarachnoid haemorrhage. *Br. J. Hosp. Med.* **19**, 138−54.

16 Skin tumours

The skin is the seat of a wide range of tumours although many are rarely encountered. They develop from the stratified squamous epithelium of the epidermis, the connective tissue elements of the dermis and from the various appendages and specialized cells present in both of these areas.

Benign tumours

Common benign skin tumours include the following.

Squamous cell papillomas. Clinically these present as skin tags and viral warts (Fig. 16.1).

Basal cell papillomas. These warty growths are not due to viruses. They are occasionally pigmented and develop in elderly patients (Fig. 16.2).
  In both these lesions there is an orderly proliferation of either squamous cells or basal cells, so producing papillary lesions covered by keratin. The squamous lesions may include a stalk but both project from the surface of the epidermis.

Epidermal cysts commonly known as *sebaceous cysts.* These lie in the dermis projecting from under the epidermis and may achieve a

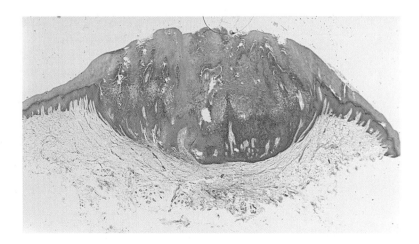

Fig. 16.1 Viral wart from the base of the foot. A mass of keratin overlies the proliferating epidermal cells.

diameter of several centimetres. They are found particularly on the scalp, face or neck.

Pigmented naevi or moles. Pigmented lesions range from freckles in which there is a local increase in melanin in the basal epidermal cells to naevi where the predominant change is an increase in the number of melanocytes or naevus cells. Melanocytes are found in similar numbers in black or white skin but in the black skin these cells are more active. The melanocytes in naevi may be confined to the epidermis or dermis or occur in both these sites (Fig. 16.3). Such naevi can be present from birth or develop during adult life. Their rate of growth parallels that of the rest of the body in that a gradual increase in size can be anticipated prior to puberty,

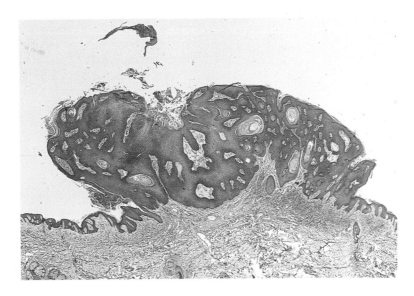

Fig. 16.2 Basal cell papilloma or seborrhoeic keratosis. The increased thickening of the epidermis is due to proliferation of the basal cells. The lesion sits above the level of the surrounding epidermis.

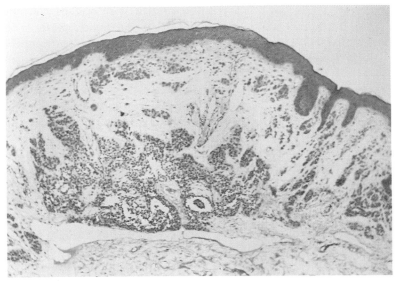

Fig. 16.3 Naevus which is papillary. Clusters of naevus cells stream towards the dermis and in the lower parts are more tightly aggregated.

with a growth spurt at puberty and subsequent slow atrophy and disappearance.

Lipomas. They lie in the dermis or subcutaneous fat and are sometimes clinically confused with epidermal cysts.

Haemangiomas or *birth marks.* They are seen as solitary small red tumours, *strawberry naevi,* or as variably sized flat or raised mauve-to-purple areas on the skin surface, *port-wine stains,* often covering large parts of the face.

Malignant tumours

Although there are potentially a substantial number of primary skin malignancies, in clinical practice only three are commonly seen. These are basal cell carcinomas, squamous cell carcinomas and melanomas. Secondary tumours occur infrequently and are most often from the common malignancies, lung, breast and stomach. Cutaneous manifestations of malignancy other than actual tumour deposits are another way in which dermatologists recognize systemic malignancy. These include skin manifestations of a disorder with a malignant potential such as neurofibromatosis and rashes and other changes that appear as a consequence of a systemic malignancy.

Basal cell carcinomas

These tumours are related to sun exposure and develop particularly in the exposed areas, mainly the face. They form the largest group of malignant skin tumours and differ from squamous cell carcinomas and melanomas in that, in practical terms, they do not produce metastases. They are locally aggressive tumours which without treatment will invade underlying tissues including bone (Fig. 16.4) and in this manner may cause death. This low-grade aggressiveness combined with surface ulceration has given rise to the alternate name of *rodent ulcer.* Early lesions are not ulcerated but firm and raised, often with a pearly appearance. The lesion gradually expands across the surface of the skin, and ulcerates with a raised and rolled firm edge. At the same time the tumour is spreading remorselessly into the dermis and underlying tissues.

Despite the name and appearances, the basal cells of the epidermis are probably not the cells of origin of these tumours. Cytologically and in its architectural pattern the tumours often bear a close resemblance to hair follicles and it is suggested that cells in these sites are the source of the tumour.

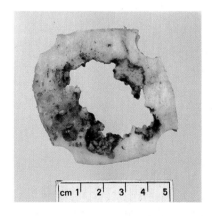

Fig. 16.4 Part of the skull which has been eroded by a basal cell carcinoma. The tumour had penetrated the dura.

APPEARANCES

Very early lesions include small clusters of basal-type cells extending from the lower border of the epidermis into the dermis. In some examples, without sections from several levels, the link between

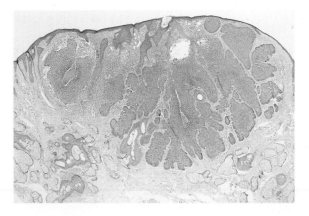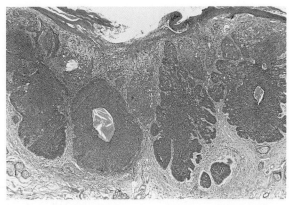

Fig. 16.5 Basal cell carcinoma. (*left*) Low power showing the irregular spread within the dermis and origin from the epidermis. There is no ulceration in this example; (*right*) the uniform nature of the tumour cells and the palisade pattern at the edges of the tumour islands is evident.

the epidermis and the tumour islands may not be appreciated. Another phenomenon dependent on the thoroughness of tissue sectioning is the presence of several islands of basal cell carcinoma lying along the length of the epidermis. When sufficient sections are cut it becomes obvious that these apparently *'multifocal basal cell carcinomas'* are all part of the same tumour. The term multifocal is nevertheless useful since the clinician then knows that he is dealing with a widespread lesion and one in which, despite an apparently adequate excision, parts may still remain in situ.

Large tumours include variably sized islands of the basal type cells spreading into the dermis as well as infiltrating strands of similar cells (Fig. 16.5). The cells are remarkably uniform with few mitoses and a characteristic feature is that those at the edge of the islands are arranged in a regular palisade. Cysts containing mucus develop within the centres of some of the cell clusters. The amount of stroma surrounding the tumour cells varies but includes fibrous and mucoid components. An artefact arising from this in paraffin sections is shrinkage of the stroma from the tumour islands, so producing a gap at this junction. Histological subclassifications of basal cell carcinomas are made according to these cell patterns and the stromal contribution but have little prognostic importance.

There is usually an infiltrate of mononuclear cells within the stroma and the surrounding dermis. The dermis may also include *solar elastosis* which involves the formation of eosinophilic masses, some including thick, partly refractile fibres (Fig. 16.6). This hyperplasia of elastic tissue, although referred to as solar elastosis, is not entirely due to sun exposure but is also a part of the natural ageing process.

Squamous cell carcinoma

Most lesions are small and recognized by the patient as a localized red papule or small non-healing area of ulceration. No region of the skin is exempt but the majority occur in the sun-exposed areas, including the face and backs of the hands. Most patients are elderly as is the involved skin, which is thin and inelastic. The tumour can

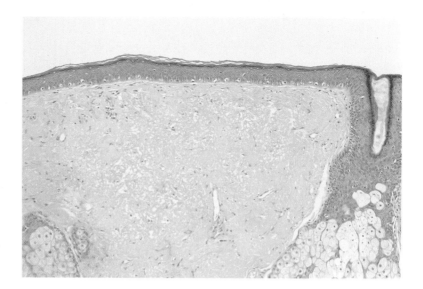

Fig. 16.6 Solar elastosis. Eosinophilic strands of elastic tissue fill the dermis. The thinning of the epidermis is further evidence of sun damage.

also appear as a complication of old burn scars and long-standing skin ulcers. Provided that squamous cell carcinomas are adequately treated metastases are rare and no reduction in life expectancy occurs, an observation not applicable to squamous cell carcinomas in other sites.

APPEARANCES

The tumour arises from the epidermal squamous cells or *keratinocytes* which are characterized by the formation of keratin. This is seen as eosinophilic material, either confined within the cytoplasm of cells or clumped in the centre of islands of keratinocytes, *keratin pearl formation*. Tumours differ in their keratin content and those with abundant keratin are regarded as well differentiated, in contrast to those with little keratin, the poorly differentiated tumours. The proliferating squamous cells extend from the epidermis into the dermis as irregular tongues, islands and infiltrating cells (Fig. 16.7).

The surrounding epidermis may be normal or include evidence of in situ carcinoma (*Bowen's disease*) (Fig. 16.8) or of a *solar keratosis* (Fig. 16.9). A solar keratosis like Bowen's disease is a potentially malignant condition. The dysplastic features, unlike Bowen's disease, do not extend through the full thickness of the epidermis but are restricted to the basal third. Also, the epidermis, in contrast to Bowen's disease, is thin. Heaped up keratin is present over the involved regions and the patient is aware of a localized, crusty, thickened area. The underlying dermis, like that adjacent to many squamous cell carcinomas, includes solar elastosis.

Melanoma

Melanomas are formed from melanocytes and are hence invariably pigmented. Although the skin is the most important primary site,

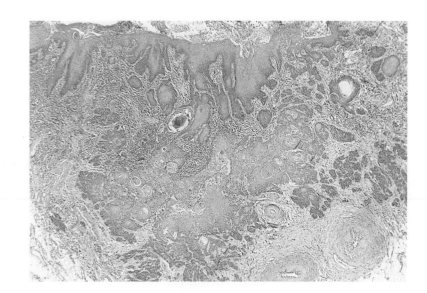

Fig. 16.7 Squamous cell carcinoma. The origin of the tumour from the epidermis is seen and the tumour is spreading in an irregular fashion in the dermis.

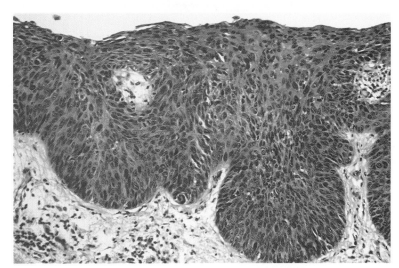

Fig. 16.8 Bowen's disease. The normal maturation of the epidermis is lost and throughout there are large and pleomorphic cells. There is no spread into the dermis.

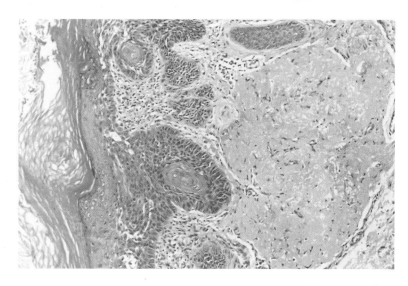

Fig. 16.9 Solar keratosis. Epidermal changes similar to those in Fig. 16.8 are confined to the lower parts of the epidermis. Filling the dermis is solar elastosis.

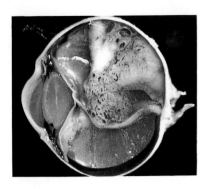

Fig. 16.10 Melanoma (top right) arising from the uveal tract in the eye.

melanomas do develop in other sites, most notably the eye (Fig. 16.10). It is customary in melanomas to refer to the cells as melanocytes and not naevus cells, although both terms embrace the same cell.

Causative factors

Melanomas are a hazard for many of the indigenous white population of Australia and South Africa, among whom those of Celtic origin and red-haired individuals are especially at risk. They are also occurring in greater numbers amongst European populations, most notably Scandinavians and women, and are tumours that are increasing yearly by at least 5%. About 3000 melanomas are diagnosed annually in the UK. Sun exposure is the all important factor. The risk is greater for any individual who tans with difficulty or burns easily in the sun. Sudden bursts of intense sunbathing, especially if the skin is burnt, are more relevant than continuous exposure without sunburn. This finding probably underlies the observation that melanomas affect indoor workers and their spouses in high socio-economic groups rather than sailors, gardeners and swimming pool attendants.

Amongst biopsies of skin exposed to sun lamps there is a decrease in the *Langerhan's cells.* These cells are macrophages and are concerned with antigen processing and presentation to T-lymphocytes. Langerhan's cells remain depleted for some weeks and then gradually assume their normal population. If a similar mechanism follows sun exposure it is possible that antigens capable directly or indirectly of triggering melanogenesis may enter the epidermis and melanoma follow. Since most melanomas appear on the trunk and can develop in areas including the soles of the feet where sun exposure does not occur, persistent sunlight may not be the only aetiological factor. Evidence implicating other agents is the short latent period between sun exposure and many melanomas. This is demonstrated by their high incidence among young adults as opposed to elderly patients and contrasts with the long latent period needed by most carcinogenic agents. Among some patients genetic predisposition may be important since 'melanoma families' are well recognized and in one-third of other patients melanomas develop from naevi.

Classification

Melanomas are often regarded as rapidly fatal tumours unresponsive to any intervention. This is untrue provided the tumour is recognized in its early stages. Melanomas develop through a series of changes from lesions confined to the epidermis to ones that progressively invade the dermis and ultimately extend into the subcutaneous tissues and beyond. The sequence is not always apparent clinically but it is possible to divide melanomas into three clinical groups according to the stage in growth they have reached (Fig. 16.11).

Melanomas restricted to the epidermis include *lentigo malignant melanomas* and *superficial spreading melanomas* (Fig. 16.12). These

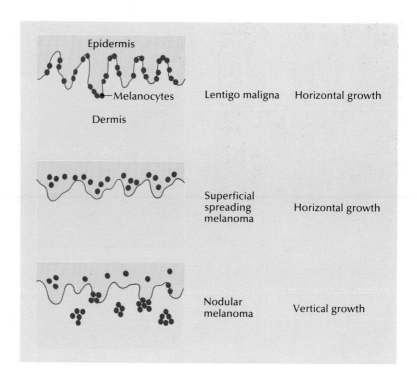

Fig. 16.11 Features underlying the clinical forms of melanoma.

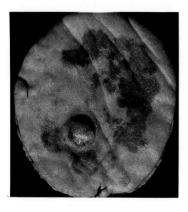

Fig. 16.12 Lentigo malignant melanoma excised from the face. Most of the pigmented area is flat (horizontal growth phase) but in the bottom left a nodule (vertical growth phase) has formed.

differ in the times they take to change from this horizontal phase of growth to a vertical growth phase with dermal invasion. The transition for the lentigo malignant melanoma takes between 10–20 years, while that for the superficial spreading melanoma 2–10 years. The long transition period for the lentigo malignant melanoma and its virtual restriction to sun-exposed areas and other coincident evidence of sun damage are all firm pointers to sun exposure as the cause of these lesions.

Melanomas invading the dermis are *nodular melanomas*. Some will include features of the other two main types, while others will have no evidence of any preceding horizontal growth phase (Fig. 16.13).

Melanomas removed before there is dermal spread will not adversely affect the patient's life expectancy and even when the tumour has just penetrated the papillary dermis this, for many patients, is not altered. In contrast only a third of the patients with melanoma extending to the subcutaneous fat will be alive after 7 years. These prognostic findings are expressed as either measurements of thickness, when a maximum thickness of less than 1.5 mm can equate with a normal life span and one of over 4 mm with a markedly reduced life span or as levels within the epidermis and dermis referred to as *Clarke's levels* (Fig. 16.14).

Both approaches are subject to error and to reduce this both are reported by the histopathologist. Subsequent therapy is significantly influenced by these methods of staging.

A phenomenon rare among most tumours is regression and disappearance. Among melanomas this reaction occurs not infrequently

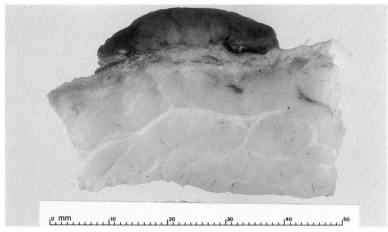

Fig. 16.13 Nodular melanoma. This is partly a papillary tumour and has also replaced much of the dermis.

in part or all of a tumour but it is not associated with any improvement in the patient's prognosis. It may explain the occasional finding of widespread metastatic melanoma in the absence of a primary tumour.

APPEARANCES

Melanomas appear on all parts of the body although lentigo melanoma predominates in the head and neck areas and superficial spreading melanoma on the trunk. They are invariably darkly pigmented, irregular or strictly localized lesions which in the horizontal growth phases are flat. With the development of vertical growth thickened areas are palpable and become visible. Nodular melanomas are raised, generally ovoid and if untreated may reach massive sizes (Fig. 16.15).

All melanomas include large melanocytes with prominent nuclei and abundant cytoplasm. The cytoplasm may be vacuolated and clear or may be filled with melanin pigment either as diffuse small particles or as large aggregates. The absence of melanin does not rule out the diagnosis and may, especially with metastases, provide

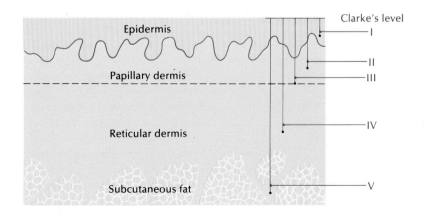

Fig. 16.14 Staging of melanoma.

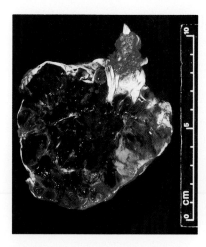

Fig. 16.15 Large melanoma. The patient was elderly and disregarded the tumour until it was knocked and bled profusely.

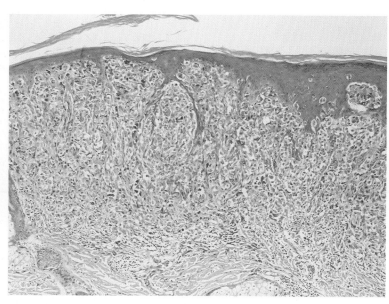

Fig. 16.16 Melanoma with obvious pigmentation of the tumour cells. The cells have infiltrated the epidermis and dermis and lie in groups.

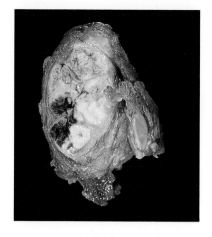

Fig. 16.17 Lymph node with metastatic melanoma. The pigmentation of part of the metastasis suggests a melanoma as the primary growth.

problems in recognizing the tumour's origin. These tumours are called *amelanotic melanomas*. Resource to electron microscopy where melanosomes are looked for and to antibody markers can, in these circumstances, sometimes provide help. Lentigo malignant melanomas include aberrant melanocytes only in the basal part of the epidermis and around the rete pegs while in superficial spreading melanomas they lie throughout the epidermis. The melanocytes remain confined to the epidermis for as long as the horizontal growth phase persists. The onset of the vertical growth phase is heralded by clusters of melanocytes at the dermo-epidermal junction and later by active spread into the dermis. Sheets and islands of melanocytes infiltrating the dermis and epidermis characterize nodular melanomas (Fig. 16.16). These tumours may project from the skin surface and become ulcerated. A variable mononuclear cell infiltrate is seen at the base of melanomas at any stage and these include many macrophages filled with melanin (*melanophages*).

Spread

Metastases develop in any organ and virtually none is exempt, including the brain. If these include melanin they are black or brown and can be recognized immediately (Fig. 16.17). Microscopically the features mimic those of the primary growth. Lymphatics provide the main pathway for metastases in the early phases and blood vessels in the terminal stages.

Further reading

Clark, W.H. Elder, D.E. and Vanhorn, M. (1986). The biologic forms of malignant melanoma. *Hum. Pathol.* **17**, 443–50.

Mackie, R.M. (1984). *Milne's Dermapathology*. Edward Arnold: London.

Index

in endocarditis 55
in inflammatory bowel disease
  115
in meningitis 301
in pneumonia 70

gall-stones 17, 161
gangrene 19–21
gaseous exchange 66–7
gastrectomy, gastritis following 108
gastric acidity and ulceration 108
gastric atrophy 108, 110–11
gastric carcinoma 111, 125–32
gastric reflux 107, 129
gastrin secretion, and peptic
  ulceration 108
gastritis 107
  acute 110, 111
  appearance 110–11, 112
  causes 107–8
  chronic 110–11
  classification 110
gastroenteropancreatic endocrine
  system 250
gastrointestinal tract 109–32
gelatinous lesions in atherosclerosis
  44, 45
germ cell tumours
  ovarian 241–2
  testicular 221–2, 223–4
  thymic 283
Ghon complex 73
Ghon focus 73, 74
giant cells 15
Giardia infection
  and immunodeficiency 125
  in inflammatory bowel disease
    115
glandular fever 270–1
glial tissue 298
glioma 313–14
glomerulonephritis 189–90
  ancillary immunological studies
    200–1
  antibody disease 200, 200–1
  appearances 203–4
  clinical presentation 188
  deposits 195–6, 197, 198
  immune complex disease 194,
    199, 200, 201–2
  immunofluorescence studies
    198–200
  injury mechanisms
    anti-glomerular basement
      membrane antibody 202–3
    immune complex 201–2
  podocyte fusion 196, 197, 198
  presentation 190
  prognostic features 194–5
  terminology

light microscopy 191–5
  ultrastructural 195–8
in transplantation 215
glomerulus 190–1
  changes in systemic disease 204,
    205
  glomerulonephritis
    ancillary immunological studies
      200
    diagnosis 190
    immunofluorescence studies
      198
    light microscopy terminology
      191
    presentation 190
    ultrastructural terminology 195
gluten enteropathy 112, 113, 128
glycogen storage disease, liver
  involvement 158
goitre, congenital 262
Goodpasture's syndrome 203
granulation tissue 9, 10, 13
granulomas 14, 15–17, 18
  in Crohn's disease 116, 118
  tuberculous 14, 15, 16, 73, 74
granulomatous hepatitis 142
granulosa cell tumours 242, 245
Grawitz tumour 217
grey hepatisation 72
ground glass cells 143, 144
gynaecomastia 139, 221, 285

haemangioma 32, 154, 318
haematemesis 106
haematuria
  in adenocarcinoma of the kidney
    217
  in glomerulonephritis 190
  in urinary tract tumours 184–5
haemochromatosis, and liver cell
  carcinoma 156, 158
haemolysis in necrosis 20
haemolytic uraemia syndrome 209
haemopericardium 62, 64
Haemophilus influenzae 301
haemoptysis 202–3
haemorrhage
  in atherosclerosis 46–7
  in cirrhosis 153
  in diverticular disease 122
  in peptic ulceration 109
  in renal failure 189
  spontaneous intracranial 307–9
  tumour-associated 31, 32–3, 36
haemosiderosis 138
Hashimoto's thyroiditis 261
head injury 309–11
healing by first/second intention 13
heart
  atrophy 41

congenital abnormalities 61
effects of rheumatic fever 52–3
failure 39, 40, 54, 58, 208
hypertrophy 39–40
neoplasms 60
heart valves
  disorders of 54, 55, 61
  effects of rheumatic fever 52, 53
  endocarditis 54
    development 56
    appearances 57
    complications 58
hepatitis 140
  acute 140
  alcohol-related 148–9
  appearances 145
  chronic 137, 138, 140–1
  non-viral 140
  in renal failure 189
  viral 142
    causative viruses 140
    course 142
    histological effects 143, 144
    mechanism of injury 144–5
    serological diagnosis 142–3
hepatitis A virus (HAV) 142
hepatitis B virus (HBV) 140, 142, 143
  antigens 142–3
  cirrhosis-associated 150, 151
  and liver cell carcinoma 154,
    155–6
  mechanism of injury 144–5
hepatocellular carcinoma 154–6, 157
  alcohol-induced 150
  appearances 157
  complications 157–8
  spread 157
hepatocytes 133
hepatorenal syndrome 139, 153
Herpes simplex encephalitis 302,
  304
Herpes simplex type 2 virus, and
  cervical carcinoma 230–1
hiatus hernia 107
Hirschsprung's disease 120, 121
histamine 163
histiocytes 8, 268
histiocytoses 283–4
histiocytosis X 283–4
histopathology, definition 1
hob-nail liver 153
Hodgkin's lymphoma 276–8
  aetiology 278–9
  appearances 279
  classification 278
  complications 279–80
  staging 278
honeycomb lung 90
hormones 251
  ectopic production 251
  gastrointestinal tract 106